Study Guide

to accompany

Maternity & Women's Health Care

D1117759

Study Guide

to accompany

Maternity & Women's Health Care

EIGHTH EDITION

DEITRA LEONARD LOWDERMILK, RNC, PHD, FAAN

SHANNON E. PERRY, RN, CNS, PHD, FAAN

prepared by
KAREN A. PIOTROWSKI, RNC, MSN

Associate Professor of Nursing
D'Youville College
Buffalo, New York

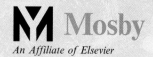

Mosby

An Affiliate of Elsevier

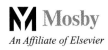

Mosby

An Affiliate of Elsevier

11830 Westline Industrial Drive
St. Louis, Missouri 63146

STUDY GUIDE TO ACCOMPANY MATERNITY & WOMEN'S HEALTH CARE
Copyright © 2004, Mosby, Inc. All rights reserved.

NOTICE

Pharmacology is an ever-changing field. Standard safety precautions must be followed, but as new research and clinical experience broaden our knowledge, changes in treatment and drug therapy may become necessary or appropriate. Readers are advised to check the most current product information provided by the manufacturer of each drug to be administered to verify the recommended dose, the method and duration of administration, and contraindications. It is the responsibility of the licensed health care provider, relying on experience and knowledge of the patient, to determine dosages and the best treatment for each individual patient. Neither the publisher nor the author assumes any liability for any injury and/or damage to persons or property arising from this publication.

Previous edition copyrighted 2000

ISBN-13: 978-0-323-02719-9
ISBN-10: 0-323-02719-9

Executive Editor: Michael S. Ledbetter
Senior Developmental Editor: Laurie K. Muench
Publishing Services Manager: Catherine Jackson
Senior Project Manager: Jeff Patterson
Designer: Teresa McBryan Breckwoldt

Printed in the United States of America

Last digit is the print number: 9   8   7   6   5

INTRODUCTION

This Student Learning Guide is designed to accompany the 8th edition of *Maternity and Women's Health Care*. It includes Chapter Review Activities, Critical Thinking Exercises, and Evolve website activities for each chapter in the textbook.

I.   **Chapter Review Activities** focus upon recall and application of critical concepts and essential terminology. These activities are specifically designed to help you to identify the important content of the chapter and to test your level of knowledge and understanding after reading the chapter. Completion of each of the activities will provide you with an excellent resource to use when you are reviewing important content before course examinations. The knowledge that you attain by completing the activities will help you to develop the theoretical foundation that you will need to answer the critical thinking exercises that follow, to successfully pass course examinations and the NCLEX-RN examination, and to manage the care of your clients in the clinical setting. Answers or answer guidelines for the activities are provided in the Answer Key located at the end of this Study Guide.

II.   **Critical Thinking Exercises** focus primarily upon the application of critical chapter content. Typical client care situations are presented and you are required to apply concepts found in the chapter to solve problems, to make decisions concerning care management, and to provide responses to a client's questions and concerns. These exercises may be completed by you on your own or with members of your study group. Completing the critical thinking exercises will help you prepare for clinical experiences, course examinations, and the NCLEX-RN examination, all of which focus on problem solving and application of nursing knowledge. Guidelines for completing the exercises and specific chapter section, box, or table where the content for the answer is found are provided in the Answer Key located at the end of this Study Guide.

III.   **Evolve Website Activities** are designed to help you to develop skill in the use of the Internet while expanding your knowledge base related to the content presented in the chapter and developing your appreciation of the value of the Internet as a resource for client information and support. These activities may provide you with ideas for issue papers or group presentations that may be required for your classes or seminars. All activities can be accessed at **http://evolve.elsevier.com/Lowdermilk/MatWmnHlth/**.

CONTENTS

UNIT FOUR

CHILDBIRTH

UNIT FIVE

POSTPARTUM

UNIT SIX

THE NEWBORN

UNIT SEVEN

COMPLICATIONS OF PREGNANCY

UNIT EIGHT

NEWBORN COMPLICATIONS

CHAPTER 1

Contemporary Maternity Nursing and Women's Health Care

CHAPTER REVIEW ACTIVITIES

MATCHING: Match the definition in Column I with the appropriate descriptive term in Column II.

COLUMN I

_____ 1. Number of live births in one year per 1000 population

_____ 2. Number of women who die as a result of problems related to pregnancy or childbirth per 100,000 live births

_____ 3. Number of stillbirths plus the number of neonatal deaths per 1000 live births

_____ 4. Number of births per 1000 women 15 to 44 years of age

_____ 5. Infant whose weight at birth is less than 2500 g (5 lb, 8 oz)

_____ 6. Number of deaths of infants younger than 1 year of age per 1000 live births

_____ 7. Number of deaths of infants younger than 28 days of age per 1000 live births

COLUMN II

A. Fertility rate
B. Infant mortality rate
C. Birth rate
D. Maternal mortality rate
E. Neonatal mortality rate
F. Perinatal mortality rate
G. Low-birth-weight infant

FILL IN THE BLANKS: Insert the term or phrase that corresponds to each of the following definitions.

8. _____ Specialty area of nursing practice that focuses on the care of childbearing women and their families through all stages of pregnancy and childbirth, as well as the first 4 weeks after birth.

9. _____ Specialty of nursing practice that focuses on the physical, psychologic, and social needs of women throughout their lives.

10. _____ Practice that is based on findings obtained through research and clinical trials.

11. _____ Method of care that measures effectiveness of care against benchmarks or standards based on results achieved by others. Quality indicators include _____, _____, and _____.

12. _____ The agenda of the United States for improving health. Its two major goals are to increase the _____ and to eliminate _____.

13. _____ Guidelines for nursing practice based on current knowledge and representative of levels of practice agreed upon by leaders in the specialty area of nursing.

14. _____ Umbrella term for the use of communication technologies and electronic information to provide or support health care when the participants are separated by distance.

15. _____ A program or service that has been recognized for excellence; it provides a better or a new way to achieve goals and be sound from operational, clinical, and financial perspectives.

16. _____ A process used to compare one's own performance against the performance of the best in an area of service; it supports and promotes continuous quality improvement.

17. _____ An evolving process that identifies risks, establishes preventive practices, develops reporting mechanisms, and delineates procedures for managing law suits.

18. _____ Form of care that encompasses complementary and alternative therapies in combination with conventional Western modalities of treatment.

19. *IDENTIFY* the factors that contribute to the infant mortality rate in the United States.

TRUE OR FALSE: Circle "T" if true or "F" if false for each of the following statements. Correct the false statements.

T F 20. The neonatal period refers to the first week of an infant's life.

T F 21. Currently the highest birth rates are for women between 20 and 29 years of age.

T F 22. Births to unmarried women are frequently related to less favorable outcomes because there are typically a large number of adolescents in this group.

T F 23. In the United States, the birth rate for unmarried women in 1997 was highest among Hispanic women.

T F 24. Infant mortality can be reduced by shifting the emphasis from high technology to improving access to preventive health care services, especially for low-income families.

T F 25. The incidence of low birth weight has steadily decreased since the 1970s.

T F 26. The greatest risk for giving birth to a low-birth-weight infant occurs among African-American women.

T F 27. The United States ranks 15th in infant mortality rate among industrialized nations.

T F 28. The maternal mortality rate is a common indicator of the adequacy of prenatal care and the health of the nation as a whole.

T F 29. The maternal mortality rate for African-American women is four times higher than the rate for Caucasian women.

T F 30. One of the four predominant causes of maternal death in the United States is pregnancy-induced hypertension.

T F 31. The percentage of all pregnant women in the United States who received early prenatal care was over 90% in 2000.

T F 32. The most significant barrier to accessible prenatal care is the inability to pay.

T F 33. The cesarean birth rate has increased to over 22% in 2000.

T F 34. The incidence of high risk pregnancies has steadily decreased since 1990.

T F 35. The two most frequently reported maternal medical risk factors are hypertension associated with pregnancy and infection.

T F 36. Although the rate of abortion among adolescents has declined, the United States still has a higher abortion rate than any other industrialized country.

37. *CITE* three major changes that have occurred in childbirth practices in the United States. For each change cited explain how the change has improved the quality of care received by pregnant women and their families.

38. *IDENTIFY* several factors and social conditions that affect the health of women. For each factor and social condition identified, describe the impact it has had on women's health.

CRITICAL THINKING EXERCISES

1. *IMAGINE* that you are the nursing director of an inner-city prenatal clinic that serves a large number of minority women, many of whom are younger than 20 years of age. *DESCRIBE* five nursing services you would provide for these women of childbearing age that would help reduce the potential for infant and maternal morbidity and mortality, and low birth weight (LBW). Use the biostatistical data and risk behaviors presented in this chapter to support the types of services you propose.

2. *SUPPORT* the accuracy of the following statement: An emphasis on high-technology medical care and lifesaving techniques will not reduce the rate of preterm and LBW infants in the United States.

3. *PROPOSE* three changes in health care and its delivery that you believe will improve the health status and well-being of mothers and their infants and reduce the rate of infant and maternal mortality. *SUPPORT* your answer by using the content presented in Chapter 1 and your own experiences with the health care system.

4. Self-care approaches in health care management are appealing to women who want to assume responsibility for their own level of wellness and to become active partners with their health care providers. *DISCUSS* the care measures that you as a nurse would implement when providing health care in order to enhance a woman's responsibility for herself and partnership with you.

5. Many barriers exist interfering with a woman's participation in early and ongoing prenatal care. *DESCRIBE* incentives and services that you would offer pregnant women to encourage their participation in early and ongoing prenatal care. State the rationale for your proposals. Your answer should reflect an understanding of the barriers.

ONLINE LEARNING ACTIVITIES

Access the Lowdermilk, Perry **Evolve** website at **http://evolve.elsevier.com/Lowdermilk/MatWmnHlth/** and enter the **Student** portion through the **Learning Resources** section. Use Chapter 1 as a starting point for a search of the Internet to gather the following information:

- Biostatistical data regarding the factors involved in infant and maternal morbidity and mortality rates
- *Healthy People 2000* and *Healthy People 2010* goals for infant and maternal morbidity and mortality rates

Write a four-page paper that includes the following:

- Summary of the information you gathered during your Internet search.
- Discussion of health care strategies that you would propose to improve the infant and maternal morbidity and mortality rates in the United States in order to reach or surpass the goals identified in the *Healthy People* report; state the rationale for each health care strategy you propose.

Use Evolve to search the Internet for information regarding female genital mutilation. Gather information regarding what the procedure involves, how it is performed, why it is done, and the effect it has on the reproductive and sexual health of women upon whom it is performed. Use the information you gathered to outline a presentation you would give to a group of nurses working in a clinic where the client population has begun to include immigrant women who have experienced genital mutilation.

CHAPTER 2

Community Care: The Family and Culture

CHAPTER REVIEW ACTIVITIES

MATCHING: Match the family described in Column I with the appropriate family form in Column II.

COLUMN I

_____ 1. Miss M. lives with her 4-year-old adopted Korean daughter, Kim.

_____ 2. Anne and Duane are married and live with their daughter, Susan, and Duane's mother, Ruth.

_____ 3. Gloria and Andy are a married couple living with their new baby girl, Annie.

_____ 4. Carl and Allan are a gay couple living with Carl's daughter, Sally, whom they are raising together.

_____ 5. This family consists of Jim, his second wife Jane, and Jim's two daughters by a previous marriage.

_____ 6. Laurie and John have been divorced for 3 years. They share custody of their four children.

COLUMN II

A. Binuclear family
B. Single parent family
C. Homosexual family
D. Nuclear family
E. Extended family
F. Reconstituted (blended) family

MATCHING: Match the description in Column I with the appropriate cultural concept in Column II.

COLUMN I

_____ 7. Mrs. M., a Mexican-American woman who just gave birth, tells the nurse not to include certain foods on her meal tray because her mother told her to avoid those foods while breastfeeding. The nurse tells her that she doesn't have to avoid any foods and should eat whatever she desires.

_____ 8. Ms. P., an immigrant from Vietnam, has lived in the United States for one year. She tells you that she enjoys the comfort of wearing blue jeans and sneakers on casual occasions such as shopping even though she never would have done so in Vietnam.

_____ 9. A Cambodian family immigrated to the United States and have been living in Denver for over 5 years. The parents express concern about their children 10, 13, and 16 years of age, stating, "The children act so differently now. They are less respectful to us, want to eat only American food and go to rock concerts. It's hard to believe they are our children."

_____ 10. The Amish represent an important ethnic community located in Lancaster, Pennsylvania.

_____ 11. The nurse is preparing a healthy diet plan for Mrs. O. In doing so, she takes the time to include the Polish foods that are favorites of Mrs. O.

COLUMN II

A. Cultural relativism
B. Ethnocentrism
C. Assimilation
D. Subculture
E. Acculturation

FILL IN THE BLANKS: Insert the term that corresponds to each of the following descriptions.

12. _____ A unified set of values, ideas, beliefs, and standards of behavior shared by a group of people. It tells the person how to view the world and how to relate to other people, supernatural forces, and the natural environment.

13. _____ A group existing within a larger cultural system that retains its own characteristics.

14. _____ Recognizing that people from different cultural backgrounds actually comprehend the same situations or objects differently. It affirms the uniqueness and value of every culture.

15. _____ Changes that can take place in one group or among several groups when people from different cultures come in contact with one another and exchange and adopt each other's mannerisms, styles, and practices.

16. _____ Process in which one cultural group loses its cultural identity and becomes a part of the dominant culture.

17. _____ Being centered in one's own cultural system, judging the world in general by the standards established in that particular system. It is the view that one's cultural way of doing things is the right and natural way—my group is best.

18. _____ Nursing practice approach that focuses on the way people of different cultures perceive life events and the health care system. It reflects the nurse's ability to think, feel, and act in ways that acknowledge, respect, and build upon ethnic, sociocultural, and linguistic diversity.

19. _____ Families with this type of time orientation may not adhere to strict schedules and may be described as "living for the moment."

20. _____ Families or persons with this type of time orientation are more likely to return for follow-up visits related to health care and to participate in primary prevention activities.

21. _____ Families or persons with this type of time orientation are more likely to strive to maintain tradition or the status quo and have little motivation for formulating future goals.

22. _____ Concept that reflects dimensions of personal comfort zones and feelings of territoriality that are developed within a cultural setting. Actions such as touching the client, placing the client in proximity to others, taking away personal possessions, and making decisions for the client affect the need for distance and can thereby decrease personal security and heighten anxiety.

23. _____ Fundamental societal unit or group related by blood, marriage, adoption, or emotional commitment who have a permanent relationship and work together to meet life goals and needs.

24. _____ Family form consisting of parents and their children living as an independent unit sharing roles, responsibilities, and economic resources.

25. _____ Family form that includes the nuclear family and other relatives (kin) such as grandparents, aunts, uncles, and cousins living in the same household.

26. _____ Family form that refers to the family after divorce, in which the children are members of both the maternal and paternal nuclear households.

27. _____ Family form in which there is only one unmarried biologic or adoptive parent as head of the household; it is becoming an increasingly recognized structure in our society. These families tend to be vulnerable both _____ and _____.

28. _____ Family form that is created as a result of divorce and remarriage. It includes unrelated family members such as stepparents, stepchildren, and stepsiblings.

29. _____ Family form in which gay or lesbian couples are the parents.

30. _____ A family theory based on a science of wholeness that is characterized by interaction among the components of the family and between the family and the environment. The family is viewed as a whole that is different from the sum of the individual members.

31. _____ A family theory that focuses on the family as it moves through stages. Each family member progresses through phases of growth and development, from dependence through active independence, and to interdependence. The family structure and function also varies over time.

32. _____ A family theory concerned with the ways families react to stressful events and suggests factors that promote adaptation to these events. The way a family responds and adapts is influenced by the stressor itself, the family's existing resources, and the family's perception of the stressor. Stress must be studied within the _____ and _____ contexts in which the family is living.

33. _____ A geographically defined area; its residents; their culture, religious, and ethnic characteristics; and the activities or functions through which the needs of the residents are met.

34. _____ Subpopulations whose needs may differ from those of the larger community.

35. _____ Health-related activities involving health promotion and disease prevention to decrease the occurrence of illness and enhance general health and quality of life. Specific activities can include _____, _____, and _____.

36. _____ Health-related activities involving early detection of health problems and prompt treatment that can shorten disease duration and severity. Specific activities can include various methods of _____.

37. _____ Health-related activities that follow occurrence of a defect or disability that is permanent and irreversible. It involves the treatment and rehabilitation of persons who have developed diseases or disabilities to prevent complications and further deterioration and maintain an optimum level of function.

38. _____ Health-related activities involving genetic modifications to prevent susceptibility to some conditions.

39. _____ Health care delivery approach with the goal of improving coordination of health care, care outcomes, communication among health care providers, and client, payer, and provider satisfaction while reducing costs.

40. _____ Public or private organizations or employer groups that pay for health care expenses.

TRUE OR FALSE: Circle "T" if true or "F" if false for each of the following statements. Correct the false statements.

T F 41. A subculture's beliefs and practices related to childbearing and parenting must be assessed for each woman and family representing that subculture because variations in beliefs and practices are possible.

T F 42. Women from Southeast Asia often vocalize while experiencing the pain and discomfort associated with the childbirth process.

T F 43. African-American women seek prenatal care early because they view pregnancy as a time when women require medical care and supervision.

T F 44. Hispanic women appreciate the opportunity to shower or bathe as soon as possible after birth.

T F 45. The nurse should recognize that a Vietnamese woman may not wish to breastfeed until her milk comes in since she believes that newborns should not be fed colostrum because it is dirty.

T F 46. European-American women typically prefer a technology-dominated childbirth approach rather than a natural approach.

T F 47. Native American women often use herbal preparations to promote uterine contractions during labor and to stop bleeding in the postpartum period.

T F 48. Hispanic-American women often desire and expect reduced activity or even bed rest for as long as 3 days after birth.

T F 49. Breast self-examination is an example of secondary prevention.

T F 50. Immunization programs are an example of tertiary prevention.

T F 51. The largest group among rural homeless is couples with children.

T F 52. Migrant laborers are considered to be episodically homeless because their shelter is often dependent upon seasonal employment.

T F 53. Most migrant laborers value their health, readily seeking health promotion and disease prevention services if offered.

T F 54. Refugees typically come to the United States for economic reasons.

T F 55. The perinatal continuum of care starts with family planning and ends when the infant is 1 year of age.

T F 56. Perinatal home health care became a viable health care alternative when third-party payers pushed for cost-containment in maternity services.

T F 57. Women who require intravenous fluids during their pregnancies must be hospitalized and therefore are not candidates for home care.

T F 58. Infection control measures are less important when care is given in the client's home.

T F 59. When documenting a home visit, the nurse should avoid statements such as "no change" or "same as last visit."

60. *DISCUSS* the maternity nursing implications for each of the following theoretical approaches to care of families:

A. Family Systems Theory

B. Family Life Cycle Theory

C. Family Stress Theory

D. Health Belief Model

61. *DISCUSS* why the nurse should take each of the following aspects of culture into consideration when providing care within a cultural context:

A. Communication

B. Space

C. Time orientation

D. Family roles

62. Nurses must avoid making stereotypical assumptions when caring for pregnant women from specific sociocultural or religious groups. *EXPLAIN* the process you would follow when providing culturally competent care that is reflective of a pregnant woman's unique values, beliefs, and behavioral patterns.

63. Women are considered to be a high risk or vulnerable population of interest to perinatal nurses working in the community.
    A. *DESCRIBE* the factors that increase the vulnerability of women.

    B. *IDENTIFY* six subgroups of women that are highly vulnerable, presenting challenges to the community-based perinatal nurse. *DESCRIBE* at least one challenge that women in each of these groups present.

64. *STATE* three characteristics of refugees that can significantly increase the difficulties they experience as they strive to adapt to a new language and culture.

65. *DESCRIBE* the ways that nurses can provide care to perinatal clients using the telephone.

MULTIPLE CHOICE: Circle the one correct option and state the rationale for the option chosen.

66. A gay couple is raising the son of one of the men. The nurse caring for this family should recognize that
    A. The son has an increased likelihood of being gay himself
    B. Research indicates that children of homosexual parents appear to grow and thrive as well as children in heterosexual families
    C. The son will have difficulty developing a sexual relationship with a female partner
    D. The gay and lesbian family form is rare in the United States

12 Chapter 2: Community Care: The Family and Culture

67. A family with open boundaries
   A. Uses available support systems to meet its needs
   B. Is more prone to crisis related to increased exposure to stressors
   C. Discourages family members from setting up channels
   D. Strives to maintain family stability by avoiding outside influences

68. Which one of the following nursing actions is most likely to reduce a client's anxiety and enhance the client's personal security as it relates to the concept of personal space needs?
   A. Touching the client before and during procedures
   B. Providing explanations when performing tasks
   C. Making eye contact as much as possible
   D. Reducing the need for the client to make decisions

69. A Native-American woman gave birth to a baby girl 12 hours ago. The nurse notes that the woman keeps her baby in the bassinet except for feeding and states that she will wait until she gets home to begin breastfeeding. The nurse recognizes that this behavior is most likely a reflection of
   A. Embarrassment
   B. Delayed attachment
   C. Disappointment that the baby is a girl
   D. A belief that babies should not be fed colostrum or handled often

CRITICAL THINKING EXERCISES

1. *IMAGINE* that you are a nurse working in a clinic that provides prenatal services to a multicultural community predominated by Hispanic, African-American, and Asian families. *DESCRIBE* how you would adapt care measures to reflect the cultural beliefs and practices of pregnant women and their families from each of the following cultural groups.
   Hispanic

   African-American

   Asian-American

2. Pamela is a 20-year-old Native American woman. She is 3 months pregnant and has come to the prenatal clinic on the reservation where she lives for her first visit in order to obtain some prenatal vitamins that her friends at work told her are important.

    A. *STATE* the questions the nurse should ask to determine Pamela's cultural explanations about childbearing.

    B. *DESCRIBE* the communication approach you would consider when interviewing Pamela.

    C. *IDENTIFY* the Native American beliefs and practices regarding childbearing that may influence Pamela's approach to her pregnancy and birth.

3. A nurse has been providing care to a Hispanic family. This family recently experienced the birth of twin girls at 38 weeks' gestation. It is the first birth experience for both parents and the first grandchildren for the extended family. Both newborns are healthy and living at home. *DESCRIBE* the cultural beliefs and practices that the family, as Hispanic, might use as guidelines to provide care to their twin girls.

4. The nurse-midwife at a prenatal clinic has been assigned to care for a refugee couple from Bosnia that has recently emigrated to the United States. The woman has just been diagnosed as 2 months' pregnant. Neither she nor her husband speak English. Outline the process that this nurse should use when working with a translator to facilitate communication with this couple thereby enhancing care management.

5. As a nurse working in home care, it would be helpful for the nurse to become familiar with the neighborhood and resources with which her or his clients interact.

    A. *DESCRIBE* the walking survey and how it can be used to assess the characteristics of a community.

B. *DISCUSS* how the nurse could use the findings from this survey to provide health care to the clients who reside in the assessed community.

6. Marie is a single parent of two young children 1 and 4 years of age. She and her children have been homeless for 3 months since her husband abandoned her and she lost her job because she had no one to help her care for her children.

   A. *DISCUSS* the types of health problems to which Marie and her children are most vulnerable.

   B. Research indicates that Marie is at increased risk for becoming pregnant again. *STATE* the factors that make Marie more vulnerable.

   C. *OUTLINE* the principles that should guide a nurse in providing care to Marie and her children should they present themselves to the homeless shelter's clinic for health care.

7. Consuelo is the wife of a migrant laborer. She and her husband, along with their two children, have been working on a California farm for 2 weeks. She has arrived at a health center established for migrant laborers. Consuelo states that she is 4 months' pregnant. As the woman's health nurse practitioner assigned to care for Consuelo, what approaches would you use to ensure that Consuelo obtains quality health care that addresses her unique health risks as a migrant worker?

8. *WRITE* a series of questions that you would ask when making a postpartum follow-up call to a woman who gave birth 3 days ago.

9. Eileen, a woman, gave birth to a son 36 hours ago. A home care nurse has been assigned to visit Eileen and her husband in their home to assess the progress of her recovery after birth, the health status of her newborn son, and the adaptation of family processes to the responsibilities of newborn care.

A. *OUTLINE* the approach the nurse should take in preparing for this visit.

B. *DESCRIBE* the nurse's actions during the visit using the care management process as a format.

C. *DISCUSS* how the nurse should end the visit.

D. *IDENTIFY* important interventions the nurse should implement at the conclusion of the visit with Eileen and her husband.

E. *SPECIFY* how the nurse should protect her personal safety both outside and inside Eileen's home.

F. *CITE* the infection control measures the nurse should use when conducting the visit and providing care in Eileen's home.

10. Angela has recently been diagnosed with hyperemesis gravidarum and has been hospitalized to stabilize her fluid and electrolyte balance. The hospital-based nurse must evaluate Angela for referral to home care.

A. State the criteria that this nurse should follow in order to determine Angela's readiness for discharge from hospital to home care.

B. Angela has been discharged and will be receiving parenteral nutrition in her home. Discuss the additional information required related to high-technology home care.

C. Identify specific home environment criteria that must be met to ensure the safety and effectiveness of Angela's treatment.

11. A nurse is seeking funding to start a home care agency designed to provide home visits to postpartum women and their families within 1 week of birth and follow-up visits as indicated. *STATE* the points the nurse should emphasize as a rationale for the importance of this health care service and the cost-effectiveness of funding such a service.

ONLINE LEARNING ACTIVITIES

Access the Lowdermilk, Perry **Evolve** website at **http://evolve.elsevier.com/Lowdermilk/MatWmnHlth/** and enter the **Student** portion through the **Learning Resources** section. Using Chapter 2 as a starting point, search the Internet for websites designed to inform persons about the values and beliefs of various cultures. Prepare a report that includes each of the following:
- List of at least one site and the web address for each of the ethnic groups described in this chapter
- Description of two of the sites in terms of:
  - Sponsor—person, agency, organization
  - Type of information provided about the ethnic group including its beliefs and values regarding health care during childbearing and childrearing
  - Value of the information related to the provision of culturally sensitive care
  - Variety of links to other similar sites
- Discussion regarding how health care providers could use these sites when managing health care for individuals and families representing these ethnic groups

Write a three- to four-page paper that describes the health of your community in terms of health status and risk factor indicators. Use Internet resources to gather the biostatistical information required to determine your community's indicators. Based on your findings propose two services that should be offered by your community to solve health problems revealed by the biostatistical data. Include a rationale for each of the services you proposed.

CHAPTER **3**

Genetics

CHAPTER REVIEW ACTIVITIES

MATCHING: Match the description in Column I with the appropriate genetic concept in Column II.

COLUMN I

_____ 1. Observable traits or characteristics.
_____ 2. Failure of chromosomes to separate.
_____ 3. Small segments of DNA.
_____ 4. An abnormality in chromosome number.
_____ 5. A person's entire genetic make-up.
_____ 6. Union of a normal gamete with a gamete containing an extra chromosome, resulting in a cell with 47 chromosomes.
_____ 7. X, Y
_____ 8. Combination of genetic and environmental factors to result in congenital malformations.
_____ 9. Common, minute variations in human DNA.
_____ 10. Single gene controls a particular trait or disorder.
_____ 11. Complete set of genetic instructions in nucleus of each human cell.
_____ 12. Disorder reflecting absent or defective enzymes.
_____ 13. Chromosomal material is exchanged between two chromosomes.
_____ 14. Thread-like packages of genes and other DNA in a cell nucleus.
_____ 15. Both genes in pair must be abnormal for disorder to be expressed.
_____ 16. Union of a normal gamete with a gamete missing a chromosome.
_____ 17. A spontaneous and permanent change in normal gene structure.
_____ 18. One copy of abnormal gene is needed for phenotypic expression.
_____ 19. Pictorial analysis of an individual's chromosomes.

COLUMN II

A. Human genome
B. Chromosome
C. Gene
D. Sex chromosomes
E. Karyotype
F. Aneuploidy
G. Trisomy
H. Nondisjunction
I. Monosomy
J. Translocation
K. Mutation
L. Unifactorial inheritance
M. Multifactorial inheritance
N. Autosomal dominant inheritance
O. Autosomal recessive inheritance
P. Inborn error of metabolism
Q. Phenotype
R. SNPs (single nucleotide polymorphisms)
S. Genotype

FILL IN THE BLANKS: Insert the term that corresponds to each of the following descriptions.

20. _____ Disorders present at birth.
21. _____ Testing that involves the analysis of DNA, RNA, chromosomes, or proteins to detect abnormalities related to an inherited condition.
22. _____ Tests used to directly examine the DNA and RNA that make up a gene.
23. _____ Tests that look at markers coinherited with a gene that causes a genetic condition.
24. _____ Tests that examine the protein products of genes.
25. _____ Tests that examine chromosomes.
26. _____ Tests used to identify individuals who have a gene mutation for a genetic condition, but do not show symptoms of the condition because it is a condition that is inherited in an autosomal recessive form.
27. _____ Tests used to clarify the genetic status of asymptomatic family members. There are two specific types of these tests, namely _____ tests (gene mutation is present and symptoms are certain to appear if the individual lives long enough) and _____ tests (gene mutation is present but this positive result does not indicate that there is a 100% risk of developing the condition).
28. _____ Tests that use a special kind of DNA chip called a microarray to differential between tumors caused by inherited genetic changes and those caused by sporadic changes.
29. _____ The use of genetic information to individualize drug therapy. A primary benefit is the potential to reduce adverse drug reactions.
30. _____ Therapeutic approach that is based on the use of genetic information to treat a health problem.

TRUE OR FALSE: Circle "T" if true or "F" if false for each of the following statements. Correct the false statements.

T   F   31. The Human Genome Project has determined that human beings are 50% identical at the DNA level.

T   F   32. Normal human somatic (body) cells contain 23 pairs of chromosomes.

T   F   33. An individual having two copies of the same allele for a given trait is said to be heterozygous for that trait.

T   F   34. Euploidy denotes the correct number of chromosomes.

T   F   35. Polyploidy is a deviation in chromosome number that is not an exact multiple of the haploid set.

T   F   36. The most common trisomal abnormality is dwarfism.

T   F   37. An individual with Down syndrome is more likely to be affected by congenital disorders than is the general population.

T   F   38. Eighty percent of children with Down syndrome are born to mothers older than 40 years of age.

T   F   39. Hemophilia is an example of X-linked dominant inheritance.

T   F   40. Neural tube defects result from a combination of genetic and environmental factors.

T   F   41. In order for a recessive trait to be expressed in their offspring, both parents must contribute the abnormal gene.

T   F   42. In autosomal dominant inheritance, if one parent is affected by the disorder, there is a 100% chance of passing the abnormal gene to an offspring during each pregnancy.

T F 43. If a couple gives birth to a child with an autosomal dominant disorder, there is a 50% reduction in risk that the next pregnancy will result in an affected child.

T F 44. Inborn errors of metabolism are an example of autosomal dominant inheritance.

T F 45. The nurse generalist should be expert in performing genetic health assessments.

T F 46. Tay-Sachs disease is an inborn error of metabolism that occurs more commonly in Ashkenazi Jews and French-Canadians from Quebec.

T F 47. Most breast cancer occurs in women who inherit the BRCA1 mutation.

48. *IDENTIFY* the five main genetics-related nursing activities.

49. *STATE* several advances in human genetics that have occurred as a direct result of the Human Genome Project.

50. *DISCUSS* the major ELSI (ethical, legal, social implications) risks associated with genetic testing.

51. *IDENTIFY* the factors that can influence a person's decision to have genetic testing or to refuse it.

52. *EXPLAIN* each of the following types of inheritance and give an example of a disorder that can be transmitted by each.

Unifactorial Inheritance

Multifactorial Inheritance

MULTIPLE CHOICE: Circle the one correct option and state the rationale for the option chosen.

53. An expectant woman, 40 years old, undergoes an amniocentesis to detect the presence of Down syndrome. The fetal chromosomes are arranged and photographed to facilitate diagnosis. The picture is called a:
    A. Genotype
    B. Phenotype
    C. Chromosome type
    D. Karyotype

54. Based on genetic testing of a newborn, a diagnosis of dwarfism was made. The parents ask the nurse if this could happen to future children. Because this is an example of autosomal dominant inheritance, the nurse would tell the parents:
    A. "For each pregnancy, there is a 50/50 chance the child will be affected by dwarfism."
    B. "This will not happen again because the dwarfism was caused by the harmful genetic effects of the infection you had during pregnancy."
    C. "For each pregnancy there is a 25% chance the child will be a carrier of the defective gene but unaffected by the disorder."
    D. "Because you already have had an affected child there is a decreased chance for this to happen in future pregnancies."

55. A female carries the gene for hemophilia on one of her X chromosomes. Now that she is pregnant she asks the nurse how this might affect her baby. The nurse should tell her:
    A. A female baby has a 50% chance of also being a carrier.
    B. A male baby can be a carrier or have hemophilia.
    C. Female babies are never affected by this disorder.
    D. Hemophilia is always expressed if a male inherits the defective gene.

56. A pregnant woman carries a single gene for cystic fibrosis, an inborn error of metabolism. The father of her baby does not carry this gene. Which of the following is true regarding the genetic pattern of the inborn error of metabolism as it applies to this family?
    A. The pregnant woman has cystic fibrosis herself.
    B. There is a 50% chance her baby will have the disorder.
    C. There is a 25% chance her baby will be a carrier.
    D. There is no chance her baby will be affected by this disorder.

CRITICAL THINKING EXERCISES

1. *SUPPORT THIS STATEMENT:* All nurses must possess a basic understanding of and expertise in genetics in order to provide holistic family-centered care.

2. Angela has come for her first prenatal visit. *IDENTIFY* the questions the nurse should ask during the health history interview to determine if factors are present that would place Angela at risk for giving birth to a baby with an inheritable disorder.

3. Mr. and Mrs. G., who are Jewish, are newly married and are planning for pregnancy. They express to the nurse their concern that Mrs. G. has a history of Tay-Sachs disease in her family. Mr. G. has never investigated his family history.
   A. *DESCRIBE* the nurse's role in the process of assisting the couple to determine their genetic risk.

   B. Both Mr. and Mrs. G. are found to be carriers of the disorder. *DISCUSS* the estimation of risk and interpretation of risk as it applies to the couple for giving birth to a child who is normal, is a carrier, or is affected by the disorder.

   C. *OUTLINE* the nurse's role in the education and emotional support of the couple now that a diagnosis and estimation of risk have been made.

ONLINE LEARNING ACTIVITIES

Access the Lowdermilk, Perry **Evolve** website at
http://evolve.elsevier.com/Lowdermilk/MatWmnHlth/ and enter the **Student** portion through the
Learning Resources section to assist you in searching the literature for research studies related to the
impact a diagnosis of an inheritable disorder can have on families and the role that genetic
counseling plays in assisting families to cope with the disorder and make informed decisions regarding
the course of action that is best for them.

- Create an annotated bibliography of at least five research studies.
- Choose one study and complete a bibliography card that includes the following:
  - Hypothesis; research question
  - Summary of the methodology used and key findings
  - Reliability of the study and its findings
  - Recommendations for further research
  - How the professional nurse can use this information to guide and support families when a
    diagnosis of an inheritable disorder is made.

CHAPTER 4

Alternative and Complementary Therapies

CHAPTER REVIEW ACTIVITIES

MATCHING: Match the description in Column I with the appropriate term from Column II.

COLUMN I

_____ 1. Massage techniques applied to specific points along certain energy pathways of the body called meridians.

_____ 2. A form of treatment using slender needles to stimulate points along energy pathways to correct, enhance, and rebalance the flow of body energy.

_____ 3. Techniques that teach the client to consciously control certain body functions usually thought of as unconscious.

_____ 4. The use of imagination and thought processes in a purposeful way to change certain physiologic and emotional conditions.

_____ 5. A combination of energetic healing techniques used by nurses and other health care professionals.

_____ 6. System of healing based on the belief that small doses of the same agent that caused a disease could cure it and that each client is a unique individual requiring a remedy specific to him or her.

_____ 7. Any activity that focuses the attention in the present moment and, in the process, quiets and relaxes the mind and body.

_____ 8. Looking within for solutions and answers to certain dilemmas, using intuition and inner wisdom as guides for attainment of healing.

_____ 9. The absence or alleviation of mental, physical, or emotional tension through purposeful activities that quiet the body and mind.

_____ 10. A modern interpretation of the laying on of hands for healing.

COLUMN II

A. Reflection
B. Biofeedback
C. Meditation
D. Healing touch
E. Acupressure
F. Guided imagery
G. Relaxation
H. Acupuncture
I. Therapeutic touch
J. Homeopathy

FILL IN THE BLANKS: Insert the term that corresponds to each of the following descriptions.

11. _____ Form of care that focuses on the correction of underlying disharmony in the interaction of _____, _____, and _____ and demonstrates concern and compassion for the whole client, not just the client's symptoms.

12. _____ Nontraditional approaches to health care and healing, often philosophically different from Western medicine. Interventions are said to induce healing from within the _____ or improve the _____ so that the _____, _____, or _____ can heal. They are often referred to as "_____."

13. _____ A variety of techniques and disciplines that are said to augment, modulate, stimulate, or remedy certain deficiencies or blocks in the human energy system.

14. _____ Philosophy that states that the whole is greater than the sum of its parts. In healing, it refers to consideration and treatment of the whole client as a unified being.

15. _____ Nursing practice that stems from the view that the client is an integrated whole and is influenced by a variety of internal and external factors including the _____ and _____ dimensions of the person as an integrated whole.

16. _____ The individual's connection to one's own values, purpose, and meaning of life. It may encompass organized religion or belief in a higher power or authority.

17. _____ Terms used to describe the current American health care system, which is often focused on one body system or disease complex and the use of pharmaceutical or surgical treatments.

18. _____ Ancient methods of healing that combine herbs, energy healing, and movement as a pathway to health. Seeks to heal on deeper levels rather that just deal with symptoms.

TRUE OR FALSE: Circle "T" if true or "F" if false for each of the following statements. Correct the false statements.

T   F   19. Alternative methods of healing are often cited as being more beneficial for the treatment of chronic illness than is standard or allopathic medicine.

T   F   20. Holistic nurses provide care that is relationship centered and seek to blend technology with holistic healing approaches.

T   F   21. Most holistic therapies and modalities used by nurses require no formal training or practice before implementation with clients.

T   F   22. Touch therapies often use an energy-based philosophy that recognizes human energy fields which are detectable and capable of modulation and change.

T   F   23. Biofeedback has been successfully used as a component of treatment for certain systemic diseases such as asthma.

T   F   24. Herbal preparations from the foxglove plant can be used to treat depression.

T   F   25. Herbal preparations containing feverfew can be effectively used to prevent migraine headaches.

T   F   26. Pressure applied to one or both temples can relieve nausea.

T   F   27. Massage has been used to enhance the progress of labor.

28. *CITE* barriers that exist which prevent the full integration of traditional and alternative approaches to health care.

29. *EXPLAIN* why touch is a powerful healing tool. *CITE* several examples of how touch is used as an alternative therapy in women's health care.

30. The mind can be used as a powerful healing tool. *DESCRIBE* how the mind affects healing when each of the following modalities are used:
   A. Guided imagery

   B. Meditation, prayer, reflection, relaxation

   C. Biofeedback

31. Herbs can be used as part of a client's therapeutic regime. *STATE* the guidelines that should be followed and the precautions taken to ensure safety and effectiveness when herbs are used as a component of treatment.

CRITICAL THINKING EXERCISES

1. Many of today's health care consumers are turning away from standard (Western or allopathic) medicine and seeking alternative and complementary therapies to promote, maintain, and restore their health.
   A. *IDENTIFY* the factors that are responsible for this trend.

B. *DISCUSS* how alternative approaches address the factors identified above.

C. *DESCRIBE* how nurses responded to the consumer demand for alternative therapies.

D. *DISCUSS* the three concepts that are shared by most alternative and complementary therapies.

2. Marie, a 52-year-old woman, has been experiencing symptoms associated with perimenopause including hot flashes, anxiety, and difficulty falling asleep at night. At a routine women's health check-up, Marie asks the nurse practitioner about what she can do to relieve these symptoms in a "natural way without using dangerous hormones." *DISCUSS* how the nurse should respond to Marie's concern.

3. A Childbirth Educator offers classes to pregnant women and their families throughout pregnancy. She encourages women to try alternative approaches to deal with the discomforts associated with pregnancy and the pain associated with childbirth. *IDENTIFY* two approaches this nurse could recommend to her clients. *EXPLAIN* the basis for the effectiveness of each of the approaches you identified.

ONLINE LEARNING ACTIVITIES

Perform an Internet search related to holistic nursing. Access one site and prepare a report that includes the following information:
- Stated mission or philosophy of the site
- Organization supporting the site
- Services offered to consumers of health care and health care providers
- Research data provided to validate the effectiveness of the alternative health care approaches described and recommended by the site
- Your reaction to the information and care measures presented on the site and how you would use this information when providing care to your clients

CHAPTER 5

Assessment and Health Promotion

CHAPTER REVIEW ACTIVITIES

FILL IN THE BLANKS: Insert the term that corresponds to each of the following definitions related to the female reproductive system and breasts.

1. _____ Fatty pad that lies over the anterior surface of the symphysis pubis.
2. _____ Two rounded folds of fatty tissue covered with skin that extend downward and backward from the mons pubis; their purpose is to protect the inner vulvar structures.
3. _____ Two flat reddish folds composed of connective tissue and smooth muscle, which are supplied with nerve endings that are extremely sensitive.
4. _____ Hoodlike covering of the clitoris.
5. _____ Fold of tissue under the clitoris.
6. _____ Thin flat tissue formed by the joining of the labia minora; it is underneath the vaginal opening at the midline.
7. _____ Small structure composed of erectile tissue with numerous sensory nerve endings; it increases in size during sexual arousal.
8. _____ Almond-shaped area enclosed by the labia minora that contains openings to the urethra, Skene's glands, vagina, and Bartholin's glands.
9. _____ Skin-covered muscular area between the fourchette and the anus that covers the pelvic structures.
10. _____ Fibromuscular, collapsible tubular structure that extends from the vulva to the uterus and lies between the bladder and rectum. Its mucosal lining is arranged in transverse folds called _____. _____, and _____ glands secrete mucus that lubricates the vagina.
11. _____ Anterior, posterior, and lateral pockets that surround the cervix.
12. _____ Muscular pelvic organ located between the bladder and the rectum and just above the vagina. The _____ is a deep pouch, or recess, posterior to the cervix formed by the posterior ligament.
13. _____ Upper triangular portion of the uterus.
14. _____ Also known as the lower uterine segment, it is the short constricted portion that separates the corpus of the uterus from the cervix.
15. _____ Dome-shaped top of the uterus.
16. _____ Highly vascular lining of the uterus.
17. _____ Layer of the uterus composed of smooth muscles that extend in three different directions.

18. _____ Lower cylindrical portion of the uterus composed of fibrous connective tissue and elastic tissue.

19. _____ Canal connecting the uterine cavity to the vagina. The opening between the uterus and this canal is the _____. The opening between the canal and the vagina is the _____.

20. _____ Location in the cervix where the squamous and columnar epithelium meet; it is the most common site for neoplastic changes; cells from this site are scraped for the _____ smear.

21. _____ Passageways between the ovaries and the uterus; they are attached at each side of the dome-shaped top of the uterus.

22. _____ Almond-shaped organs located on each side of the uterus; their two functions are _____ and the production of the hormones _____, _____, and _____.

23. _____ The paired mammary glands.

24. _____ Segment of mammary tissue that extends into the axilla.

25. _____ Mammary papilla.

26. _____ Pigmented section of the breast that surrounds the nipple.

27. _____ Sebaceous glands that cause the areola to appear rough.

28. _____ Breast structures which are lined with epithelial cells that secrete colostrum and milk.

29. _____ Milk reservoirs.

TRUE OR FALSE: Circle "T" for true or "F" for false for each of the following statements. Correct each of the false statements.

T F 30. Most women enter the heath care system for the first time to seek assistance regarding a gender-related concern.

T F 31. The biologic marker on which both serum and urine pregnancy tests are based is estrogen.

T F 32. Approximately 25% of pregnancies in the United States each year are unintended.

T F 33. Approximately 15% of couples in the United States have some degree of infertility.

T F 34. Sexual orientation can be a significant barrier for women seeking health care.

T F 35. A sexually active adolescent who does not use contraception has a 50% chance of pregnancy within 2 years.

T F 36. The rate of teen pregnancies steadily increased between 1991 and 2000.

T F 37. A woman's ethnicity influences her health risks and behaviors.

T F 38. Preconception counseling and care is a health care service designed primarily for women of childbearing age who have chronic health problems.

T F 39. Women tend to use primary care services more often than men.

T F 40. Smoking increases the risk for osteoporosis after menopause.

T F 41. Smoking has little to no effect on fertility.

T F 42. Women are more likely than men to abuse drugs.

T F 43. No method of contraceptive offers complete protection from contracting a sexually transmitted infection.

T F 44. It is recommended that the first Pap smear take place at the age of 21.

T F 45. Clinical breast examination by a health care provider is recommended every 1 to 3 years for women starting at the age of 30.

T   F   46. Annual mammograms should begin at age 35.

T   F   47. Swimming should be recommended to perimenopausal women as an exercise that can help to prevent osteoporosis.

T   F   48. Kegel exercises help to strengthen abdominal muscles.

T   F   49. Cigarette smoking among adolescents and young adult women is higher than for men.

T   F   50. The breasts of a healthy, mature woman should be symmetrical.

T   F   51. Progesterone is the hormone responsible for the maturation of mammary gland tissue, specifically the lobules and acinar structures.

T   F   52. The breasts often change in size and nodularity during the menstrual cycle.

T   F   53. Breast swelling, tenderness, and leakage from the nipple are expected assessment findings during the postmenstrual period.

T   F   54. In North America, girls experience menarche at approximately 15 years of age.

T   F   55. Menstruation usually begins at about 14 days after ovulation.

T   F   56. The last day of bleeding or menses is day one of a new menstrual cycle.

T   F   57. Pregnancy is possible at any time after menarche occurs.

T   F   58. Variations in the length of the follicular phase account for almost all variations in ovarian cycle length.

T   F   59. Implantation (nidation) of a fertilized ovum usually occurs about 14 days after ovulation.

T   F   60. Mittelschmerz refers to the stretchable quality of cervical mucus that occurs in response to estrogen secretion prior to ovulation.

T   F   61. Dysmenorrhea (painful menstruation) is most often associated with the production of progesterone.

T   F   62. The average age for menopause is approximately 60 years.

T   F   63. Men and women are more alike than different in terms of their physiologic response to sexual excitement and orgasm.

T   F   64. Sexual arousal is characterized by increased muscular tension called myotonia.

T   F   65. The acidity of vaginal secretions is an important body defense against infection.

T   F   66. For many women, modesty, fear, and anxiety can make the health history interview and the physical examination an ordeal.

T   F   67. Vulvar self-examination (VSE) should be performed at least once a month between menstrual periods.

68. A nurse working in the field of women's health must have knowledge of the female reproductive systems including the internal and external structures, the interrelationship of these structures, and their normal characteristics. *LABEL* each of the following illustrations as indicated and *DESCRIBE* on a separate sheet of paper the normal characteristics and functions of each structure (use the figures in Chapter 5 and those found in a physical assessment or anatomy textbook to assist you with the labels and descriptions).

A. **External female genitalia:**

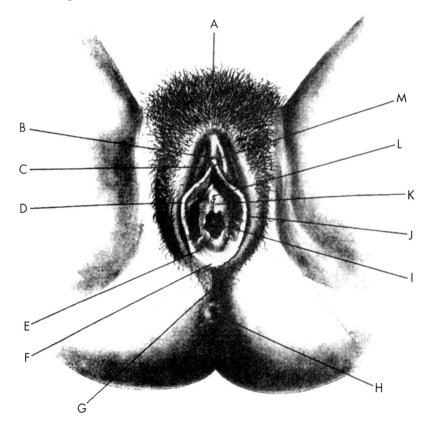

B. **Perineal body with surrounding tissues and organs**

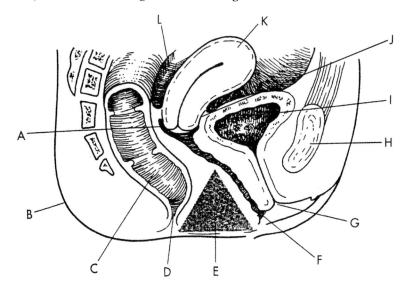

C. Cross section of uterus, adnexa, and upper vagina

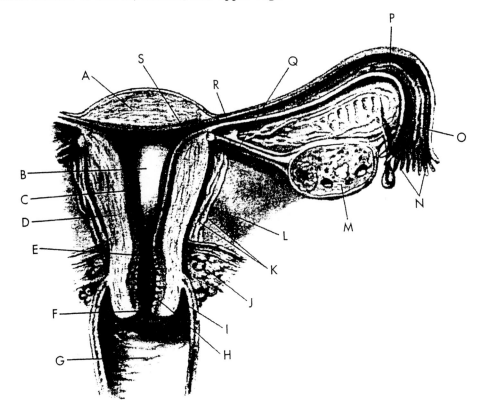

D. Female breast

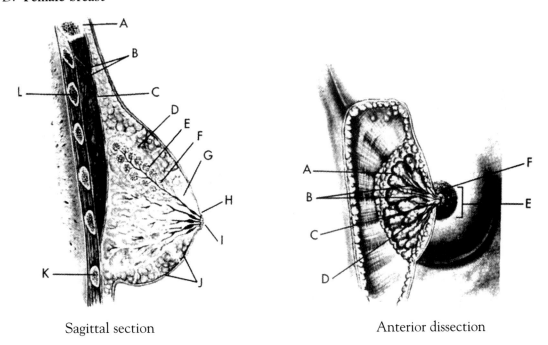

Sagittal section   Anterior dissection

E. **Female pelvis**

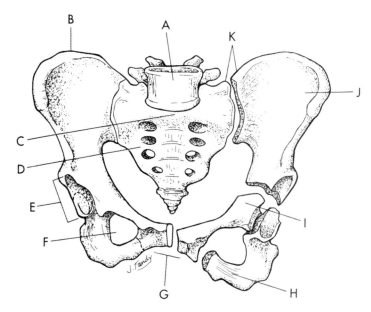

69. The diagram below illustrates the cyclical changes that occur during the menstrual cycle of a woman of childbearing age. *LABEL* the diagram as indicated in terms of hormones, phases and cycles, and specific ovarian structures.

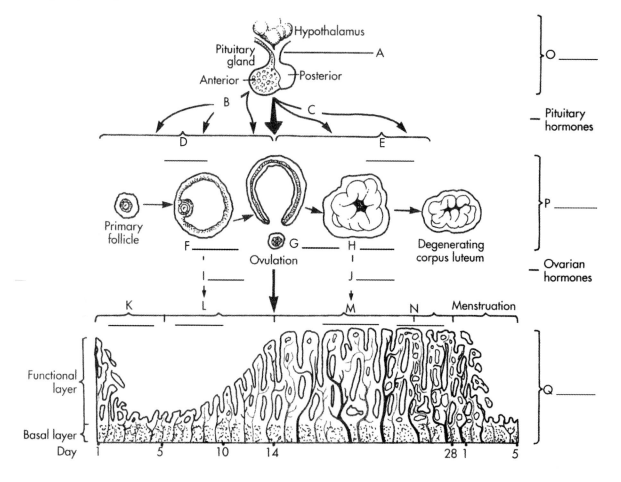

70. It is essential that guidelines for laboratory and diagnostic procedures be followed exactly in order to ensure the accuracy of the results obtained. *OUTLINE* the guidelines that should be followed when performing a Papanicolaou smear in terms of each of the following:

Client preparation

Timing during examination when the specimen is obtained

Sites for specimen collection

Handling of specimens

Frequency of performance

71. During a clinical examination of a woman's breasts the nurse identifies a lump in one of the breasts. *CITE* the characteristics that the nurse should document regarding the palpated lump.

72. Sara, a 20-year-old woman, tells the nurse that she performs breast self-examination (BSE) on a regular basis. The nurse evaluates Sara's understanding of BSE and ability to perform the technique correctly. The nurse's findings are documented below. *INDICATE* with a "+" those findings that reflect accurate knowledge and correct technique and with a "–" those findings that require further instruction and demonstration. *STATE* the nursing instruction for those findings requiring further teaching and demonstration.

A. Performs examination every 1 to 2 months.

B. Performs BSE about 4 days after menstruation begins.

C. Begins BSE by standing in front of a mirror and observing characteristics of her breasts with her arms in at least two positions: at rest at her sides and above her head.

D. Observes the size of her breasts, the direction of her nipples, appearance of her skin, and if there are dimples or lumps anywhere when looking at her breasts in the mirror.

E. Lies down on her bed and puts a pillow under the shoulder of the breast she is going to palpate. Then she places the arm on that side under her head.

F. Uses the tips of her four fingers to palpate her breast.

G. Palpates her breasts using an overlapping, circular pattern around her entire breast.

H. Squeezes her nipple between her thumb and forefinger after palpation, to check for discharge.

I. Palpates her breasts and up into her axilla while taking a shower.

MULTIPLE CHOICE: Circle the one correct option and state the rationale for the option chosen.

73. When palpating the small breasts of a young slender woman, the nurse should:
    A. Wear sterile gloves
    B. Lift hands when moving from one segment of the breast to another
    C. Use both hands
    D. Follow a systematic, overlapping pattern

74. A nurse instructed a female client regarding self-examination of the external genitalia. Which of the statements made by the client will require further instruction? I will:
    A. Perform this examination at least once a month especially if I change sexual partners or am sexually active
    B. Become familiar with how my genitalia look and feel so that I will be able to detect changes
    C. Use the examination to determine when I should get medications at the pharmacy for yeast infections
    D. Wash my hands thoroughly before and after I examine myself

75. A women's health nurse practitioner is going to perform a pelvic examination on a female client. Which of the following nursing actions would be least effective in enhancing the client's comfort and relaxation during the examination?
    A. Encourage the client to ask questions and express feelings and concerns before and after the examination
    B. Ask the client questions as the examination is performed
    C. Allow the client to keep her shoes and socks on when placing her feet in the stirrups
    D. Instruct the client to place her hands over her diaphragm and take deep, slow breaths

76. When assessing women, it is important for the nurse to keep in mind the possibility that they are victims of violence. The nurse should:
    A. Use an abuse assessment screen during the assessment of every woman
    B. Recognize that abuse rarely occurs during pregnancy
    C. Assess a woman's legs and back as the most commonly injured areas
    D. Notify the police immediately if abuse is suspected

77. A 50-year-old woman asks the nurse practitioner about how often she should be assessed for the common health problems women of her age could experience. The nurse would recommend:
    A. An endometrial biopsy every 3 to 4 years
    B. A fecal occult blood test annually
    C. A mammogram every other year
    D. Bone mineral density testing annually

78. Which of the following statements is most accurate regarding persons who should participate in preconception counseling?
    A. All women and their partners as they make decisions about their reproductive future including becoming parents
    B. All women during their childbearing years
    C. Sexually active women who do not use birth control
    D. Women with chronic illnesses such as diabetes who are planning to get pregnant

CRITICAL THINKING EXERCISES

1. A nurse is teaching a group of young adult women about health promotion activities. As part of the discussion the nurse identifies preconception care as an important health promotion activity. One woman in the class asks, "I know you need to go for check-ups once you are pregnant but why would you need to see a doctor before you get pregnant? Isn't that a big waste of time and money?" EXPLAIN how the nurse should respond to this woman's question.

2. A group of nurse practitioners and midwives is establishing a women's health clinic in a large metropolitan area of New York. They will be serving a multiethnic population that consists of women from adolescence to old age.
   A. Using an awareness that women most often initially seek health care for reproductive concerns, IDENTIFY the services the nurses at this new clinic should plan to offer.

   B. CITE the factors (barriers) that could interfere with the women in this community seeking health care at the clinic. Based on these barriers, DESCRIBE strategies these nurses could use to reduce the barriers to care and encourage the women to participate in the services offered at the clinic.

   C. Major goals of the nurses at this clinic are to promote the health of women in the community and prevent the occurrence of illness. DISCUSS the types of services the nurses should place a high priority on offering in order to achieve their goals. Include a rationale for each service proposed.

3. During a routine check-up for her annual Pap smear, Julie, a 26-year-old woman, asks the nurse for advice regarding nutrition and exercise. Her BMI is 29 and she wants to "lose weight sensibly and keep it off." DISCUSS the advice the nurse should give to Julie.

4. Alice, a 30-year-old woman, comes to the women's health clinic complaining of fatigue, insomnia, and feeling anxious. She works as a stockbroker for a major Wall Street brokerage firm. Alice states that, although she enjoys the challenge of her job, she never can seem to find time for herself or to socialize with her friends. Alice tells the nurse practitioner that she has been drinking more and started to smoke again to help her to relax. She is glad that she has lost some weight, attributing this occurrence to her diminished appetite.

A. STATE the physical and emotional signs of stress that the nurse should take note of when assessing Alice.

B. DISCUSS how the nurse can help Alice cope with stress and its consequences in a healthy manner.

C. Alice expresses interest in attempting to stop smoking. "I felt so much better when I stopped the first time. That was over 2 years ago and now, here I am back at it again." DESCRIBE an approach the nurse could use to help Alice achieve a desired change in health behavior that is long lasting.

5. During a routine women's health check-up a woman expresses concern to the nurse practitioner about the increase in violence against women. She states, "One of my friends was raped and a colleague at work was beaten by her boyfriend." DISCUSS how the nurse practitioner should respond to this woman's concern, including measures she could use to protect herself from violence and injury.

6. An inner-city women's health clinic serves a diverse population in terms of age, ethnic background, and health problems. DESCRIBE how each of the following factors should influence a women's health nurse practitioner's approach when assessing the health of the women who come to the clinic for care.

Culture

Age

Physical and emotional disorders

Abuse

7. *IMAGINE* that you are a nurse working at a clinic that provides health care to women. *DESCRIBE* how you would respond to each of the following concerns or questions of women who have come to the clinic for care.

   A. Serena, a 17-year-old woman, has just been scheduled for her first women's health check-up, which will include a pelvic examination and Pap smear. She nervously asks if there is anything she needs to do to get ready for the examination.

   B. Andrea is trying to get pregnant. She wonders if there are signs she could observe in her body that would indicate that she is ovulating and therefore able to conceive a baby with her partner.

   C. When you are teaching a group of women of various ages about breast self-examination (BSE), they ask you to describe the normal characteristics of the female breast and how these characteristics change as a woman gets older.

   D. Anne, a 24-year-old woman, asks the nurse about a recommended douche to use a couple of times a week to stay "nice and clean down there."

8. Julie, a 21-year-old woman, has come to the women's health clinic for a women's health check-up. During the health history interview she becomes very anxious and states "I have to tell you this is my first examination. I am very scared—my friends told me that it hurts a lot to have this examination." DESCRIBE how the nurse should respond in an effort to reduce Julie's anxiety.

9. As a nurse working in a women's health clinic, you have been assigned to interview Angie, a 25-year-old new female client, in order to obtain her health history.
   A. LIST the components that should be emphasized in gathering Angie's history.

   B. WRITE a series of questions that you would ask to obtain data related to Angie's reproductive and sexual health and practices.

   C. DISCUSS the therapeutic techniques that you would use to facilitate communication. GIVE an example of each technique.

10. Self-examination of the breasts and vulva (genitalia) are important assessment techniques to teach a woman. OUTLINE the procedure that you would use to teach each technique to one of your clients. INCLUDE the teaching methodologies that you would use to enhance learning.
    Breast self-examination

    Vulvar (genital) self-examination

11. Lu Chen is a 25-year-old exchange student from China who has been living in the United States for 3 months. This is the first time that she is away from home. She comes to the university women's health clinic for a "check-up" and to obtain birth control. *DESCRIBE* how the nurse assigned to Lu Chen would approach and communicate with her in a culturally sensitive manner.

12. Nurses working in women's health care must be aware of the growing problem of violence against women. All women should be screened when being assessed during health care for the possibility of abuse.

   A. *DESCRIBE* how you as a nurse would adjust the environment where the health history interview and physical examination will take place to elicit a woman's confidence and trust.

   B. *IDENTIFY* indicators of possible abuse that you would look for before the appointment and then during the health history interview and physical examination.

   C. *STATE* the questions you would ask to screen for abuse.

   D. *DISCUSS* the approach you would take if abuse is confirmed during the assessment.

13. When teaching a group of preadolescent girls about menstruation, one student asks the nurse "what will happen to me when all of this stuff starts?" *DESCRIBE* what the nurse should tell the girls about the changes that they can expect and what is happening to their bodies during each of the following components of the menstrual cycle:
   Hypothalamic-pituitary cycle

Ovarian cycle

Endometrial cycle

14. As a student you may be assigned to assist a health care provider during the performance of a pelvic examination for one of your clients.
   A. *DESCRIBE* how you would:
   Prepare your client for the examination

   Support your client during the examination

   Assist your client after the examination

   B. DESCRIBE how you would assist the health care provider who is performing the examination.

ONLINE LEARNING ACTIVITIES

Access the Lowdermilk, Perry **Evolve** website at **http://evolve.elsevier.com/Lowdermilk/MatWmnHlth/** and enter the **Student** portion through the **Learning Resources** section. Using Chapter 5 as a starting point, search the Internet for information regarding the pelvic examination. Based on the information you gathered:
- Prepare a list of Internet resources that provide information regarding the pelvic examination
- Use the information you gathered to write a set of guidelines that health care providers can use when performing pelvic examinations; the guidelines should address issues related to:

- Accuracy of results
- Client comfort and privacy
- Stress reduction
- Education of women regarding their bodies

Use the Centers for Disease Control and Prevention (CDC) and the National Center for Health Statistics (NCHS) websites to gather statistical data regarding the incidence of:
- Substance use and abuse among women
- Morbidity and mortality rates for the most common health problems among women

Create a chart that depicts the statistical data according to the characteristics of women including age and racial/ethnic background.

Use Evolve to assist you in searching the literature for nursing articles related to preconception care, substance use and abuse among women, or eating disorders.
- Compile an annotated bibliography related to your chosen topic
- Choose one article and complete a bibliography card that includes the following:
  - Summary of the article's key points
  - Personal reaction to the ideas presented in the article
  - How the professional nurse can use the article's ideas to enhance and improve the quality of health care for women

CHAPTER 6

Violence Against Women

CHAPTER REVIEW ACTIVITIES

FILL IN THE BLANKS

1. _____ refers to the actual or threatened physical, sexual, psychologic, or emotional abuse by a current or ex-spouse, boyfriend, or girlfriend, date, or cohabitating partner. It can include _____, _____, and _____.

2. _____, _____, and _____ or _____ are terms applied to a pattern of assaultive and coercive behaviors inflicted by the male partner in a marriage or other heterosexual, significant, intimate relationship. Common elements are _____ deprivation, _____ abuse, _____, _____, and _____ and _____ victims and their children.

3. According to the cycle of violence theory, battering occurs in _____ cycles. The three-phase cyclic pattern that occurs begins with a period of _____ leading to the _____, which is then followed by a period of _____ and _____ known as the _____ phase.

4. _____ or compulsive masculinity is associated with wife abuse. It encompasses the traditional male values of _____ and _____.

5. Childhood sexual abuse is defined as any type of sexual exploitation that involves a child younger than _____ years of age at the time of the first molestation, at least a _____ age difference between the victim and perpetrator, and a variety of behaviors between the victim and perpetrator that may include _____, _____, _____, _____, _____, and _____, _____, or _____ penetration.

6. _____ is any type of sexual exploitation between blood relatives or surrogate relatives before the victim reaches the age of _____. If a stranger commits the sexual abuse it is considered to be _____.

7. _____ encompasses a wide range of sexual victimization, including _____ and unwanted or uncomfortable _____, _____, _____, _____, _____, or other sexual acts.

8. _____ is an act of violence rather than a sexual act and in its strictest sense it is forced _____ or the _____ of the female _____ or _____ without the woman's consent. It is called _____ when the perpetrator is 18 or older and the victim is under the age of consent as defined by the individual state. Forms of this act of violence include _____, _____, _____, _____, and _____.

9. _____ consists of noncoital sexual activity between a child and an adolescent or adult.

10. _____ is the use of power and control tactics to victimize women sexually particularly in the workplace.

11. _____ syndrome may be experienced by women after they have been sexually assaulted. It is characterized by extreme _____ and _____ resulting in _____ and _____ reactions and _____ complaints. The three phases of this syndrome are _____, _____, and _____.

12. IDENTIFY psychologic, sociologic, and biologic factors that are associated with and may increase the risk for abusive behavior patterns against women.
    Psychologic factors

    Sociologic factors

    Biologic factors

13. STATE how cultural beliefs and values can affect violence against women: its occurrence, how it is viewed, and the help sought by and provided to women who are abused. CITE examples from specific cultures.

14. Nurses working in women's health care should be aware of the characteristics typical of women who are abused and the men who abuse them.
    A. CONTRAST the characteristics of women who are most likely to be in abusive relationships with the characteristics of women who are most likely to be in nonviolent relationships.

    B. CITE the characteristics of women who are most likely to seek assistance when they are abused.

C. *EXPLAIN* why women may not seek help when they are in an abusive relationship.

D. *IDENTIFY* the characteristics of men who are most likely to become abusive husbands (partners).

E. *DESCRIBE* the forms of abuse that a man can inflict on his wife (partner).

15. Clarise is a victim of intimate partner violence (IPV) by her male partner. *DESCRIBE* how the nurse caring for Clarise could use the ABCDEs tool to provide Clarise with the support she needs.

16. *DESCRIBE* the strategies nurses can use to prevent the cycle of violence against women in our society.

17. *INDICATE* the factors that can deter women from reporting that they have been raped.

TRUE OR FALSE: Circle "T" if true or "F" if false for each of the following statements. Correct the false statements.

T F 18. Race, religion, social background, age, and educational level are all significant factors in differentiating women at risk for abuse.

T F 19. The key feature to establish rape is the absence of consent.

T F 20. More than 25% of women are beaten when they are pregnant.

T F 21. In the United States, violence is the second leading cause of injuries to women 15 to 44 years of age.

T F 22. Mental illness accounts for nearly 50% of all violence.

T F 23. Approximately 30% of abused children become abusers as adults.

T   F   24. Battering follows a cyclic pattern.

T   F   25. Nurses should assess all women entering the health care system for abuse.

T   F   26. The majority of states have mandatory reporting laws specific to domestic violence or adult abuse.

T   F   27. The majority of victims of childhood sexual abuse are male.

T   F   28. The peak age for childhood sexual abuse is from 7 to 12 years of age.

T   F   29. About one half of rape victims report their sexual assault.

T   F   30. Most of the perpetrators in a rape are known to their victims.

T   F   31. Emergency contraception with progestin only or combined with estrogen must be used within 24 hours of a sexual assault.

T   F   32. Nausea is a common side effect of progestin- and estrogen-based emergency contraception.

MULTIPLE CHOICE: Circle the one correct option and state the rationale for the option chosen.

33. Men who are likely to abuse their female partner often exhibit:
    A. Low self-esteem
    B. High degree of assertiveness
    C. Ability to express feelings verbally
    D. Lack of interest in spending time doing things with the partner that they are abusing

34. A characteristic of women in abusive relationships would be:
    A. Masochism
    B. Willingness to take a stand no matter what the cost
    C. Absence of typical feminine characteristics such as nurturing and compassion
    D. Tendency to isolate themselves from social relationships

35. A nurse caring for pregnant women needs to be aware that physical abuse during pregnancy can result in:
    A. Excessive weight gain as a result of the inappropriate intake of food to reduce stress
    B. Use of alcohol or tobacco as a means of coping
    C. Postterm pregnancy
    D. Pregnancy-induced hypertension

36. Which of the following woman is most likely to seek assistance when battered?
    A. Woman with a career
    B. Woman battered for the first time
    C. Woman who as a child saw her mother being abused by her father
    D. Woman who has been abused herself

37. After being raped, a woman often progresses through the three stages of the rape-trauma syndrome. A characteristic behavior of the outward adjustment phase would be:
    A. Rapid mood swings
    B. Desire to discuss the rape with someone
    C. Efforts to ensure personal safety including buying a gun
    D. Nightmares and eating disorders

CRITICAL THINKING EXERCISES

1. *SUPPLY* the facts to disprove each of the following myths concerning violence against women.
   A. Spousal (partner) abuse is primarily a problem of families who are at a low socioeconomic level and poorly educated.

   B. Violence affects only a small percentage of women in this country.

   C. Battered women and their abusers cannot change their patterns of behavior.

   D. Battered women usually provoke their attack because they have a need to be beaten.

   E. Women are rarely battered when they are pregnant.

2. Research has identified a cyclic nature to battering—a cycle of violence.
   A. IDENTIFY the characteristic behaviors of each of the following phases of the cycle of violence:
   Phase I: Tension—Building State

   Phase II: Acute Battering Incident

B. *DESCRIBE* how the nurse working in women's health could use this information in providing anticipatory guidance for a battered woman who elects to stay with the partner who abuses her.

3. As a nurse working in a woman's health clinic you must be alert to cues indicative of physical abuse.

A. *IDENTIFY* the cues you would look for.

B. Carol, a 24-year-old married woman, comes to the clinic to confirm her belief that she is pregnant. During the assessment phase of the visit, you note cues that lead you to suspect that Carol is being abused by her husband. *DISCUSS* the approach you would take to confirm your suspicion that Carol is being abused.

C. Carol admits to you that her husband "beats her sometimes and it has been increasing." Now she is afraid it will get worse because she "was not supposed to get pregnant." *DISCUSS* the nursing actions that you could take in order to help Carol.

D. *LIST* the possible reasons why Carol, now that she is pregnant, is experiencing an escalation of battering/abuse from her husband.

E. *SPECIFY* what you should avoid as you work with Carol.

F. *DISCUSS* how Carol's pregnancy could be adversely affected by the abuse she is experiencing.

G. *DESCRIBE* the behaviors Carol would most likely exhibit as an indication of her readiness to leave the abusive relationship.

H. *IDENTIFY* your legal responsibilities regarding confirmation that Carol is indeed being abused.

4. Susan is a 23-year-old who was sexually abused by her father when she was a teenager.
   A. *DESCRIBE* the behaviors that might suggest to the nurse that Susan is experiencing physical and psychosocial effects related to the abuse she experienced as a teenager including delayed-onset posttraumatic stress disorder.
   Physical effects

   Psychosocial effects

   Delayed-onset posttraumatic stress syndrome

   B. DISCUSS the activities that the nurse could suggest to Susan that might help her to deal with the past abuse, to heal and to grow.

5. Marie has been raped. She is admitted to the emergency room for examination.
   A. *DESCRIBE* the nurse's responsibility in assessing Marie and in collecting and preserving the physical evidence of her rape.

   B. *DISCUSS* the nursing actions that should be used to meet the emotional needs of Marie at this time.

   C. *INDICATE* during which phase of the rape-trauma syndrome the following manifestations by Marie are likely to have occurred:

COLUMN I

_____ Fear of being alone

_____ Rapid changes in mood

_____ Anger, humiliation, embarrassment

_____ Desire to talk about the experience

_____ Denial and suppression of thoughts and feelings

_____ Recognition that the experience helped her to grow

_____ Blames herself for the rape and cites things she "could have done to avoid it"

_____ Physiologic discomfort

_____ Initiates self-protection measures by enrolling in a self-defense class and buying a weapon

_____ Physical distress and memories of the rape diminish

_____ Returns to her job and starts socializing with her friends again

_____ Experiences nightmares and anorexia

_____ Feels unclean and may destroy evidence by bathing and douching

COLUMN II

A. Acute phase: disorganization

B. Outward adjustment phase

C. Long-term process: Reorganization phase

   D. *SPECIFY* the interventions required prior to discharging Marie.

Online Learning Activities

Access the Lowdermilk, Perry **Evolve** website at
http://evolve.elsevier.com/Lowdermilk/MatWmnHlth/ and enter the **Student** portion through the
Learning Resources section to assist you in searching the literature for research studies related to
violence in women—its consequences on women and their families and effective support measures to
assist victims.

- Create an annotated bibliography of at least five studies
- Choose one study and complete a bibliography card that includes:
  - Hypothesis; research question
  - Summary of the methodology used and key findings
  - Reliability of the study and its findings
  - Recommendations for further research
  - How the professional nurse can use the study's findings to enhance and improve the quality of
    health care provided to women who are victims of violence

CHAPTER 7

Reproductive System Concerns

CHAPTER REVIEW ACTIVITIES

FILL IN THE BLANKS: Insert the term that corresponds to each of the following descriptions related to menstrual disorders and experiences.

1. _____ refers to the absence of menstrual flow. It is a clinical sign of a variety of disorders but it is most commonly a result of _____. It is one of the classic signs of _____. Hypogonadotropic _____ is often related to the suppression of the hypothalamus by _____ or a sudden and severe _____, _____ disorders, strenuous _____, or _____.

2. _____ or painful menstruation is one of the most common gynecologic problems for women of all ages. Pain usually occurs during or shortly after _____. _____ is a type of painful menstruation that occurs as a result of a physiologic alteration in some women. It usually appears within _____ after menarche when _____ is established because both _____ and _____ are necessary for it to occur. _____ is acquired menstrual pain that develops later in life and is associated with pelvic pathology. Pain often begins _____.

3. _____ is a cluster of physical, psychologic, and behavioral symptoms beginning in the luteal phase of the menstrual cycle. A diagnosis is only made if the following three criteria are met: _____, _____, and _____. _____ is a severe variant, characterized by marked irritability, dysphoria, mood lability, anxiety, fatigue, appetite changes, and feeling overwhelmed.

4. _____ is a menstrual disorder that is characterized by the presence and growth of endometrial tissue outside of the uterus. This tissue responds to hormonal stimulation by growing during the _____ and _____ phases of the menstrual cycle and bleeding during or immediately after _____, resulting in an _____ response with subsequent _____ and _____ to adjacent organs. The major symptoms of this disorder are _____ and deep pelvic _____. Many women also experience bowel symptoms such as _____, _____, and _____. Impaired _____ may result from adhesions around the uterus and uterine tubes.

5. _____ refers to infrequent menstrual periods characterized by intervals of 40 to 45 days or longer. _____ refers to scanty bleeding at normal intervals. One of the most common causes of scanty menstrual flow is the use of _____.

6. _____ or _____ refers to any episode of bleeding (spotting, menses, hemorrhage) that occurs at a time other than the normal menses. _____, a small amount of bleeding at the time of ovulation, is considered to be normal.

7. _____ refers to the bleeding that occurs when the contraceptive pill does not sufficiently maintain a hypoplastic endometrium, resulting in shedding of the endometrium in small amounts at a time.

8. _____ or _____ is defined as excessive menstrual bleeding, either in duration or amount. The causes may include _____ disturbances, _____ diseases, _____, _____, and _____. _____ and _____ provide objective indicators to actual blood loss and should always be assessed.

9. _____ is any form of uterine bleeding that is irregular in amount, duration, or timing and not related to regular menstrual bleeding.

10. _____ is excessive uterine bleeding with no demonstrable organic cause. It is most frequently caused by _____ where there is no surge of _____ or if insufficient _____ is produced by the _____ to support the endometrium. As a result the endometrium begins to involute and shed. This most often occurs at the extremes of a woman's reproductive years when the menstrual cycle is just becoming established at _____ or when it draws to a close at _____.

TRUE OR FALSE: Circle "T" if true or "F" if false for each of the following statements. Correct the false statements.

T   F   11. A pregnancy test is recommended as an important initial step when a woman experiences amenorrhea.

T   F   12. Premature osteoporosis can occur as a consequence of low levels of progesterone associated with hypogonadotropic amenorrhea.

T   F   13. The exact cause of PMS is unknown.

T   F   14. Oral contraceptive pills (OCP) are the first-line medications for the treatment of primary dysmenorrhea.

T   F   15. Endometriosis is a menstrual disorder primarily affecting Caucasian women.

T   F   16. Nafarelin (Synarel) is a gonadotropic-releasing hormone agonist administered to treat hot flashes associated with perimenopause.

T   F   17. The only definitive cure for endometriosis is a total abdominal hysterectomy (TAH).

T   F   18. The length of menstrual cycles is most irregular in the first year after menarche and the 2 years prior to menopause when anovulatory cycles are most common.

T   F   19. Primary dysmenorrhea most often is related to excessive prostaglandin secretion during an ovulatory cycle.

T   F   20. Women often experience a decrease in primary dysmenorrhea after a full term pregnancy.

T   F   21. Women who experience primary dysmenorrhea should avoid physical activity including exercising for the first few days of menstrual bleeding.

T   F   22. The pain associated with secondary dysmenorrhea is often sharp, radiating over the abdomen from umbilicus to symphysis pubis.

T   F   23. Lifestyle changes usually have little effect in the treatment of premenstrual syndrome.

T   F   24. Evening primrose oil taken daily has been found to be effective in relieving breast symptoms associated with premenstrual syndrome.

T   F   25. Pregnancy is contraindicated for women who are being treated with Danazol for endometriosis.

T   F   26. A common side effect of the use of contraceptive implants such as Norplant is menorrhagia.

T   F   27. One of the most common causes of scanty menstrual flow is the use of oral contraceptives.
T   F   28. African-American women who are obese have a high probability of developing osteoporosis during the perimenopause and postmenopause.
T   F   29. Obese women are more likely to experience dysfunctional uterine bleeding than slender women.
T   F   30. The occurrence of perimenopausal mental health problems is closely associated with estrogen deficiency.
T   F   31. Menopausal hormone therapy using a combination of estrogen and progestin is the best approach for preventing the development of cardiovascular disease.
T   F   32. Adequate calcium and vitamin D intake is essential to prevent osteoporosis in menopausal women.
T   F   33. Menopausal estrogen therapy should be used when a woman still has her uterus in order to reduce her risk for endometrial cancer.
T   F   34. Soy-rich foods can reduce symptoms experienced by perimenopausal women.
T   F   35. Women should be taught to take alendronate sodium with meals to reduce gastric distress and enhance absorption.

36. The perimenopause is a period of approximately _____ years. The majority of women experience its onset between ages _____ and _____. This period of time in a woman's life encompasses the transition from normal _____ to cessation of _____ and is marked by _____. _____ refers to the complete cessation of menses and is said to occur when a woman has not experienced menstrual flow or spotting for _____ year(s). The _____ is another term used when referring to this transitional period. COMPLETE the following table related to perimenopausal changes, their manifestations and physiologic and/or psychologic basis.

Change	Manifestations	Physiologic and Psychologic Basis
Bleeding		
Genital Changes		
Vasomotor Instability		
Mood and Behavioral Responses		

37. Postmenopausal women are at risk for coronary artery disease (CAD) because of changes in _____. There is a decline in serum levels of _____ and an increase in serum levels of _____. *IDENTIFY* additional factors that increase a woman's risk for developing and dying from cardiovascular disease in the postmenopause.

38. Menopausal hormone therapy (MHT) is a treatment option chosen by many perimenopausal women.
    A. *STATE* the therapeutic uses for MHT.

    B. *IDENTIFY* the side effects/adverse reactions women may experience when taking MHT.

    C. *SPECIFY* the risks associated with MHT.

    D. *DESCRIBE* several nonhormonal approaches that can be used in place of MHT to relieve menopausal discomforts/symptoms. Indicate the therapeutic effect of each approach identified.

MULTIPLE CHOICE: Circle the one correct option and state the rationale for the option chosen.

39. Which of the following women is at greatest risk for developing hypogonadotropic amenorrhea?
    A. 48-year-old woman experiencing perimenopausal changes
    B. 13-year-old figure skater
    C. 18-year-old softball player
    D. 30-year-old (G3 P3003) breastfeeding woman

40. Pharmacologic preparations can be used to treat primary dysmenorrhea. Choose the preparation that would be least effective in relieving the symptoms of primary dysmenorrhea.
    A. Oral contraceptive pill (OCP)
    B. Naproxen sodium (Anaprox)
    C. Acetaminophen (Tylenol)
    D. Ibuprofen (Motrin)

41. Women experiencing primary dysmenorrhea should be advised to avoid which of the following foods?
    A. Red meats
    B. Asparagus
    C. Cranberry juice
    D. Whole-grain cereals

42. The nurse counseling a 30-year-old woman regarding effective measures to use to relieve symptoms associated with premenstrual syndrome (PMS) could suggest:
    A. Decrease intake of fruits especially peaches and watermelon
    B. Reduce exercise during the luteal phase of the menstrual cycle when symptoms are at their peak
    C. Maintain a salt intake of 6 g/day or less
    D. Avoid tobacco, alcohol, and caffeine

43. A 28-year-old woman has been diagnosed with endometriosis. She has been placed on a course of treatment with danazol (Danocrine). The woman exhibits understanding of this treatment when she says:
    A. "Since this medication stops ovulation I do not need to use birth control."
    B. "I will need to take this medication until I reach menopause."
    C. "I can experience a decrease in my breast size, oily skin, and hair growth on my face as a result of taking this medication."
    D. "I will need to spray this medication into my nose twice a day."

44. A female client, age 26, describes scant bleeding between her menstrual periods. The nurse would record this finding as
    A. Metrorrhagia
    B. Oligomenorrhea
    C. Menorrhagia
    D. Hypomenorrhea

45. Dysfunctional uterine bleeding (DUB) is most likely to occur when women:
    A. Experience ovulatory cycles
    B. Are less than their expected body weight
    C. Are experiencing signs of the onset of perimenopause
    D. Secrete high levels of prostaglandin

46. A 55-year-old woman tells the nurse that she has started to experience pain when she and her husband have intercourse. The nurse would record that this woman is experiencing:
    A. Dyspareunia
    B. Dysmenorrhea
    C. Dysuria
    D. Dyspnea

CRITICAL THINKING EXERCISES

1. Maria is a 16-year-old gymnast who has been training vigorously for a placement on the United States Olympic team. She has been experiencing amenorrhea and the development of her secondary sexual characteristics has been limited. Maria expresses concern because her nonathletic friends have all been menstruating for at least 1 year and have well-developed breasts. After a health assessment, Maria was diagnosed with hypogonadotropic amenorrhea.

   A. *STATE* the risk factors for this disorder that Maria most likely exhibited during the assessment process.

   B. *STATE* one nursing diagnosis reflective of Maria's concern.

   C. *WRITE* two expected outcomes for a plan of care for Maria.

   D. *OUTLINE* a typical care management plan for Maria that will address the issues associated with hypogonadotropic amenorrhea.

2. Mary, a 17-year-old who experienced menarche at age 16, comes to the Women's Health Clinic for a routine check-up. She complains to the nurse that her last few periods have been very painful. "I have missed a few days of school because of it. What can I do to reduce the pain that I feel during my periods?" Physical examination and testing reveal normal structure and function of Mary's reproductive system. A medical diagnosis of primary dysmenorrhea is made.

   A. *COMPARE AND CONTRAST* the medical diagnoses of primary and secondary dysmenorrhea in terms of etiology and characteristics of the pain and discomfort experienced.

   B. *STATE* the priority nursing diagnosis appropriate for Mary.

C. *IDENTIFY* appropriate relief measures for primary dysmenorrhea that the nurse could suggest to Mary.

3. Susan experiences physical and psychologic signs and symptoms associated with premenstrual syndrome (PMS) during every ovulatory menstrual cycle.
   A. *LIST* the signs and symptoms most likely described by Susan that lead to the diagnosis of PMS.

   B. *IDENTIFY* one nursing diagnosis that may be appropriate for Susan when she is experiencing the signs and symptoms of PMS.

   C. *DESCRIBE* the approach the nurse would use in helping Susan to deal with this menstrual disorder.

4. Lisa is 26 years old and has been diagnosed recently with endometriosis.
   A. *LIST* the signs and symptoms Lisa most likely exhibited to lead to this medical diagnosis.

   B. Lisa asks the nurse, "What is happening to my body as a result of this disease?" *DESCRIBE* the nurse's response.

   C. Lisa asks about her treatment options. "Are there medications I can take to make me feel better?" *DESCRIBE* the action/effect and potential side effects for each of the following pharmacologic approaches to treatment.
   Oral contraceptive pills

Gonadotropin-releasing hormone (GnRH) agonists

Androgen derivatives

   D. *IDENTIFY* support measures the nurse can suggest to assist Lisa to cope with the effects of endometriosis.

5. Jane, a 45-year-old slender white woman who works as a secretary, is at the beginning of the perimenopausal period. Her health history reveals a high intake of fast foods, coffee, and diet soft drinks especially Pepsi, along with a smoking habit of one pack per day. Jane states that her favorite leisure activities are reading, needlework, and playing Bingo two evenings a week. She expresses concern about the development of osteoporosis because her mother experienced the stress fractures and dowager's hump characteristic of this disorder. Jane requests information concerning what she can do to prevent this from happening to her.
   A. *IDENTIFY* the risk factors for osteoporosis present in this situation.

   B. *DISCUSS* the information you should give Jane regarding prevention measures that would reduce her risk for developing osteoporosis and its sequelae.

   C. *LIST* the signs Jane would exhibit if she begins to develop osteoporosis.

6. Heidi is a 50-year-old woman experiencing the changes typical of perimenopause. During a routine GYN check-up at the women's health clinic she tells her nurse practitioner that she is having a hard time coping with hot flashes, stress incontinence, and insomnia. Heidi also expresses concern about the vaginal dryness she is experiencing because it has resulted in discomfort and even pain when she and her husband have intercourse. Heidi asks the nurse if there is anything she could suggest to reduce the discomfort associated with all these problems. She tells the nurse that several of her friends have been taking hormones and seem to be doing better.

A. *DESCRIBE* the relief measures the nurse practitioner should suggest to Heidi regarding:

Hot flashes (flushes)

Insomnia

Headache

Urogenital symptoms (e.g., vaginal dryness, incontinence, dyspareunia)

B. *DISCUSS* the approach the nurse practitioner should use to help Heidi decide about menopausal hormone therapy.

C. Heidi decides to begin MHT using a combination of estrogen and progestin transdermal patch (CombiPatch). *SPECIFY* the instructions that Heidi should be given regarding this treatment to ensure its safety and effectiveness.

D. Heidi is a computer expert and enjoys using the Internet to research a variety of topics and "chat" with persons who share her interests in quilting and mystery novels. *DESCRIBE* how the nurse could use Heidi's interest in and expertise with computers to direct her to appropriate websites that would provide her with reliable information and support during the perimenopause period.

ONLINE LEARNING ACTIVITIES

Access the Lowdermilk, Perry **Evolve** website at
http://evolve.elsevier.com/Lowdermilk/MatWmnHlth/ and enter the **Student** portion through the **Learning Resources** section. Using Chapter 7 as a starting point, search the Internet for websites designed to educate and support women during the perimenopausal and postmenopausal years. Prepare a report that includes the following:
- List of at least five relevant websites
- Description of two of the sites in terms of:
  - Sponsoring person, agency, or organization
  - Clarity, accuracy, accessibility (ease of use), value, and depth of the information provided
  - Currency—frequency of site updates
  - Variety of links to other relevant sites
  - Ability of persons visiting the site to obtain additional information and individualized support through services such as e-mail and chat rooms
  - Discussion regarding how the professional nurse could use these sites and the information provided to enhance and improve the quality of health care

CHAPTER 8

Sexually Transmitted and Other Infections

CHAPTER REVIEW ACTIVITIES

FILL IN THE BLANKS: Insert the infection or prevention measure that corresponds to each of the following descriptions.

1. _____ Infections or infectious disease syndromes primarily transmitted by close intimate contact. The most common infections of this type in women are _____, _____, _____, _____, _____, and _____.

2. _____ Precautions used during sexual activity to prevent the transmission of pathogens. These precautions include _____, _____, _____, and _____.

3. _____ The physical barrier promoted for the prevention of sexual transmission of human immunodeficiency virus (HIV) and other sexually transmitted infections (STIs). Another effective physical barrier is the _____.

4. _____ Bacterial infection that is the most common and fastest spreading STI in American women. This infection is often silent and highly destructive to the female reproductive tract.

5. _____ The oldest communicable disease in the United States. Because it is a reportable communicable disease, health care providers are legally responsible for reporting all cases to health authorities.

6. _____ One of the earliest STIs. It is caused by *Treponema pallidum*, a spirochete. _____ is characterized by a lesion or _____ that appears _____ days after infection. _____ occurs _____ after the appearance of the primary lesion and is characterized by a widespread _____ on the _____ and _____ and general _____. The infected individual may experience _____, _____, _____, and _____. _____ may develop on the vulva, perineum, and anus. If left untreated the client enters a _____ that is asymptomatic for most persons. _____ is characterized by neurologic, cardiovascular, musculoskeletal, and multiorgan system complications.

7. _____ Infectious process that most commonly involves the uterine tubes, uterus, and more rarely ovaries and peritoneal surfaces. The greatest risk for this infection occurs during the _____ or following an _____, _____, or _____.

8. _____ Infection previously named genital or venereal warts. It is now the most prevalent viral STI seen in ambulatory health care settings. The visible lesions caused by the infection are called _____.

9. _____ A viral infection that is transmitted sexually and is characterized by distinctive vesicle type lesions on the genitalia. Clients with a primary genital infection exhibit multiple _____, _____, _____, _____, and severe _____.

10. _____ Viral infection acquired primarily through a fecal-oral route by ingestion of contaminated food, particularly _____, _____, or _____, or _____ contact.

11. _____ Viral infection involving the liver that is transmitted parenterally and through intimate contact. It is 50 to 100 times more contagious than HIV and is often a "silent" infection. A vaccine is available to protect infants, children, and adults.

12. _____ Viral infection of the liver that is transmitted parenterally and through intimate contact. There is no vaccine available to provide protection against this infection.

13. _____ A retrovirus that is transmitted primarily though exchange of body fluids. Severe depression of the _____ system is associated with this infection.

14. _____ A normal vaginal flora that is present in 10% to 30% of healthy pregnant women. It has been suggested as a factor in preterm labor, chorioamnionitis, urinary tract infections during pregnancy, and postpartum infections. Vertical transmission to the newborn during birth has been implicated as an important factor in perinatal and neonatal morbidity and mortality.

15. _____ Vaginal infection formerly called nonspecific vaginitis, Haemophilus vaginitis, or Gardnerella. It is the most common type of vaginitis today. It is characterized by a profuse, thin, and white, gray, or milky discharge that has a characteristic _____ odor.

16. _____ This yeast infection is the second most common type of vaginal infection in the United States. Vulvar and possible vaginal _____, _____, and _____ are common symptoms. The discharge is _____, _____, _____, and _____. It appears as patches on the _____, _____, and _____.

17. _____ A vaginal infection caused by an anaerobic one-celled protozoan with characteristic flagellae. The typically copious discharge is yellowish-green, frothy, mucopurulent, and malodorous.

18. _____ A group of infections that can affect a pregnant woman and her fetus. The infecting organisms are capable of crossing the placenta and adversely affecting the development of the fetus.

19. _____ A protozoan infection associated with the consumption of infested raw or undercooked meat and with poor handwashing after handling infected cat litter.

20. _____ German or 3-day measles transmitted by droplets.

21. _____ Viral infection that may begin as a mononucleosis-like syndrome. It is primarily transmitted by respiratory droplets but the virus has also been found in other body fluids. It can lead to profound neurologic and sensory disorders if transmitted to the newborn.

TRUE OR FALSE: Circle "T" if true or "F" if false for each of the following statements. Correct false statements.

T F 22. Sexually transmitted diseases are among the most common health problems in the United States today.

T F 23. Safer sex practices are secondary prevention activities.

T F 24. Anal intercourse is a safe alternative to vaginal intercourse if a condom is not available.

T F 25. It is an unfounded assumption that older persons have few if any sexual partners and infrequent sexual encounters.

T F 26. The most common sexually transmitted bacterial pathogen in American women is gonorrhea.

T F 27. The majority of women contracting gonorrhea are 30 years of age or older.

T F 28. Chlamydia can be transmitted by direct sexual contact or exposure at birth.

T F 29. The Centers for Disease Control and Prevention (CDC) recommends that all women between the ages of 18 and 40 be screened for chlamydia every year at the time of the Papanicolaou (Pap) smear.

T F 30. Women older than 30 years of age have the lowest rate of infection with chlamydia.

T F 31. Chlamydia is the most common infectious cause of ophthalmia neonatorum.

T F 32. Gonorrhea can be spread by direct contact with infected lesions and indirectly by transfer from inanimate objects, or fomites.

T F 33. The most common manifestation of neonatal gonorrheal infection is pneumonia.

T F 34. The Venereal Disease Research Laboratories (VDRL) test will be positive within 1 week of infection.

T F 35. Even without treatment, the chancres from primary syphilis may heal, thus allowing the disease to progress to the next stage.

T F 36. Erythromycin is the primary treatment for syphilis.

T F 37. *Chlamydia trachomatis* is estimated to cause at least one half of all cases of pelvic inflammatory disease (PID).

T F 38. Ascending spread of microorganisms from vagina to the upper genital tract most often occurs just before menstruation.

T F 39. Visible warts characterize the type of human papillomavirus (HPV) with the highest potential for cervical cancer.

T F 40. Human papillomavirus (HPV) infections are thought to be more frequent in pregnant women than in nonpregnant women.

T F 41. Colposcopy is the most commonly used screening technique for HPV infection.

T F 42. Lesions characteristic of recurrent episodes of herpes simplex virus II (HSV II) infections are unilateral, beginning as vesicles and progressing rapidly to ulcers.

T F 43. Vaginal birth is acceptable if visible HSV II lesions are not present at the onset of labor.

T F 44. Women who test positive for hepatitis B should not breastfeed their newborn.

T F 45. Women are the fastest growing population of individuals with human immunodeficiency virus (HIV) infection and acquired immunodeficiency syndrome (AIDS).

T F 46. Once HIV enters the body, seroconversion to HIV positivity occurs within 2 to 4 weeks.

T F 47. Presence of HIV antibodies in infants younger than 18 months of age is not diagnostic of infection.

T F 48. HIV can be transmitted to the newborn via the breast milk of an infected mother.

T F 49. Zidovudine (AZT) has been found to be a safe and effective treatment method for women who are HIV-positive during pregnancy.

T F 50. Tuberculosis is the most commonly seen opportunistic infection in persons with HIV and AIDS.

T F 51. Vaccination of a woman for hepatitis B during pregnancy can infect the fetus and is therefore contraindicated until after birth.

T F 52. The recommended treatment for women in labor who test positive for Group B streptococcus is the intravenous administration of penicillin G.

T F 53. Women who receive the rubella vaccine must avoid pregnancy for at least 3 months after vaccination.

T F 54. Standard precautions are to be used as soon as a client is diagnosed with a blood-borne infection.

MULTIPLE CHOICE: Circle the one correct option and state the rationale for the option chosen.

55. Infections of the female mid-reproductive tract such as chlamydia are dangerous primarily because these infections:
    A. Are asymptomatic
    B. Cause infertility
    C. Lead to pelvic inflammatory disease
    D. Are difficult to treat effectively

56. A finding associated with human papillomavirus (HPV) infection would include which of the following?
    A. White, curd-like, adherent discharge
    B. Soft papillary swelling occurring singly or in clusters
    C. Vesicles progressing to pustules and then to ulcers
    D. Yellow to green frothy malodorous discharge

57. A recommended medication effective in the treatment of vulvovaginal candidiasis would be
    A. Metronidazole
    B. Clotrimazole
    C. Penicillin
    D. Acyclovir

58. A woman is determined to be group B streptococcus (GBS) positive at the onset of her labor. The nurse should prepare this woman for
    A. Cesarean birth
    B. Intravenous administration of penicillin during labor
    C. Isolation of her newborn after birth
    D. Application of acyclovir to her labial lesions

59. When providing a woman, recovering from primary herpes, with information regarding the recurrence of herpes infection of the genital tract, the nurse would tell her:
    A. Fever and flu-like symptoms will precede a recurrent infection
    B. Little can be done to control the recurrence of infection
    C. Transmission of the virus is only possible when lesions are open and draining
    D. Itching and tingling often occur prior to the appearance of vesicles

60. *IDENTIFY* two sexual behaviors that apply to each of the following categories:
    Safest behaviors

    Low risk behaviors

    Possibly risky (possible exposure) behaviors

    High risk (unsafe) behaviors

61. *CITE* several common risk factors for sexually transmitted infections.

62. *STATE* two specific precautions for each of the following categories:
    Standard Precautions

    Precautions for invasive procedures

63. *COMPLETE THE FOLLOWING TABLE* related to common reproductive tract infections.

Infection	Clinical Manifestations	Management Guidelines
Chlamydia		
Gonorrhea		
Syphilis		
Human Papillomavirus		
Herpes Simplex Virus		
Bacterial Vaginosis		
Candidiasis		
Trichomoniasis		

64. Heterosexual transmission is the most common means of infecting women with the human immunodeficiency virus (HIV).
   A. *STATE* the mode of transmission for HIV.

   B. *LIST* the clinical manifestations that may be exhibited during seroconversion to HIV positivity.

C. *OUTLINE* the care management approach that should be used by nurses who care for women who test HIV positive.

65. *STATE* the infection represented by the group of infections known collectively as TORCH.

CRITICAL THINKING EXERCISES

1. Terry, a 20-year-old woman, comes to a women's health clinic for her first visit.
   A. During the health history interview, it is imperative that the nurse practitioner determine Terry's risk for contracting a sexually transmitted infection including HIV. *WRITE* one question for each of the following risk categories.
   Sexual risk

   Drug use–related risk

   Blood-related risk

   HIV concerns

   B. Terry asks the nurse about measures she could use to protect herself from STIs. *CITE* the major points that the nurse practitioner should emphasize when teaching Terry about prevention measures.

C. Terry tells the nurse that she does not know if she could ever tell a partner that he must wear a condom. *DESCRIBE* the approach the nurse can take to enhance Terry's assertiveness and communication skills.

2. Martha is 4 weeks' pregnant. As part of her prenatal assessment it was discovered that she was HIV positive. *IDENTIFY* the measures that can be used to reduce the risk of transmission of HIV from Martha to her baby.

3. Suzanne, a 20-year-old woman, is admitted for suspected severe, acute pelvic inflammatory disease (PID).
   A. *IDENTIFY* the risk factors for PID that the nurse would be looking for in Suzanne's health history.

   B. A complete physical examination is performed to determine if the criteria for PID are met. *SPECIFY* the criteria that Suzanne's health care provider would be alert for during the examination.

   C. Suzanne is hospitalized when the diagnosis of PID secondary to chlamydial infection is confirmed. Intravenous antibiotics will be used as the primary medical treatment followed by oral antibiotics at the time of discharge. *STATE* three priority nursing diagnoses that are likely to be present during the acute stage of Suzanne's infection and treatment.

   D. *OUTLINE* a nursing management plan for Suzanne in terms of each of the following:
   Position and activity

Comfort measures

Support measures

Health education in preparation for discharge

E. *LIST* the recommendations for Suzanne's self-care during the recovery phase.

F. *IDENTIFY* the reproductive health risks that Suzanne may face as a result of the pelvic infection she experienced.

4. Laura has just been diagnosed with gonorrhea, a sexually transmitted infection.
   A. *STATE* the essential areas of assessment the nurse should keep in mind when interviewing Laura during the health history.

   B. Laura is very upset by the diagnosis stating, "This is just awful—what kind of sex life can I have now?" *CITE* a nursing diagnosis that reflects Laura's concern.

   C. *OUTLINE* a management plan that will assist Laura to take control of her self-care and prevent future infections.

5. Cheryl, a 27-year-old woman, is being treated for human papillomavirus (HPV). A primary diagnosis identified for Cheryl is acute pain related to lesions on the vulva and around the anus secondary to HPV infection. *STATE* the measures the nurse could suggest to Cheryl to reduce the pain from the condylomata and enhance their healing.

6. Mary, a 20-year-old woman, has just been diagnosed with a primary herpes simplex II infection. In addition to the typical systemic symptoms, Mary exhibits multiple, painful genital lesions.
   A. Relief of pain and healing without the development of a secondary infection are two expected outcomes for care. *IDENTIFY* several measures that the nurse can suggest to Mary in an effort to help her achieve the expected outcomes of care.

   B. Mary asks the nurse if there is anything she can do so that this infection does not return. *DISCUSS* what the nurse should tell Mary about the recurrence of herpes infection II and the influence of self-care measures.

7. Gloria tested positive for hepatitis B. *DESCRIBE* the measures that the nurse should teach Gloria in an effort to decrease the risk for transmission of the virus to other persons in Gloria's life.

8. Sonya is concerned that she has been exposed to HIV and has come to the women's health clinic for testing.
   A. During the health history the nurse questions Sonya about behaviors that could have placed her at risk for HIV transmission. *CITE* the behaviors that the nurse would be looking for.

   B. *EXPLAIN* the testing procedure that will most likely be followed to determine Sonya's HIV status.

C. *OUTLINE* the counseling protocol that should guide the nurse when caring for Sonya before and after the test.

D. Sonya's test result is negative. *DISCUSS* the instructions the nurse should give Sonya regarding guidelines she should follow to reduce her risk for the transmission of HIV with future sexual partners.

ONLINE LEARNING ACTIVITIES

Access the website related to the Surgeon General's report entitled *Healthy People 2010*. Prepare a report that includes the following:
- Goals for reducing the incidence of STIs in the United States
- Identification of strategies that should be effective in making progress toward goal achievement
- Your proposal for additional strategies that will be effective in fully meeting and even surpassing the stated goals. Give the rationale for the strategies that you propose.

CHAPTER 9

Contraception and Abortion

CHAPTER REVIEW ACTIVITIES

FILL IN THE BLANKS: Insert the term that corresponds to each of the following descriptions.

1. _____ Method that requires the male partner to withdraw his penis from the woman's vagina prior to ejaculation.
2. _____ Group of contraceptive methods that rely on avoidance of intercourse during fertile periods.
3. _____ Methods that combine the charting of signs and symptoms of the menstrual cycle with the use of abstinence or other contraceptive methods during fertile periods.
4. _____ Method based on the number of days in each cycle counting from the first day of menses. The fertile period is determined after accurately recording lengths of menstrual cycles for 6 months.
5. _____ Method based on variations in a woman's lowest body temperature, which is determined immediately after waking and before getting out of bed.
6. _____ Term used to refer to the stretchiness of cervical mucus.
7. _____ Method that combines the basal body temperature (BBT) and cervical mucus methods with awareness of secondary cycle, phase-related symptoms. The woman gains fertility awareness as she learns the physiologic and psychologic changes that occur during each phase of her menstrual cycle.
8. _____ Chemical that destroys sperm. When inserted into the vagina it acts as both a chemical and physical barrier to sperm.
9. _____ Thin, stretchable sheath that covers the penis or is inserted into the vagina.
10. _____ Shallow, dome-shaped rubber device with a flexible rim that covers the cervix.
11. _____ A 22- to 31-mm soft natural rubber dome with a firm but pliable rim that fits snugly around the base of the cervix close to the junction of the cervix and vaginal fornices.
12. _____ A small round polyurethane device that contains spermicide. It fits over the cervix and has a woven polyester loop to facilitate its removal.
13. _____ Form of oral contraceptive pill that provides a fixed dosage of estrogen and progesterone.
14. _____ Form of oral contraceptive pill that has varying amounts of progestin and sometimes estrogen within each cycle.
15. _____ Form of hormonal contraception in which six flexible, nonbiodegradable Silastic capsules containing progestin are implanted subdermally into the inner aspect of the upper arm.

16. _____ Progesterone antagonist that prevents the implantation of a fertilized ovum.
17. _____ Small, T-shaped device inserted into the uterine cavity. It is loaded with copper or a progestational agent.
18. _____ Surgical procedures intended to render the person infertile. For the female the _____ are occluded. It is accomplished by _____, _____, or the application of _____ or _____. For the male, the _____ are occluded, with _____ being the most commonly used method.
19. _____ Purposeful interruption of a pregnancy before 20 weeks' gestation. If it is performed at the woman's request, it is termed an _____. If it is performed for reasons of maternal or fetal health or disease it is termed a _____.

TRUE OR FALSE: Circle "T" if true or "F" if false for each of the following statements. Correct the false statements.

T   F   20. Despite the large number of persons who use contraception, almost one third of pregnancies in the United States are unintended.

T   F   21. Contraception failure rate refers to the percentage of contraceptive users expected to experience an accidental pregnancy during the first year of use, even when they use the method consistently and correctly.

T   F   22. The fertile period extends from 4 days before to 3 to 4 days after ovulation.

T   F   23. Coitus interruptus is similar to barrier methods with regard to effectiveness.

T   F   24. The typical failure rate for all fertility awareness methods is about 25% during the first year of use.

T   F   25. Variations in the length of menstrual cycles are usually the result of differences in the length of the period from ovulation to the onset of menstruation.

T   F   26. When preparing to use the calendar rhythm method, a woman needs to accurately record the lengths of the previous two menstrual cycles.

T   F   27. The LH surge in urine just prior to ovulation can be affected if the woman is ill at the time of the test.

T   F   28. Nonoxynol 9 provides protection against the transmission of human immunodeficiency virus (HIV).

T   F   29. Research has demonstrated that polyurethane condoms are as effective as latex condoms in protecting against sexually transmitted infections and HIV infections.

T   F   30. The female condom can be inserted up to 8 hours before intercourse.

T   F   31. Use of a diaphragm can increase the risk for urethritis and recurrent cystitis.

T   F   32. An advantage of using a cervical cap is that it can be left in place longer than a diaphragm.

T   F   33. When using a cervical cap, the woman must apply spermicide prior to each act of intercourse.

T   F   34. A new contraceptive sponge needs to be inserted for each act of sexual intercourse.

T   F   35. Use of oral contraceptives may lower a woman's risk for ovarian and endometrial cancer.

T   F   36. Women using the combined oral contraceptive pill should expect decreased menstrual blood loss.

T   F   37. Oral contraceptives are considered to be a safe option for older, nonsmoking women until menopause.

T F 38. A diabetic woman using oral contraceptives may require a decrease in her daily insulin dosage.
T F 39. Antibiotics can decrease the effectiveness of the oral contraceptive pill.
T F 40. Women should delay pregnancy at least 6 months after discontinuing the use of oral contraceptives.
T F 41. The Norplant system provides up to 3 years of contraceptive effectiveness.
T F 42. Norplant completely suppresses ovulation.
T F 43. After injecting Depo-Provera intramuscularly, the nurse should massage the injection site to fully distribute the progestin.
T F 44. Depo-Provera injections must be repeated every 6 months.
T F 45. An antiemetic taken 1 hour before each oral dose of estrogen and progesterone used for emergency contraception will help to minimize nausea.
T F 46. The intrauterine device (IUD) is more appropriate than oral contraceptives for women older than 35 years of age who are heavy smokers.
T F 47. Following a vasectomy, another form of birth control should be used until the sperm count is zero for at least two consecutive semen analyses.
T F 48. Although a vasectomy has no effect on potency, it does result in a reduction in the volume of ejaculate.
T F 49. No change in the menstrual cycle should occur following a tubal ligation.
T F 50. Approximately 90% of abortions are performed during the first trimester of pregnancy.
T F 51. Mifepristone (RU 486) can be taken up to 5 weeks after conception to terminate a pregnancy.
T F 52. Oxytocin administered as a gel or parenterally is the most common medical technique to terminate a pregnancy in the second trimester.

MULTIPLE CHOICE: Circle the one correct option and state the rationale for the option chosen.

53. A single, young adult woman received instructions from the nurse regarding the use of an oral contraceptive. The woman would demonstrate a need for further instruction if she:
   A. Stops asking her sexual partners to use condoms with spermicide
   B. Enrolls in a smoking cessation program
   C. Takes a pill every morning
   D. Uses a barrier method of birth control if she misses two or more pills

54. Oral contraception in the form of a combination of low-dose estrogen and progesterone:
   A. Reduces the pH of cervical mucus, thereby destroying sperm
   B. Protects against iron deficiency anemia by reducing blood loss with menses
   C. Prevents the transmission of sexually transmitted diseases
   D. Is 90% effective in preventing pregnancy when used correctly

55. The most common, and for some women the most distressing side effect of Norplant, is
   A. Irregular menstrual bleeding
   B. Headache
   C. Nervousness
   D. Nausea

56. A woman with an IUD should confirm its placement by checking the IUD's string:
    A. Before each menstrual period
    B. After intercourse
    C. At the time of ovulation
    D. During menstrual bleeding

57. When teaching women about the effective use of chemical barriers, the nurse should tell them to:
    A. Insert foams at least 1 hour prior to coitus
    B. Insert suppositories just prior to penile contact with the vagina
    C. Douche immediately after last intercourse
    D. Reapply before each act of coitus

58. When using a cervical cap, the woman should:
    A. Apply spermicide inside the cap and around the rim
    B. Leave it in place for a minimum of 8 hours and maximum of 48 hours after the last act of coitus
    C. Continue to use the cap during menstrual periods
    D. Check the position of the cap and insert additional spermicide before each act of coitus

59. A nurse is working with a couple to help them choose a method of contraceptive that is right for them.
    A. *LIST* the factors that can influence the effectiveness of the contraceptive method they choose.

    B. Informed consent is a vital component when helping this couple to choose a contraceptive. *STATE* the elements of an informed consent that need to be met and documented as part of the decision-making process. Use the letters below to organize your response.

       B   R   A   I   D   E   D

60. A woman is a little uncomfortable about checking her cervical mucus and asks the nurse what she could possibly find out about doing this assessment. *STATE* the useful purpose of self-evaluation of cervical mucus.

61. June's religious and cultural beliefs prohibit her from using any artificial method of birth control. She is interested in learning about periodic abstinence or natural family planning as a method of contraception. *FILL IN THE BLANKS* in each of the following statements concerning this method.

A. The two principal problems with fertility awareness methods are difficulty in determining the exact time of _____ and difficulty in _____ for several days before and after ovulation. Women with _____ have the greatest risk for failure.

B. Using the calendar method, June and her husband would abstain from day _____ to _____ of her menstrual cycle because her shortest cycle was 23 days and the longest cycle was 33 days.

C. Basal body temperature (BBT) will _____ about _____ C at about the time of ovulation. After ovulation, because of increasing levels of _____, the BBT will _____ about _____ C. This change in BBT will last until _____ before menstruation. These changes in BBT are termed the _____.

D. The _____ method would require June to recognize and interpret the cyclical changes in the characteristics of her _____ such as _____ and _____.

E. The Symptothermal Method combines _____ and _____ methods with awareness of secondary cycle phase-related symptoms such as increased _____, midcycle _____, _____, pelvic _____ or _____, and vulvar _____. The woman is taught to palpate her _____ to assess for changes indicating ovulation such as slight _____, _____, and _____ in the vagina.

F. The predictor test for ovulation detects the sudden surge of _____ in the urine that occurs approximately _____ hours before ovulation.

62. Alice and Bob use nonprescription chemical and mechanical contraceptive barriers. *LABEL* each of the following actions with "C" if correct or "I" if incorrect. *INDICATE* how the action should be changed for those actions labeled "I".

A. _____ When using a vaginal suppository form of spermicide, Alice waits about 30 minutes after insertion before beginning intercourse.

B. _____ When using a spermicidal vaginal foam, Alice shakes the container prior to application.

C. _____ Alice reapplies the spermicide before each act of intercourse.

D. _____ Alice douches within 2 hours of intercourse because she finds the spermicidal foam sticky and uncomfortable.

E. _____ Bob applies a condom over his erect penis leaving an empty space at the tip.

F. _____ Bob often lubricates the outside of a latex condom with Vaseline, a petroleum-based lubricant.

G. _____ Alice and Bob occasionally use the vaginal sheath instead of a male condom. Because they are more expensive, Alice and Bob reuse it if they have intercourse more than once.

63. Joyce has chosen the diaphragm as her method of contraception. *LABEL* each of the following actions with "C" if correct or "I" if incorrect. *INDICATE* how the action should be changed for those actions labeled "I".

A. _____ Joyce came to be refitted after healing was complete following the term vaginal birth of her son.

B. _____ Joyce applies a spermicide only to the rim of the diaphragm just prior to insertion because she dislikes the stickiness of the spermicide.

C. _____ Joyce empties her bladder before inserting the diaphragm.

D. _____ Joyce inserts the diaphragm about 3 to 4 hours before intercourse to increase spontaneity.

E. _____ Joyce applies more spermicide for each act of intercourse.

F. _____ Joyce removes the diaphragm within 1 hour of intercourse.

G. _____ After removal, Joyce washes the diaphragm with warm water and an antiseptic-type soap, dries it, and then applies baby powder.

H. _____ Joyce always uses the diaphragm during her menstrual periods.

64. *CITE* four factors that can contribute to a woman's decision to seek an induced abortion.

CRITICAL THINKING EXERCISES

1. A nurse working in a women's health clinic should be aware that toxic shock syndrome (TSS) is a possible complication for women who use a diaphragm as their method of contraception.

A. *CITE* the prevention measures that the nurse should teach women to use to reduce their risk for TSS.

B. *IDENTIFY* the clinical manifestations of TSS that the nurse should be alert for when assessing women who use diaphragms.

2. Kathy, an 18-year-old woman, has come to Planned Parenthood for information on birth control methods and assistance with making her choice. She tells the nurse that she is planning to become sexually active with her boyfriend of 6 months and is worried about getting pregnant. "I know I should know more about all of this but I just don't."
    A. *STATE* the nursing diagnosis that reflects Kathy's concern.

    B. *OUTLINE* the approach the nurse should use to help Kathy make an informed decision in choosing contraception that is right for her.

3. June plans to use a combination estrogen-progestin oral contraceptive.
    A. *DESCRIBE* the mode of action for this type of contraception.

    B. *LIST* the advantages of using oral contraception.

    C. *IDENTIFY* the factors that, if present in June's health history, would constitute absolute or relative contraindications to the use of oral contraception with estrogen and progesterone.

    D. *CITE* the side effects that can occur in terms of estrogen excess and deficiency and progestin excess and deficiency.
    Estrogen excess

    Estrogen deficiency

Progestin excess

Progestin deficiency

E. Using the acronym ACHES, *IDENTIFY* the signs and symptoms that would require June to stop taking the pill and notify her health care provider.

A

C

H

E

S

F. *SPECIFY* the instructions the nurse should give June about taking the pill to ensure maximum effectiveness.

4. Beth has decided to try the cervical cap as her method of contraception.
   A. *IDENTIFY* factors that if present in Beth's health history would make her a poor candidate for this contraceptive method.

   B. Following assessment, Beth is determined to be a good candidate for using the cervical cap. *DESCRIBE* the principles that the nurse should teach Beth to guide her in the safe and effective use of this method.

5. Anita has just had a Copper-T 380 A IUD inserted. *SPECIFY* the instructions that the nurse should give Anita before she leaves the women's health clinic after the insertion.

6. Judy (6-4-0-2-4) and Allen, both aged 36, are contemplating sterilization now that their family is complete. They are seeking counseling regarding this decision.
   A. *DESCRIBE* the approach a nurse should use in helping Judy and Allen make the right decision for them.

   B. They decide that Allen will have a vasectomy. *DISCUSS* the preoperative and postoperative care and instructions required by Allen.

7. Anne and her husband, Ian, will be using the symptothermal method of fertility awareness.
   A. *LIST* the assessment components of this method.

   B. *OUTLINE* the points the nurse should emphasize when teaching Anne and Ian in order to ensure that they will accurately:
   Measure basal body temperature (BBT)

   Evaluate cervical mucus characteristics

   C. *STATE* the effectiveness of this method of contraception.

8. Edna is a 20-year-old, unmarried woman. She is 9 weeks' pregnant and is unsure about what to do. She comes to the Women's Health Clinic and asks for the nurse's help in making her decision, stating, "I just cannot support a baby right now. I am alone and trying to finish my education. What can I do?"
   A. *CITE* the nursing diagnosis reflective of Edna's current dilemma.

B. *DESCRIBE* the approach the nurse should take in helping Edna to make a decision that is right for her.

C. Edna elects to have an abortion. A vacuum aspiration will be performed in the morning. Laminaria will be used in preparation for the procedure. Edna asks what will happen to her as part of the abortion procedure. *DESCRIBE* how the nurse should respond to Edna's question.

D. *IDENTIFY* three nursing diagnoses related to Edna's decision and the procedure she is facing.

E. *DESCRIBE* the nursing measures related to the physical care and emotional support that Edna will require as part of this procedure.

F. *OUTLINE* the discharge instructions that Edna should receive.

9. Marlee comes to the women's health clinic to report that she had unprotected intercourse last night. She is worried about getting pregnant since she is at mid-cycle and has already noticed signs of ovulation. Marlee tells the nurse that she hardly knows her partner and that her emotions just got the best of her. She is very anxious and asks the nurse what her options are. *DESCRIBE* the approach this nurse should use to assist Marlee with her concerns.

ONLINE LEARNING ACTIVITIES

Access the Lowdermilk, Perry **Evolve** website at
http://evolve.elsevier.com/Lowdermilk/MatWmnHlth/ and enter the **Student** portion through the
Learning Resources section. Using Chapter 9 as a starting point, search the Internet for websites
designed to provide birth control information. Prepare a report that includes the following:
- List of relevant sites
- Description of two sites in terms of:
  - Sponsoring person(s), agency, or organization
  - Target population of the site: health care professional and/or consumer
  - Clarity, accuracy, accessibility (ease of use), value, and depth of information provided
  - Currency—frequency of site updates
  - Variety of links to other relevant sites
  - Ability of persons visiting the site to obtain further information through services such as e-mail
    and chat rooms
- Discussion as to how you would use this information when assisting individuals and couples to
  make informed decisions regarding the method of contraception that is right for them; which of
  the sites would you recommend for their use
- Create a chart that summarizes statistical data concerning the most commonly used methods and
  the characteristics of persons using them

CHAPTER *10*

Infertility

CHAPTER REVIEW ACTIVITIES

MATCHING: Match the description in Column I with the appropriate test in Column II.

COLUMN I

_____ 1. Immunologic test to determine sperm and cervical mucus interaction and compatibility.

_____ 2. Basic test for male infertility.

_____ 3. Examination of the lining of the uterus to detect secretory changes and receptivity to implantation.

_____ 4. Test for adequacy of coital technique, cervical mucus, sperm, and degree of sperm penetration through cervical mucus.

_____ 5. Examination of uterine cavity and tubes using radiopaque contrast material instilled through the cervix. It is often used to determine tubal patency and to release a blockage if present.

_____ 6. Visualization of pelvic internal structures by inserting a small endoscope through an incision in the anterior abdominal wall.

COLUMN II

A. Laparoscopy
B. Postcoital Test (PCT)
C. Endometrial Biopsy
D. Hysterosalpingo-graphy
E. Sperm Immobilization Antigen-Antibody Reaction
F. Semen Analysis

FILL IN THE BLANKS: Insert the term that corresponds to each of the following descriptions of assisted reproductive therapies (ARTs).

7. _____ A woman's eggs are collected from her ovaries, fertilized in the laboratory with sperm, and transferred into her uterus once normal embryo development has occurred.

8. _____ Selection of one sperm cell that is injected directly into the egg to achieve fertilization.

9. _____ Oocytes are retrieved from the ovary, placed in a catheter with sperm, and immediately transferred into the fimbriated end of the uterine tube.

10. _____ After in vitro fertilization the ova are placed in one uterine tube during the zygote stage.

11. _____ Sperm from a person other than the male partner are used to inseminate the female partner.

12. _____ Embryo(s) from one couple are transferred into the uterus of another woman who has contracted with the couple to carry the baby to term. This woman has no genetic investment in the child.

13. _____ Process by which a woman is inseminated with the semen from the infertile woman's partner and then carries the baby till birth.

14. _____ The zona pellucida is penetrated chemically or manually to create an opening for the dividing embryo to hatch and to implant into the uterine wall.

TRUE OR FALSE: Circle "T" if true or "F" if false for each of the following statements. Correct the false statements.

T F 15. Infertility is a problem for 25% of reproductive age couples in the United States.

T F 16. Infertility that is solely a result of female factors is responsible for approximately 70% of infertility cases.

T F 17. Unknown factors and unusual causes account for 15% of infertility cases.

T F 18. Unexplained infertility may be related to immune system dysfunction.

T F 19. A high level of stress can influence a woman's fertility by causing the release of excess prolactin.

T F 20. Acidity of cervical mucus supports sperm, thereby facilitating their upward transport through the cervix.

T F 21. Vaginal-cervical infections can destroy or reduce the number of viable, motile sperm by altering the pH of reproductive tract secretions.

T F 22. Clinical tests for the detection of ovulation such as basal body temperature and secretory endometrial changes are based on the secretion of large amounts of estrogen.

T F 23. Mumps, especially after adolescence, can result in permanent damage to the testes.

T F 24. Substance abuse is considered to be a major factor in male infertility.

T F 25. An increase in scrotal temperature when using hot tubs and saunas may lessen fertility by interfering with spermatogenesis.

T F 26. Hysterosalpingography is scheduled for 2 to 5 days after menstruation.

T F 27. Referred shoulder pain associated with a hysterosalpingogram indicates the presence of an infection in the uterus and/or the fallopian tubes.

T F 28. An endometrial biopsy is typically performed in the luteal phase of the menstrual cycle about 2 to 3 days before expected menses.

T F 29. A history of impaired fertility is considered to be a risk factor for pregnancy-related complications.

T F 30. The use of condoms during genital intercourse for 2 months will reduce the female antibody production in most women who have elevated antisperm antibody titers.

T F 31. The multifetal pregnancy rate with the use of pharmacologic therapy for female infertility is less than 10%.

T F 32. Pergonal is administered orally twice a day beginning on the first day of a menstrual cycle.

MULTIPLE CHOICE: Circle the one correct option and state the rationale for the option chosen.

33. A woman must assess herself for signs that ovulation is occurring. Which of the following is a sign associated with ovulation?
    A. Reduction in level of luteinizing hormone (LH) in the urine 12 to 24 hours prior to ovulation
    B. Spinnbarkeit
    C. Drop in basal body temperature (BBT) following ovulation
    D. Increase in amount and thickness of cervical mucus

34. A couple is to undergo a postcoital test. The nurse should tell the couple that:
    A. Intercourse should occur daily for 3 days prior to the test
    B. The test will be used to determine how sperm penetrate and survive in cervical mucus
    C. The test will be scheduled for the day after menstruation ceases
    D. The examination of cervical mucus must be performed within 30 minutes of intercourse

35. Lifestyle and sexual practices can affect fertility. Which of the following practices could enhance a couple's ability to conceive?
    A. Male wears boxer shorts instead of briefs
    B. Female assumes a supine position with hips elevated for 1 hour after intercourse
    C. Couple only uses water-soluble lubricants if needed during intercourse
    D. Male relaxes in a hot tub every day after work

36. A woman taking human menopausal gonadotropin (Pergonal) for infertility should understand that:
    A. She should take the medication orally, once a day after breakfast
    B. The medication stimulates the pituitary gland to produce follicle stimulating (FSH) and luteinizing (LH) hormones
    C. She must report for ultrasound testing as scheduled to monitor follicular development
    D. Clomiphene (Clomid) should be taken daily, along with the Pergonal, until ovulation occurs

37. An infertile woman may be given danazol (Danocrine) in order to:
    A. Stimulate her pituitary gland
    B. Treat endometriosis
    C. Induce ovulation
    D. Help her to relax prior to intercourse

38. Mary and Jim have come for their first visit to the fertility clinic. The nurse needs to instruct them about the interrelated structures, functions, and processes essential for conception, emphasizing that they are a biologic unit of reproduction.
    A. *IDENTIFY* and *DESCRIBE* each component required for normal fertility.

    B. *SUPPORT* the statement: Assessment of infertility must involve both partners.

39. *EXPLAIN* why a male should stop smoking if he and his partner are planning a pregnancy.

40. *STATE* the mode of action and purpose for each of the following medications used in the treatment of infertility.
   Clomiphene citrate (Clomid, Serophene)

   Purified FSH (Metrodin)

   Bromocriptine (Parlodel)

   Progesterone (Progesterol)

   Human menopausal gonadotropin (Pergonal)

   Human chorionic gonadotropin (Profasi)

41. *CITE* several surgical procedures that could be helpful in treating the causes of infertility.

42. Infertility implies _____, a prolonged time to _____. _____ refers to an inability to conceive. Primary infertility applies to a woman who has never been _____ or the man who has never _____. Secondary infertility applies to a woman who has been _____ in the past.

   A. *LIST* the probable causes for female and male infertility:
      Female infertility

Male infertility

B. *GIVE* several examples of how religious and cultural beliefs, values, and practices can influence an individual's fertility or explain the basis for infertility.

CRITICAL THINKING EXERCISES

1. Mark and his wife, Mary, are undergoing testing for impaired fertility.
   A. *DESCRIBE* the nursing support measures that should be used when working with this couple.

   B. *LIST* the components of the assessment for both Mary and Mark.
      Assessment for the woman

      Assessment for the man

   C. Mark must provide a specimen of semen for analysis. *DESCRIBE* the procedure he should follow to ensure accuracy of the test.

   D. *STATE* the semen characteristics that will be assessed.

E. A postcoital test will be part of the diagnostic process for Mary and Mark. *DESCRIBE* the instructions you would give them to maximize the effectiveness and accuracy of the test.

2. Assisted reproductive therapies (ARTs) are being developed and perfected, creating a variety of ethical, legal, financial, and psychosocial concerns. *DISCUSS* the issues and concerns engendered by these alternative technologies.

3. Suzanne has been scheduled for a diagnostic laparoscopy to determine the basis of her infertility.
   A. *INDICATE* when during the menstrual cycle this test should be performed.

   B. *SPECIFY* the measures required to prepare Suzanne for this procedure.

   C. Suzanne asks the nurse why the test is needed and what will be done during the test. *DESCRIBE* the nurse's response.

   D. *SPECIFY* the postprocedure care measures required including the discharge instructions that Suzanne should receive.

4. Sara and Ben have been trying to conceive for three years. They have come to an infertility clinic to find out what is wrong. They are distraught because they have been trying so long to get pregnant. They tell the nurse that they just cannot believe what is happening to them. "None of our friends and no one in our family is having a problem—what's wrong with us?" A diagnosis of infertility is made, necessitating that Sara and Ben make decisions about treatments, use of alternative birth technologies, and adoption.

A. *IDENTIFY* the responses that Sara and Ben might exhibit related to the diagnosis of infertility. *DESCRIBE* one nursing action for each of the responses you have identified.

B. *DISCUSS* how you would guide this couple through the decision-making process required to determine a course of action that is right for both of them.

ONLINE LEARNING ACTIVITIES

Contact the websites for each of the infertility resources listed at the end of the chapter. Write a report that includes the following:

- Summary of the information and services offered at each of the sites and the populations served, for example health care professionals, consumers, or both
- Choose the site that you feel offers the most information and support for infertile couples; state the rationale for your choice
- Description regarding how you would use your chosen website as a tool when counseling and supporting an infertile couple

CHAPTER 11

Problems of the Breast

CHAPTER REVIEW ACTIVITIES

MATCHING: Match the description in Column I with the appropriate breast disorder in Column II.

COLUMN I

_____ 1. Lumpiness in both breasts with or without tenderness, usually associated with changes in the menstrual cycle.

_____ 2. Fatty breast tumor that is soft, nontender, mobile with discrete borders. It is most often found in women older than 45 years of age.

_____ 3. Breast hyperplasia characterized by very large, heavy breasts.

_____ 4. Unilateral, solid, encapsulated, nontender, breast mass that is unresponsive to dietary changes or hormone therapy.

_____ 5. Spontaneous, bilateral milky breast discharge.

_____ 6. Very small breasts.

_____ 7. Inflammatory process in the breast characterized by a thick, sticky, white or colored discharge. Burning pain and itching may be experienced. A mass may be palpated behind the nipple.

_____ 8. Small, nonpalpable lesions behind the nipple. This disorder, which occurs most often in women 30 to 50 years of age, is characterized by a unilateral, spontaneous discharge that can be serous, serosanguineous, or sanguinous.

COLUMN II

A. Fibroadenoma
B. Fibrocystic change
C. Intraductal papilloma
D. Mammary duct ectasia
E. Lipoma
F. Galactorrhea
G. Macromastia
H. Micromastia

TRUE OR FALSE: Circle "T" if true or "F" if false for each of the following statements. Correct the false statements.

T   F   9. At least 50% of women will experience a breast problem at some point in their adult life.

T   F   10. Fibrocystic breast changes characterized by proliferative lesions without atypia are associated with an increase in risk for breast cancer.

T   F   11. Typically fibrocystic change is noted as lumpiness in both breasts.

T F 12. Clinical manifestations associated with fibrocystic change are rarely related to the menstrual cycle.

T F 13. When a breast lump is palpated, a fine-needle aspiration (FNA) is performed to determine if the lump is fluid filled or solid.

T F 14. The tenderness associated with fibrocystic breast change may be reduced when caffeine is eliminated from the diet.

T F 15. The most common benign condition of the breast is fibroadenoma.

T F 16. Fibroadenomas tend to increase in size when a woman is pregnant.

T F 17. Bilateral serous drainage expressed during nipple stimulation requires a microscopic analysis to determine causation.

T F 18. Risk factors help to identify less than 30% of women who will eventually develop breast cancer.

T F 19. The most important predictor of risk for breast cancer is a family history of breast cancer.

T F 20. The United States has one of the lowest rates of breast carcinoma in the world.

T F 21. The risk of an American woman developing breast cancer in her lifetime is 1 in 8.

T F 22. The mortality rate for breast cancer is higher in Caucasian women.

T F 23. Fewer menstrual cycles and early childbearing seem to protect a woman from breast cancer.

T F 24. Most of the breast lumps detected by women during breast self-examination are malignant.

T F 25. Ultrasonography can be used to distinguish between cysts and solid tumors found in the breast.

T F 26. Involvement of the lymph nodes and breast tumor size are the most significant prognostic criteria for long-term survival.

T F 27. Lumpectomy and modified radical mastectomy have similar survival rates.

T F 28. Adjuvant hormone therapy using tamoxifen is effective if a woman's breast cancer cells are found to have estrogen and/or progesterone receptors.

T F 29. Women of childbearing age who are receiving chemotherapy for breast cancer should use oral contraceptives to prevent pregnancy.

30. Breast cancer is a major health problem facing women in the United States. Nurses are often responsible for educating women about breast cancer.
    A. *OUTLINE* the information the nurse should give women about the risk factors associated with breast cancer.

    B. *SPECIFY* the breast screening examinations the nurse should recommend for each of the following women. *INDICATE* the frequency at which each examination should be performed, according to the American Cancer Society.
       Jane (age 17)

Marion (age 29)

Denise (age 45)

C. *IDENTIFY* factors that can inhibit women from participating in breast screening examinations. Based on the factors identified, *SUGGEST* several strategies that can be used by nurses to increase compliance with breast screening examination guidelines.

D. *LIST* the clinical manifestations that are strongly suggestive of breast cancer.

E. *SPECIFY* the tests that can be performed to screen for and diagnose breast cancer.

31. *DEFINE* each of the following treatment approaches used in the care of women with breast cancer.
A. **Lumpectomy**

B. **Mastectomy (partial, modified radical, total [simple], radical)**

C. **Autologous flap reconstruction**

D. **Breast reconstruction using implants**

E. **Radiation**

F. **Adjuvant (chemotherapy; hormonal treatment) therapy**

32. Jane's mother died from breast cancer at the age of 36. Now at 30 years of age, Jane is concerned about her chances of developing breast cancer herself. She asks you about tests that are currently available to detect the gene for breast cancer and wonders if she should have this test performed especially since it is so expensive. Should women try alternative therapies as one means of treating breast cancer? *DISCUSS* your response to Jane's concern.

MULTIPLE CHOICE: Circle the one correct option and state the rationale for the option chosen.

33. When teaching women about breast cancer the nurse should emphasize that:
    A. The incidence of breast cancer is highest among African-American women
    B. Breast cancer is most prevalent among women in their thirties and forties
    C. Most women diagnosed with breast cancer exhibited clear and identifiable risk factors
    D. Early menarche and late menopause may increase the risk for breast cancer

34. The physician of a 46-year-old premenopausal woman with breast cancer has prescribed tamoxifen beginning in the postoperative period following lumpectomy. The nurse should understand that this medication:
    A. Relieves postoperative discomfort
    B. Is usually taken in an oral dose of 100 mg four times a day
    C. Must be taken for a lifetime
    D. Can cause hot flashes and menstrual irregularities

35. When providing discharge instructions to a woman who had a modified right radical mastectomy, the nurse should emphasize the importance of:
    A. Reporting any tingling or numbness in her incisional site or right arm immediately
    B. Telling health care providers not to take a blood pressure or draw blood from her right arm
    C. Learning how to use her left arm to write and accomplish the activities of daily living such as combing her hair
    D. Wearing clothing that snugly supports her right arm

36. A 26-year-old woman has just been diagnosed with fibrocystic change in her breasts. Nonproliferative lesions have been noted in both breasts. Which of the following nursing diagnoses would be a priority for this woman?
    A. Acute pain related to cyclical enlargement of breast cysts or lumps
    B. Risk for infection related to altered integrity of the areola associated with leakage from the nipples
    C. Anxiety related to anticipated surgery to remove the cysts in her breasts
    D. Fear related to high risk for breast cancer

37. When assessing a woman with a diagnosis of fibroadenoma, a characteristic the nurse would expect to find would be:
    A. Bilateral tender lumps behind the nipple
    B. Milky discharge from one or both nipples
    C. Soft and nonmovable lumps
    D. Small, well-delineated lump in the upper outer quadrant of one breast

CRITICAL THINKING EXERCISES

1. Mary Anne comes to the women's health clinic complaining that her breasts feel lumpy.
    A. OUTLINE the assessment process that should be used to determine the basis for Mary Anne's complaint.

    B. A diagnosis of fibrocystic breast changes is made. DESCRIBE the clinical manifestations Mary Anne most likely exhibited to support this diagnosis.

    C. STATE one nursing diagnosis that the nurse would identify as a priority when preparing a plan of care for Mary Anne.

    D. IDENTIFY measures the nurse could suggest to Mary Anne for lessening the symptoms she experiences related to fibrocystic changes.

E. Mary Anne expresses fear that she is now at very high risk for breast cancer. *DESCRIBE* how the nurse should respond to Mary Anne's expressed fear.

2. Molly, a 50-year-old woman, found a lump in her left breast during a breast self-examination. She comes to the women's health clinic for help.

A. *DESCRIBE* the diagnostic protocol that should be followed to determine the basis for the lump Molly found in her breast.

B. Molly's lump is diagnosed as cancerous. *DESCRIBE* the emotional impact that this diagnosis and the treatment is likely to have on Molly and her family.

C. Molly elects to have a simple mastectomy based on the information provided by her health care providers and in consultation with her husband. *IDENTIFY* two priority nursing diagnoses and *OUTLINE* the nursing care management for each of the following phases of Molly's treatment.
    Nursing diagnoses

    Preoperative-phase care measures

    Immediate postoperative-phase care measures

D. Molly will be discharged within 48 hours after her surgery. *DESCRIBE* the instructions that the nurse should give Molly to prepare her for self-care at home.

E. *DISCUSS* support measures the nurse should use to address the concerns that Molly and her husband will most likely experience and express.

3. Susan has been diagnosed with breast cancer. Her initial treatment included a lumpectomy. In addition, Susan's physician has prescribed adjuvant hormonal therapy using tamoxifen. *EXPLAIN* to Susan and her family what this medication is and how it works. *USE* a drug manual to obtain information regarding administration, dosage, and side effects that you will incorporate into a teaching plan to ensure that Susan takes the medication effectively and safely.

4. Annie is a 36-year-old woman about to begin chemotherapy for treatment of breast cancer.
   A. *OUTLINE* a teaching plan the nurse would use to prepare Annie and her family for what to expect regarding this treatment method.

   B. *IDENTIFY* two priority nursing diagnoses the nurse should address when developing a plan of care for Annie during her treatment.

ONLINE LEARNING ACTIVITIES

Imagine that you are teaching a group of women who are beginning treatment for breast cancer. Prepare a handout that describes several Internet resources designed to provide information and support for women being treated for breast cancer. The Internet resources you include in your handout should be carefully evaluated in terms of each of the following (include this information in your description of each site in your handout):
- Sponsoring person(s), agency, organization
- Quality of the information provided in terms of accuracy, clarity, accessibility (ease of use), depth, currency (frequency of site updates)
- Nature of the support offered including ability of persons visiting the site to obtain additional information and individualized support through such services as e-mail and chat rooms
- Variety of links to other relevant sites

CHAPTER 12

Structural Disorders and Neoplasms of the Reproductive System

CHAPTER REVIEW ACTIVITIES

MATCHING: Match the description in Column I with the appropriate disorder in Column II.

COLUMN I

_____ 1. The most common malignancy of the reproductive system usually seen in women between the ages of 50 and 65 years.

_____ 2. Herniation of the anterior rectal wall through the relaxed or ruptured vaginal fascia and rectovaginal septum.

_____ 3. A group of disorders that includes hydatidiform mole, invasive mole, and choriocarcinoma.

_____ 4. Pedunculated tumors usually originating from the mucosa of the cervix or endometrium.

_____ 5. Perforations between genital tract organs with most occurring between the bladder and the vagina.

_____ 6. Protrusion of the bladder downward into the vagina that develops when supporting structures in the vesicovaginal septum are injured.

_____ 7. Benign tumors arising in uterine muscle tissue and dependent upon ovarian hormones for growth.

_____ 8. The most common benign lesion of the vulva.

_____ 9. Form of cancer that is strongly linked to the human papillomavirus (types 16 and 18).

_____ 10. Reproductive cancer with a high mortality rate as a result of frequent late-stage diagnosis.

COLUMN II

A. Cystocele
B. Leiomyomas (fibroid tumors)
C. Endometrial cancer
D. Cervical cancer
E. Ovarian cancer
F. Rectocele
G. Uterine polyps
H. Genital fistulas
I. Bartholin cyst
J. Gestational trophoblastic disease (GTD)

Chapter 12: Structural Disorders and Neoplasms of the Reproductive System   105

Copyright © 2004 by Mosby, Inc. All rights reserved.

FILL IN THE BLANKS: Insert the treatment that corresponds to each of the following descriptions.

11. _____ Device used to support the uterus and hold it in the correct position.
12. _____ Surgery used to repair a cystocele.
13. _____ Surgery used to repair a rectocele.
14. _____ Surgical removal of a leiomyoma (fibroid).
15. _____ Injection of polyvinyl alcohol (PVA) pellets into selected blood vessels to block the blood supply to a leiomyoma in order to cause its shrinkage and resolution of symptoms.
16. _____ Surgical removal of the entire uterus.
17. _____ Surgical removal of both ovaries and both uterine tubes.
18. _____ Examination of the cervix using a stereoscopic binocular microscope that magnifies the view of the cervix.
19. _____ Removal of a wedge of tissue from the exocervix and endocervix in order to establish a diagnosis or effect a cure.
20. _____ Treatment that involves destroying abnormal cells by freezing them. Cells slough off and are replaced with the regeneration of normal tissue.
21. _____ Treatment for cervical dysplasia that involves use of a wire loop electrode that can excise and cauterize with minimal tissue damage.
22. _____ Surgical procedure involving the removal of the uterus, tubes, ovaries, upper third of the vagina along with certain pelvic ligaments and lymph nodes and a portion of the parametrium.
23. _____ Surgical removal of the perineum, pelvic floor, levator muscles, all reproductive organs, pelvic lymph nodes, rectum, sigmoid colon, urinary bladder, and distal ureters. A colostomy and ileal conduit are constructed.
24. _____ Surgical removal of the vulva, labia majora and minora, and possibly the clitoris.
25. _____ Surgical removal of superficial vulvar skin without clitoral removal followed by split-thickness skin grafts. Fat, muscles, and glands are preserved.
26. _____ Surgical removal of entire vulva, skin, clitoris, labia, subcutaneous tissue, and inguinal and femoral lymph nodes.

27. IDENTIFY the risk factors that, if present, increase a woman's vulnerability to the following:
A. Endometrial cancer

B. Cervical cancer

C. Ovarian cancer

28. *EXPLAIN* why ovarian cancer is called the "silent" disease.

TRUE OR FALSE: Circle "T" if true or "F" if false for each of the following statements. Correct the false statements.

T F 29. The most common type of uterine displacement is anteflexion.

T F 30. Symptoms of pelvic relaxation most often appear during the perimenopausal period as a result of the effect of decreasing ovarian hormone secretion on pelvic tissue.

T F 31. Urge incontinence occurs as a result of a sudden increase in intraabdominal pressure such as sneezing or coughing.

T F 32. Good hygiene of the genital area is critical when a pessary is being used.

T F 33. An anterior colporrhaphy is performed to surgically repair a uterine prolapse.

T F 34. A vesicovaginal fistula is the most common type of reproductive tract fistula.

T F 35. A corpus luteum cyst causes pain, ovarian tenderness, delayed menses, and irregular or prolonged menstrual flow.

T F 36. A follicular cyst requires increased progesterone secretion for growth and development.

T F 37. Multiparous Caucasian women are most vulnerable to the development of fibroid tumors of the uterus.

T F 38. A myomectomy should be performed in the proliferative phase of the menstrual cycle to avoid interrupting a possible pregnancy.

T F 39. Endometrial cancer is commonly associated with hormone imbalance such as unopposed estrogen stimulation in postmenopausal women.

T F 40. The cardinal sign of endometrial cancer is abdominal pain.

T F 41. The rate of invasive cervical cancer increased by 50% over the last 25 years.

T F 42. The single most reliable method to detect preinvasive cervical cancer is the Papanicolaou test.

T F 43. The average age range for the occurrence of cervical cancer is 30 to 40 years.

T F 44. Preinvasive lesions of the cervix are most effectively treated with internal radiation therapy.

T F 45. The most common symptom of invasive cervical carcinoma is abnormal bleeding especially after intercourse.

T F 46. Following cryosurgery of the cervix, a woman could experience a thick, bloody mucoid discharge for several weeks.

T F 47. A woman can receive no visitors during the course of internal radiation therapy.

T F 48. Treatment of ovarian cancer most often requires surgery combined with multiagent chemotherapy.

T F 49. Cancer is an uncommon occurrence during pregnancy.

T F 50. Pregnancy makes the diagnosis of breast cancer more difficult.

T F 51. Pregnancy slows the speed at which breast cancer metastasizes.

T F 52. Chemotherapy must be avoided as long as a woman is pregnant.

T F 53. Women who have been successfully treated for cancer should wait approximately 2 years after ending treatment before attempting a pregnancy.

T F 54. Vulvar cancer grows slowly with a late metastasis, thus improving survival rates.

T F 55. Estrogen and progesterone levels are used to monitor the effectiveness of treatment for gestational trophoblastic neoplasia.

MULTIPLE CHOICE: Circle the one correct option and state the rationale for the option chosen.

56. A 60-year-old woman has been diagnosed with a mild prolapse of her uterus. The nurse practitioner could suggest that this woman
    A. Assume a knee-chest position for a few minutes several times a day
    B. Use a specially fitted pessary to support her uterus and hold it in the correct position
    C. Begin progestin-only hormone replacement therapy
    D. See a surgeon to discuss the possibility of having an anterior repair (colporrhaphy) performed

57. A 35-year-old woman has recently been diagnosed with two leiomyomas (fibroid tumors) in the body of her uterus. This woman can expect to experience which of the following clinical manifestations?
    A. Shrinkage of tumors if she becomes pregnant
    B. Diarrhea
    C. Acute abdominal pain
    D. Menorrhagia

58. Which of the following measures would be LEAST effective in relieving the stress urinary incontinence experienced by a 60-year-old woman with pelvic relaxation:
    A. Performing Kegel exercises
    B. Reducing her intake of oral fluids to one liter or less per day
    C. Emptying her bladder on a regular basis every 2 hours
    D. Participating in a smoking cessation program to relieve her smoker's cough

59. A 38-year-old premenopausal woman has had an abdominal hysterectomy performed as a result of fibroid tumors that have been increasing in size and causing excessive menstrual bleeding. Postoperative care for this woman would include instructions regarding:
    A. Beginning hormone replacement therapy (HRT) prior to discharge
    B. Importance of avoiding vigorous exercise and heavy lifting for at least 6 weeks
    C. Performing a Betadine douche daily for the first week postoperatively
    D. Turning, coughing, and deep breathing every 4 hours for the first 24 hours

60. A woman has been diagnosed with carcinoma in situ (CIS) of the cervix. The nurse should prepare this woman for which of the following treatment measures?
    A. Pelvic exenteration
    B. Radical hysterectomy
    C. Cervical conization with follow-up Pap smears and colposcopy
    D. Intracavity and external radiation therapy

CRITICAL THINKING EXERCISES

1. Denise (6-5-0-1-5), a 60-year-old postmenopausal woman, has been diagnosed with a moderate uterine prolapse along with cystocele and rectocele.
   A. *DESCRIBE* the clinical manifestations Denise most likely exhibited to lead to this diagnosis.

   B. *IDENTIFY* two priority nursing diagnoses related to the signs and symptoms Denise is most likely experiencing. *WRITE* one expected outcome for each of the nursing diagnoses identified.

   C. *OUTLINE* the care management approach recommended for Denise's health problem.

   D. Denise will use a pessary during the day until a surgical repair can be accomplished.
      1) *IDENTIFY* one nursing diagnosis associated with pessary use.

      2) *SPECIFY* the instructions the nurse would give to Denise regarding the use and care of a pessary.

   E. Denise has a vaginal hysterectomy and an anterior and posterior colporrhaphy. *OUTLINE* the postoperative care Denise will require in order to heal without complications.

2. Marie, age 40, has been diagnosed with two large leiomyomas (fibroid tumors).
   A. *DESCRIBE* the clinical manifestations most likely exhibited by Marie.

B. Therapeutic management for benign uterine tumors depends on severity of _____, _____ of the woman, and desire to preserve _____. Therapeutic approaches can include medical management using _____ or _____ to reduce the size of the leiomyomas. Surgical management can include _____, _____ or _____, or _____.

3. Louise, age 60, has been diagnosed with endometrial cancer. Because of the early stage of the carcinoma, a total abdominal hysterectomy and bilateral salpingo-oophorectomy is the form of treatment chosen.
   A. *IDENTIFY* one nursing diagnosis relevant for the preoperative period and one nursing diagnosis relevant for the postoperative period. *STATE* an expected outcome for each nursing diagnosis identified.

   B. *OUTLINE* the nursing care and support required for each of the following stages in Louise's treatment.
   Preoperative stage

   Postoperative stage

   C. *SPECIFY* the instructions that Louise should receive in preparation for discharge about caring for herself once at home.

   D. *DISCUSS* how Louise's cultural beliefs could affect her responses to her diagnosis of cancer and the need to have her reproductive organs removed.

E. *IDENTIFY* one nursing diagnosis associated with Louise's likely emotional response to her diagnosis and treatment.

F. *DISCUSS* the support measures the nurse could use to meet Louise's emotional and psychosocial needs as she recovers.

4. Laura has been diagnosed with invasive carcinoma of the cervix and is about to begin a course of radiation therapy.
   A. *IDENTIFY* two priority nursing diagnoses associated with the course of treatment that Laura is about to undergo. Write one expected outcome for each nursing diagnosis identified.

   B. *COMPLETE* the following table to summarize the care and support Laura will require at each stage of her treatment regimen.

Period of Treatment	Internal Radiation	External Radiation
Pretreatment care		
Care during treatment		
Posttreatment care and discharge instructions		

   C. *DESCRIBE* the nursing precautions for self-protection the nurse should use when caring for a woman receiving internal radiation therapy.

5. Pat is recovering from a radical vulvectomy that was performed to treat invasive vulvar cancer.
   A. *IDENTIFY* three nursing measures related to the expected outcome: Pat will heal without the development of infection.

   B. *IDENTIFY* three nursing measures related to the expected outcome: Pat will maintain appropriate sexual functioning.

   C. *DISCUSS* the discharge instructions Pat should receive.

6. *DISCUSS* the issues and emotions that can confront a pregnant woman, her family, and her health care providers when the woman is diagnosed with cancer.

7. Angela has been diagnosed with advanced ovarian cancer. Metastasis has occurred and as a result she will be beginning chemotherapy.
   A. *OUTLINE* the measures you would recommend to relieve the following anticipated problems associated with chemotherapy:
   Anorexia

   Nausea and vomiting

   Stomatitis

Diarrhea

B. *DESCRIBE* the approach you would use to support Angela and her family as they cope with the effects of the chemotherapy and the diagnosis of advanced cancer.

ONLINE LEARNING ACTIVITIES

Imagine that one of your clients is going to be discharged in 2 days following surgery for ovarian cancer. She faces a long course of chemotherapy. Her family gave her a new computer to provide her with "something to do while she is recovering." Develop a set of written guidelines that she can use to find and to evaluate Internet sites that could offer her support and information about her diagnosis, the treatment regimen that she is undergoing, possible alternative therapies, and an opportunity to "chat" with other women facing the same crisis. List several websites that you have found to be helpful and reliable to get her started.

CHAPTER 13

Conception and Fetal Development

CHAPTER REVIEW ACTIVITIES

FILL IN THE BLANKS: Insert the term that corresponds to each of the following descriptions related to conception and fetal development.

1. _____ Union of a single egg and sperm. It marks the beginning of a pregnancy.
2. _____ Male and female germ cell. The male germ cell is a _____ and the female germ cell is an _____.
3. _____ The process whereby body (somatic) cells replicate to yield two _____ cells each with _____ single chromosomes or _____ pairs.
4. _____ The process whereby germ cells divide. It results in _____ cells each containing _____ single chromosomes.
5. _____ Process whereby gametes are formed and mature. For the male, the process is called _____ and for the female, the process is called _____.
6. _____ Process of penetration of the membrane surrounding the ovum by a sperm. It takes place in the _____ of the uterine tube. The membrane becomes impenetrable to other sperm, a process termed _____. The _____ number of chromosomes is restored when this union of sperm and ovum occurs.
7. _____ The first cell of the new individual. Within 3 days it becomes a 16-cell solid ball of cells called a _____. This developing structure becomes known as the _____ when a cavity becomes recognizable within it. The outer layer of cells surrounding this cavity is called the _____.
8. _____ Attachment process whereby the blastocyst burrows into the _____. _____, finger-like projections develop out of the _____ and extend into the blood-filled spaces of the uterine lining. The uterine lining is now called the _____. The portion of this lining directly under the blastocyst is called the _____ and the portion of this lining that covers the blastocyst is called the _____.
9. _____ The term used to refer to the developing baby from day 15 until about 8 weeks from conception.
10. _____ The term used to refer to the developing baby from 9 weeks' gestation to the end of pregnancy. It will develop in a _____ or crown-to-rump direction.
11. _____ Membranes that surround the developing baby and the fluid. The _____ is the outer layer of these membranes and the _____ is the inner layer.

Copyright © 2004 by Mosby, Inc. All rights reserved.

12. _____ Fluid that surrounds the developing baby in utero. _____ refers to a decreased amount of the fluid (e.g., <300 ml). _____ refers to an excessive amount of the fluid (e.g., 2 L).

13. _____ Structure that connects the developing baby to the placenta. It contains three vessels, namely two _____ and one _____. _____ is the connective tissue that prevents compression of the blood vessels to ensure continued nourishment of the developing baby. When it is wrapped around the fetal neck it is called a _____.

14. _____ Structure composed of 15 to 20 lobes/areas called _____. It produces _____ essential to maintain the pregnancy, supplies the _____ and _____ needed by the developing baby for survival and growth, and removes _____ and _____.

15. _____ Capability of fetus to survive outside the uterus.

16. _____ Special circulatory pathway that allows fetal blood to bypass the lungs.

17. _____ Shunt that allows most of fetal blood to bypass the liver and pass into the inferior vena cava.

18. _____ Opening between the fetal atria.

19. _____ Formation of blood.

20. _____ Surface-active phospholipid that needs to be present in fetal/newborn lungs to facilitate breathing after birth. The _____ ratio can be performed using amniotic fluid as one means of determining the degree to which surfactant is present in fetal lungs.

21. _____ Maternal perception of fetal movement that occurs sometime between _____ and _____ weeks' gestation.

22. _____ Dark green to black tarry substance that contains fetal waste products. It accumulates in the fetal intestines.

23. _____ Twins that are formed from two zygotes. They are also called _____ twins.

24. _____ Twins that are formed from one fertilized ovum that then divides. They are also called _____ twins.

25. _____ Substance or exposure that causes abnormal development of the embryo/fetus.

26. Each of the following structures plays a critical role in fetal growth and development. *LIST* the functions of each of the structures listed below.
    Yolk sac

    Amniotic membranes and fluid

    Umbilical cord

Placenta

TRUE OR FALSE: Circle "T" if true or "F" if false for each of the following statements. Correct the false statements.

T F 27. The stage of the fetus lasts from 6 weeks' gestation until the end of pregnancy.

T F 28. The umbilical cord is composed of two veins, one artery, Wharton's jelly, ligaments, and nerves.

T F 29. Human chorionic gonadotropin (hCG) is first detected in maternal blood 8 to 10 days after conception.

T F 30. The corpus luteum produces estrogen and progesterone to maintain the pregnancy until the placenta is mature enough to take over as an endocrine gland.

T F 31. The placenta functions as an effective barrier to substances such as viruses and drugs, thereby protecting the fetus from their potentially harmful effects.

T F 32. Oligohydramnios often indicates fetal renal abnormalities.

T F 33. Meconium may be passed into the amniotic fluid if fetal hypoxia occurs.

T F 34. Fetal viability is first reached at 30 weeks' gestation.

T F 35. A human pregnancy reaches term by 40 weeks or 280 days.

T F 36. The fetal hemoglobin concentration is approximately 50% greater than that of the mother.

T F 37. The occurrence of multifetal pregnancies with three or more fetuses has steadily decreased as a result of increased maternal exposure to teratogens.

38. COMPLETE THE FOLLOWING TABLE by naming the three primary germ layers and identifying the tissues or organs that develop from each layer.

Primary Germ Layer	Tissue/Organ Formation

MULTIPLE CHOICE: Circle the one correct option and state the rationale for the option chosen.

39. When teaching a class of pregnant women about fetal development, the nurse would include:
    A. The sex of your baby is determined by the 9th week of pregnancy.
    B. The baby's heart begins to pump blood during the 10th week of pregnancy.
    C. The baby's heart beat will be audible using a special ultrasound stethoscope as early as the 18th week of pregnancy.
    D. You should be able to feel your baby move by week 16 to 20 of pregnancy.

40. The results of an amniocentesis indicates that the pregnant woman's L/S ratio is 2:1. This result indicates that:
    A. The woman is in her 2nd trimester of pregnancy.
    B. The newborn should be able to maintain effective respiration after birth.
    C. The fetus has most likely developed a renal problem.
    D. An open neural tube defect is present.

41. If a pregnant woman's intake of iron is sufficient, her newborn will have enough iron stored in its liver to last approximately:
    A. 1 month
    B. 3 months
    C. 5 months
    D. 9 months

42. When caring for pregnant women, the nurse would recognize that a woman with which of the following disorders has the greatest risk for giving birth to a macrosomic newborn?
    A. Diabetes
    B. Anemia
    C. Hyperthyroidism
    D. Hypertension

CRITICAL THINKING EXERCISES

1. *IMAGINE* that you are a nurse-midwife working in partnership with an obstetrician. *FORMULATE* a response to each of the following concerns or questions directed to you from some of your prenatal clients.
   A. June (2 months' pregnant), Mary (5 months' pregnant) and Alice (7 months' pregnant) each ask for a description of their fetus at the present time.
   June

   Mary

Alice

B. Jessica states that a friend told her that babies born after about 35 weeks have a better chance to survive because they can breathe easier. She asks if this is true.

C. Beth, who is 1 month pregnant, states that she heard that women who are pregnant experience quickening. She wants to know what that could mean and if it hurts.

D. Susan, who is 6 months' pregnant, states that she read in a magazine that a fetus can actually hear and see. She feels that this is totally unbelievable!

E. Alexa is 2 months' pregnant. She asks how the sex of her baby was determined and if a sonogram could tell if she is having a boy or a girl.

F. Karen is pregnant for the first time. She reveals that she has a history of twins in her family. She wants to know what causes twin pregnancies to occur and what the difference is between identical and fraternal twins.

G. Louise is beginning her 2nd trimester. She tells the nurse that a friend who just had a baby told her that her position and activity can affect how her baby grows and develops. Louise asks if this is true.

ONLINE LEARNING ACTIVITIES

Access the Lowdermilk, Perry **Evolve** website at
http://evolve.elsevier.com/Lowdermilk/MatWmnHlth/ and enter the **Student** portion through the
Learning Resources section. Use Chapter 13 as a starting point for a search of the Internet for
websites that illustrate the process of fetal development. Choose the site that is most appealing to you
and prepare a report that includes the following:
- Description of the site chosen in terms of:
  - Sponsoring person(s), agency, or organization
  - Clarity, accuracy, accessibility (ease of use), visual appeal, and depth of information provided
  - Currency—frequency of site updates
  - Various links to other relevant sites
  - Ability of person visiting the site to obtain additional information through services such as
    e-mail and chat rooms
- Discussion of how you would use this site or others like it when conducting classes for expectant
  parents

CHAPTER 14

Anatomy and Physiology of Pregnancy

CHAPTER REVIEW ACTIVITIES

MATCHING: Match the assessment finding in Column I with the appropriate descriptive term in Column II.

COLUMN I

_____ 1. Menstrual bleeding no longer occurs.
_____ 2. Fundal height decreased, fetal head in pelvic inlet
_____ 3. Cervical and vaginal mucosa violet-bluish in color
_____ 4. Swelling of ankles and feet at the end of the day
_____ 5. Cervical tip softened
_____ 6. Lower uterine segment soft and compressible with palpation
_____ 7. Fetal head rebounds with gentle, upward tapping through the vagina
_____ 8. White mucoid vaginal discharge with faint, musty odor
_____ 9. Enlarged sebaceous glands in areola on both breasts
_____ 10. Plug of mucus fills endocervical canal
_____ 11. Pink stretch marks on breasts and abdomen
_____ 12. Creamy, yellowish fluid expressed from nipples
_____ 13. Cheeks, nose, and forehead blotchy, hyperpigmented
_____ 14. Pigmented line extending up abdominal midline
_____ 15. Red raised nodule on gum
_____ 16. Heartburn experienced after supper
_____ 17. Lumbosacral curve increased
_____ 18. Paresthesia and pain in right hand radiating to elbow
_____ 19. Spotting following cervical palpation or intercourse
_____ 20. Hematocrit decreased from 40% to 36%
_____ 21. Vascular spiders on neck and thorax
_____ 22. Palms pinkish red, mottled
_____ 23. Abdominal wall muscles separated

COLUMN II

A. Colostrum
B. Operculum
C. Amenorrhea
D. Telangiectasis (angioma)
E. Pyrosis
F. Friability
G. Striae gravidarum
H. Physiologic anemia
I. Linea nigra
J. Ballottement
K. Chadwick sign
L. Diastasis recti abdominis
M. Lordosis
N. Leukorrhea
O. Chloasma (mask of pregnancy)
P. Lightening
Q. Epulis
R. Palmar erythema
S. Goodell sign
T. Physiologic edema
U. Hegar sign
V. Montgomery tubercles
W. Carpal tunnel syndrome

FILL IN THE BLANKS: Insert the term that corresponds to each of the following descriptions related to pregnancy.

24. _____ Pregnancy.

25. _____ The number of pregnancies in which the fetus or fetuses have reached viability, not the number of fetuses (e.g., twins) born. Whether the fetus is born alive or is stillborn (fetus who shows no signs of life at birth) after viability is reached has no effect on the numerical designation.

26. _____ A woman who is pregnant.

27. _____ A woman who has never been pregnant.

28. _____ A woman who has not completed a pregnancy with a fetus or fetuses who have reached the stage of fetal viability.

29. _____ A woman who is pregnant for the first time.

30. _____ A woman who has completed one pregnancy with a fetus or fetuses who have reached the stage of fetal viability.

31. _____ A woman who has had two or more pregnancies.

32. _____ A woman who has completed two or more pregnancies to the stage of fetal viability.

33. _____ Capacity to live outside the uterus, about 22 to 24 weeks since the last menstrual period, or a fetal weight greater than 500 g.

34. _____ A pregnancy that has reached 20 weeks of gestation but before completion of 37 weeks of gestation.

35. _____ A pregnancy from the beginning of the 38th week of gestation to the end of the 42nd week of gestation.

36. _____ A pregnancy that goes beyond 42 weeks of gestation. The term _____ is also used to refer to this pregnancy.

37. _____ Presence of this biochemical marker in maternal urine or serum results in a positive pregnancy test result.

38. COMPLETE the following table related to the three categories of signs and symptoms of pregnancy by filling in the blanks and listing the appropriate signs and symptoms for each category.

_____, those changes felt by the woman.	_____, those changes observed by an examiner.	_____, those signs attributed only to the presence of the fetus.

39. *DESCRIBE* the obstetrical history for each of the following women, using the 4-digit and 5-digit system.

A. Nancy is pregnant. Her first pregnancy resulted in a stillbirth at 36 weeks' gestation and her second pregnancy resulted in the birth of her daughter at 42 weeks' gestation.

4-digit

5-digit

B. Marsha is 6 weeks' pregnant. Her previous pregnancies resulted in the live birth of a daughter at 40 weeks' gestation, the live birth of a son at 38 weeks' gestation, and a spontaneous abortion at 10 weeks' gestation.

4-digit

5-digit

C. Linda is experiencing her fourth pregnancy. Her first pregnancy ended in a spontaneous abortion at 12 weeks, the second resulted in the live birth of twin boys at 32 weeks, and the third resulted in the live birth of a daughter at 39 weeks.

4-digit

5-digit

TRUE OR FALSE: Circle "T" if true or "F" if false for each of the following statements. Correct the false statements.

T   F   40. Human chorionic gonadotropin (hCG) can be detected in the urine of a pregnant woman as early as 14 days after conception.

T   F   41. Serum pregnancy tests are more accurate and sensitive than urine pregnancy tests, thereby providing earlier results.

T   F   42. Drugs such as diuretics can contribute to a false-positive pregnancy test result.

T   F   43. Fetal movements palpated by an examiner are an example of a positive sign of pregnancy.

T   F   44. The uterine fundus should be above the level of the symphysis pubis by the 8th week of gestation.

T   F   45. Cervical mucus present during pregnancy exhibits ferning.

T   F   46. During pregnancy, a woman's vulnerability for yeast infections increases.

T   F   47. Lactation does not occur during pregnancy as a result of the inhibiting effect of high prolactin levels.

T   F   48. Physiologic anemia is diagnosed in a pregnant woman when the hemoglobin value falls to 10 g/dl or less or if the hematocrit value falls to 35% or less.

T   F   49. A woman is more vulnerable to thrombus formation during pregnancy as a result of increases in certain clotting factors and depression of fibrinolytic activity.

T   F   50. A pregnant woman is more likely to experience epistaxis as a result of increased vascularity and congestion of the upper respiratory tract.

T   F   51. A supine position with head elevated is the best maternal position to facilitate renal perfusion.

T   F   52. A proteinuria of 1+ or less is acceptable during pregnancy.

T   F   53. Hypercalcemia is common during pregnancy and can result in leg cramps and tetany.

T   F   54. Perspiration is increased during pregnancy as a result of increased peripheral circulation and increased sweat gland activity.

T   F   55. Carpal tunnel syndrome can occur during the third trimester of pregnancy as a result of edema compressing the median nerve beneath the carpal ligament in the wrist.

T   F   56. Increased triglyceride levels as a result of higher estrogen secretion may account for the tendency to develop gallstones during pregnancy.

T   F   57. During the second half of pregnancy, the woman's ability to use her own insulin is decreased to ensure an ample supply of glucose for the developing fetus.

T   F   58. Glycosuria can be exhibited in a normal pregnancy.

59. When assessing the pregnant woman, the nurse should keep in mind that baseline vital sign values will change as she progresses through her pregnancy.
   A. *DESCRIBE* how each of the following would change:
      Blood pressure

Heart rate and patterns

Respiratory rate and patterns

Body temperature

60. CALCULATE the mean arterial pressure (MAP) for each of the following BP readings:
120/76

114/64

110/80

150/90

61. *SPECIFY* the value changes that occur in the following laboratory tests as a result of expected physiologic adaptations to pregnancy:
CBC: hematocrit, hemoglobin, white blood cell count

Clotting activity

Acid/base balance

Urinalysis

62. *EXPLAIN* the expected adaptations in elimination that occur during pregnancy. *INCLUDE* in your answer the basis for the changes that occur.
Renal

Bowel

63. *DISCUSS* how and why the levels of each of the following substances changes during pregnancy.
Parathyroid hormone

Insulin

Estrogen

Progesterone

Thyroid hormones

Human chorionic gonadotropin (hCG)

MULTIPLE CHOICE: Circle the one correct option and state the rationale for the option chosen.

64. A pregnant woman at 10 weeks' gestation exhibits the following signs of pregnancy during a routine prenatal check-up. Which one would be categorized as a probable sign of pregnancy?
    A. Human chorionic gonadotropin in the urine
    B. Breast tenderness
    C. Morning sickness
    D. Fetal heart sounds

65. A pregnant woman with four children reports the following obstetric history: a stillbirth at 32 weeks' gestation, triplets (2 sons and a daughter) born via cesarean section at 30 weeks' gestation, a spontaneous abortion at 8 weeks' gestation, and daughter born vaginally at 39 weeks' gestation. Which of the following accurately expresses this woman's current obstetric history using the 5-digit system?
    A. 5–1–4–1–4
    B. 4–1–3–1–4
    C. 5–2–2–0–3
    D. 5–1–2–1–4

66. An essential component of prenatal health assessment of pregnant women is the determination of vital signs. An expected change in vital signs findings as a result of pregnancy would be:
    A. Increase in systolic blood pressure by 30 mm Hg or more after assuming a supine position
    B. Increase in diastolic BP by 5–10 mm Hg beginning in the first trimester
    C. Increased awareness of the need to breathe as pregnancy progresses
    D. Gradual decrease in baseline pulse rate of approximately 20 beats per minute

67. A woman exhibits understanding of instructions for performing a home pregnancy test to maximize accuracy if she:
    A. Uses urine collected at the end of the day, just before going to bed
    B. Avoids using Tylenol or aspirin for a headache for about 1 week prior to performing the test
    C. Performs the test on the day after she misses her first menstrual period
    D. Records the day of her last normal menstrual period and her usual cycle length

68. During an examination of a pregnant woman the nurse notes that her cervix is soft on its tip. The nurse would document this finding as
  A. Friability
  B. Goodell sign
  C. Chadwick sign
  D. Hegar sign

CRITICAL THINKING EXERCISES

1. *DESCRIBE* how the nurse should respond to each of the following client concerns and questions.
  A. Tina is 14 weeks' pregnant. She calls the prenatal clinic to report that she noticed slight, painless spotting this morning. She reveals that she did have intercourse with her partner the night before.

  B. Lisa suspects she is pregnant because her menstrual period is already 3 weeks' late. She asks her friend, who is a nurse, how to use the pregnancy test that she just bought so that she obtains the best results.

  C. Joan is 3 months' pregnant. She tells the nurse that she is worried because a friend told her that vaginal and bladder infections are more common during pregnancy. She wants to know if this could be true and if so why.

  D. Tammy, who is 20 weeks' pregnant, tells the nurse that she has noted some "problems" with her breasts: There are "little pimples" near her nipples and her breasts feel "lumpy and bumpy" and "leak a little" when she does BSE.

  E. Tamara is concerned because she read in a book about pregnancy that a pregnant woman's position could affect her circulation, especially to the baby. She asks what positions are good for her circulation now that she is pregnant.

F. Beth, a pregnant woman, calls to tell the nurse that she had a nosebleed this morning and has noticed occasional feelings of fullness in her ears. She asks if these occurrences are anything to worry about.

G. Karen is 7 months' pregnant and works as a secretary full time. She asks the nurse if she should take a "water pill" that a friend gave her because she has noticed that her ankles "swell up" at the end of the day.

H. Jan is in her third trimester of pregnancy. She tells the nurse that her posture seems to have changed and that she occasionally experiences low back pain.

I. Monica, who is 36 weeks' pregnant with her first baby, calls the clinic stating that she knows the baby is coming since she felt some uterine contractions before getting out of bed in the morning. Monica confirms that they seem to have decreased in intensity and frequency since she has gotten out of bed and walked around.

J. Nina is a primigravida who is at 32 weeks' gestation. When she comes for a prenatal visit she reports that she has been experiencing occasional periods of shortness of breath during the day and sometimes has to use an extra pillow to sleep comfortably. Nina expresses concern that she is developing a breathing problem.

2. Accurate blood pressure readings are critical, if significant changes in the cardiovascular system are to be detected as a woman adapts to pregnancy during the prenatal period. WRITE a protocol for blood pressure assessment that can be used by nurses working in a prenatal clinic to ensure accuracy of the results obtained during blood pressure assessment.

ONLINE LEARNING ACTIVITIES

Access the Lowdermilk, Perry **Evolve** website at
http://evolve.elsevier.com/Lowdermilk/MatWmnHlth/ and enter the **Student** portion through the
Learning Resources section to assist you in searching the medical literature for nursing research
studies related to how women and their families (support system) respond to the physiologic and
anatomic changes associated with pregnancy.

- Create an annotated bibliography of at least five research studies.
- Choose one study and complete a bibliography card that includes the following:
  - Hypothesis; research question
  - Summary of the methodology used and key findings
  - Reliability of the study and its findings
  - Recommendations for further research
- Describe how you would use the findings of these studies to assist women and their families to cope
  effectively with the changes encountered with pregnancy.

CHAPTER 15

Maternal and Fetal Nutrition

CHAPTER REVIEW ACTIVITIES

FILL IN THE BLANKS: Insert the term that corresponds to each of the following descriptions.

1. A _____ before conception is the best way to ensure that adequate nutrients are available for the developing fetus. Adequate intake of _____ is important for decreasing risk for _____ or failures in the closure of the neural tube. An intake of _____ daily is recommended.

2. Inadequate maternal nutrition and inadequate weight gain may impair fetal growth and development resulting in _____. _____ is defined as a birth weight of 2500 g (5½ pounds) or less. LBW infants may be _____ and/or _____. Poor weight gain early in pregnancy increases the risk for giving birth to a _____ infant whereas inadequate gains during the last half of pregnancy increase the risk for _____.

3. Obesity, either preexisting or developed during pregnancy, increases the likelihood of _____ and _____, _____ birth, emergency _____, postpartum _____ and _____, birth _____, and late _____.

4. When individualizing the recommended daily allowances for pregnant and lactating women, nurses need to consider variations in a pregnant woman's situation including such factors as stage of _____, and number of _____, and maternal _____, _____, and current _____. _____ needs are met by carbohydrates, fats, and protein in the diet and should be increased during the second and third trimesters _____ Kcal above prepregnancy needs. Longitudinal assessment of maternal _____ during pregnancy is the best way to determine if the kilocalorie intake is adequate.

5. Woman at greatest risk for inadequate protein intake would include _____, _____, and _____.

6. Inadequate intake of iron can lead to the development of _____ during pregnancy, a nutritional health problem. In the United States, it is more common among _____, _____ women, and women of _____.

7. _____ is the inability to digest milk sugar because of the lack of the lactase enzyme in the small intestine.

8. _____ is the practice of consuming nonfood substances such as _____, _____, and _____ or excessive amounts of food stuffs low in nutritional value such as _____ or _____, _____, or _____, and _____. Women who follow this practice have been found to have lower _____ levels and may develop _____. _____ is the urge to consume specific types of foods such as ice cream, pickles, and pizza and are thought to be caused by an innate drive to consume _____ missing from the diet.

9. Assessment of nutritional status begins with a diet history which should include _____, _____, and _____. Physical examination includes _____ measurement such as _____ and _____. Calculation of the _____ is a method of evaluating the appropriateness of weight for height and is used to guide a woman's weight gain during pregnancy.

10. Vegetarian diets can vary in terms of the foods allowed. Basic to almost all vegetarian diets are _____, _____, _____, _____, _____, and _____. A _____ diet includes fish, poultry, eggs, and dairy products but does not allow beef or pork. _____ consume dairy products and plant products. _____ or _____ consume only plant products.

11. COMPLETE the following table by stating the importance of each of the following nutrients for healthy maternal adaptation to pregnancy and optimum fetal growth and development. INDICATE the major food sources for each nutrient.

Nutrient	Importance for Pregnancy	Major Food Sources
Protein		
Iron		
Calcium		
Zinc		
Fat-soluble vitamins (A, D)		
Water-soluble vitamins (folic acid, B_6, C)		

12. When assessing pregnant women it is critical that nurses are alert for factors that could place women at nutritional risk so that early intervention can be implemented. *STATE* five of these indicators or risk factors of which the nurse should be aware.

13. At her first prenatal visit, Marie, a 20-year-old primigravida, reports that she has been a strict vegetarian for the past 3 years. *IDENTIFY* two major guidelines that the nurse should follow when planning menus with Marie.

14. Evaluation of nutritional status is an essential part of a thorough physical assessment of pregnant women. *CITE* four signs of good nutrition and four signs of inadequate nutrition that the nurse should observe for during the assessment of a pregnant woman.

15. *IDENTIFY* three nursing measures appropriate for each of the following nursing diagnoses:
    A. Imbalanced nutrition: less than body requirements related to inadequate intake associated with moderate nausea and vomiting (morning sickness).

    B. Constipation, related to decreased intestinal motility associated with increased progesterone levels during pregnancy.

    C. Acute pain related to reflux of gastric contents into esophagus following dinner.

16. *DETERMINE* the approximate body mass index (BMI) for each of the following pregnant women and *INDICATE* the recommended weight gain and pattern for each woman based on her calculated BMI.

Woman	BMI	Weight Gain
June: 5 feet 3 inches, 124 pounds		
Alice: 5 feet 8 inches, 190 pounds		
Ann: 5 feet 5 inches, 95 pounds		

TRUE OR FALSE: Circle "T" if true or "F" if false for each of the following statements. Correct the false statements.

T   F   17. Good maternal nutrition before and during pregnancy is considered to be one of the most important preventive measures for low birth weight (LBW).

T   F   18. A series of 24-hour diet recalls is the best way to determine the appropriateness of a woman's kcal intake.

T   F   19. A woman whose BMI is 29 (overweight/high) should gain approximately 0.3 kg/per week during the second and third trimesters of pregnancy.

T   F   20. During pregnancy, women should drink at least 6 to 8 glasses of fluid each day.

T   F   21. A caloric increase of 600 kcal per day is recommended for pregnant women beginning in the first trimester.

T   F   22. A weight gain of more than 2 kg in a month after the 30th week of gestation is strongly suggestive of pregnancy-induced hypertension (PIH).

T   F   23. Iron deficiency anemia increases the risk for postpartum infection and poor wound healing.

T   F   24. Pregnant women should avoid caffeine because an intake of more that 300 mg daily increases the risk for spontaneous abortion and intrauterine growth restriction (IUGR).

T   F   25. Women should begin taking an iron supplement starting at 12 weeks' gestation.

T   F   26. All pregnant women require a supplement of 60 mg of ferrous iron daily.

T   F   27. If moderate peripheral edema occurs during pregnancy, the woman's sodium intake should be reduced.

T   F   28. Excessive intake of vitamin A, a fat-soluble vitamin, during pregnancy can cause congenital malformations of the fetus.

T F 29. Development of neural tube defects appears to be more common in the fetuses of pregnant women whose diets are low in vitamin B_6.

T F 30. Dehydration may increase the risk for contractions of the uterus and preterm labor.

T F 31. Lactating women need to consume at least 2500 kcal/day.

T F 32. Lactating women should be told that loss of the weight gained during pregnancy will begin after they stop breastfeeding.

T F 33. The most common nutrition-related laboratory test for a pregnant woman is a hematocrit and hemoglobin measurement.

T F 34. A 1200-mg calcium supplement daily may be required if the lactating woman consumes a diet that is low in calcium.

T F 35. Smoking may impair the production of milk in lactating women.

T F 36. Caffeine intake can lead to a reduction in the concentration of iron in the milk of lactating women.

T F 37. Iron and folic acid requirements for breastfeeding mothers increase above pregnancy requirements.

38. Jean is going to be breastfeeding her infant until she returns to work in 6 months. *STATE* three guidelines that the nurse should teach Jean to follow to ensure adequate nutrition during lactation.

39. Mary asks the nurse why her nutrient needs increase during pregnancy. *STATE* four factors that the nurse should explain to Mary as reasons why her needs increase.

MULTIPLE CHOICE: Circle the one correct option and state the rationale for the option chosen.

40. A nurse teaching a pregnant woman about the importance of iron in her diet would tell her to avoid consuming which of the following foods at the same time as her iron supplement because it will decrease iron absorption?
    A. Tomatoes
    B. Strawberries
    C. Meat
    D. Eggs

41. A 25-year-old pregnant woman is at 10 weeks' gestation. Her BMI is calculated to be 24. Which one of the following is recommended in terms of weight gain during pregnancy?
    A. Total weight gain of 18 kg
    B. First trimester weight gain of 1 to 2.5 kg
    C. Weight gain of 0.4 kg each week for 40 weeks
    D. Weight gain of 3.0 kg per month during the second and third trimester

42. A pregnant woman at 6 weeks' gestation tells her nurse-midwife that she has been experiencing nausea with occasional vomiting every day. The nurse could recommend which of the following as an effective relief measure?
    A. Eat starchy foods such as buttered popcorn or peanut butter with crackers in the morning before getting out of bed
    B. Avoid eating before going to bed at night
    C. Alter eating patterns to small meals every 2 to 3 hours
    D. Skip a meal if nausea is experienced

43. A woman demonstrates an understanding of the importance of increasing her intake of foods high in folic acid when she includes which of the following foods in her diet?
    A. Seafood
    B. Legumes
    C. Corn
    D. Cheese

44. A 30-year-old woman at 16 weeks' gestation comes for a routine prenatal visit. Her 24-hour dietary recall is evaluated by the nurse. Which of the following entries would indicate that this woman needs further instructions regarding nutrient needs during pregnancy?
    A. Servings up to 10 ounces total from the meat, poultry, fish, dry beans, eggs, and nuts group
    B. Total kcal intake is 300 kcal above her calculated prepregnancy needs
    C. Daily iron supplement taken at bedtime with a glass of orange juice
    D. Four servings from the milk, yogurt, cheese group

CRITICAL THINKING EXERCISES

1. Nutrition and weight gain are important areas of consideration for nurses who care for pregnant women. In addition, weight gain is often a source of stress and body image alteration for the pregnant woman. *DISCUSS* the approach you would use in each of the following situations.
    A. Kelly (5' 8" and 130 pounds) complains to you that her physician recommended a weight gain of approximately 30 pounds during her pregnancy. She states, "Babies only weigh about 7 pounds when they are born! Why do I have to gain much more than that?"

    B. Kate (5' 4" and 122 pounds) has just found out that she is pregnant. She states, "I am so glad to be pregnant. I love to eat, and now I can start eating for two. It will be great not to have to watch the scale or what I eat."

C. June tells you that she does not have to worry about her nutrient intake during her pregnancy. "I take plenty of vitamins—everything from A to Z!!"

D. Erin is 7 months' pregnant. She asks you what she can do to relieve the heartburn she experiences after meals, especially dinner.

E. Sara (BMI = 28.7) is 1 month pregnant. She asks you for dietary guidance, including a weight reduction diet because she does not want to gain too much weight with this pregnancy.

F. Beth is 2 months' pregnant. She states, "I have cut down on my water intake. I do get a little thirsty but it is worth it since I do not have to urinate so often."

G. Hedy is 2 months' pregnant and has come for her second prenatal visit. During a discussion about nutrition needs during pregnancy she states, "I know I will never get enough calcium because I get sick when I drink milk."

H. Lara is 36 weeks' pregnant. She states that she would like to breastfeed her baby but is concerned about getting back into shape and losing weight after the baby is born. "My friends told me that I will lose weight more slowly since I will not be able to start on a weight reduction diet as long as I am breastfeeding."

2. Yvonne's hemoglobin is 13 g/dl and her hematocrit is 37% at the onset of her pregnancy. She asks the nurse if she will have to take iron during her pregnancy if she tries to follow a good diet. "My friend took iron when she was pregnant and it made her sick to her stomach." *DISCUSS* the appropriate response by the nurse.

3. Gloria is an 18-year-old Native American woman (5' 6" and 98 pounds) who has just been diagnosed as 8 weeks' pregnant. In her discussions with you at her first prenatal visit, she expresses a lack of knowledge regarding the nutritional requirements of pregnancy and an interest in learning about what to eat because she wants to have a healthy baby.
   A. *OUTLINE* the approach that you would use in order to help Gloria learn about and meet the nutritional requirements of her pregnancy.

   B. *PLAN* a 1-day menu that incorporates Gloria's nutritional needs and reflects the traditions of her culture.

ONLINE LEARNING ACTIVITIES

Access the Lowdermilk, Perry **Evolve** website at **http://evolve.elsevier.com/Lowdermilk/MatWmnHlth/** and enter the **Student** portion through the **Learning Resources** section to assist you in searching the medical literature for nursing research studies related to effective measures pregnant women can use to relieve nausea and vomiting associated with pregnancy.
- Create an annotated bibliography of at least five research studies
- Choose one study and complete a bibliography card that includes the following:
  - Hypothesis; research question
  - Summary of the methodology used and key findings
  - Reliability of the study and its findings
  - Recommendations for further research
  - How the professional nurse can use the study's findings to teach pregnant women more effective, evidence-based measures to relieve morning sickness

CHAPTER 16

Nursing Care During Pregnancy

CHAPTER REVIEW ACTIVITIES

FILL IN THE BLANKS: Insert the term that corresponds to each of the following descriptions.

1. Pregnancy can be diagnosed by assessing a woman for the presence of specific signs and symptoms associated with pregnancy. _____ indicators of pregnancy can be caused by conditions other than gestation and are not reliable for diagnosis. _____ indicators of pregnancy are those that can be detected by an examiner and are mainly related to changes in the uterus. _____ indicators are directly attributed to the fetus.

2. _____ rule is used to determine the _____ by subtracting _____ from and adding _____ and _____ (if appropriate) to the first day of the _____. Pregnancy is divided into three 3-month periods called _____. The duration of a full term pregnancy is _____ to _____ weeks.

3. _____ can occur when a woman lies on her back for an examination of her abdomen. The _____ and the _____ are compressed by the weight of the abdominal contents, including the uterus. Signs and symptoms that this has occurred would include _____, _____, _____, _____, _____, _____, and _____.

4. A variety of assessment methods are used to evaluate the progress of pregnancy. _____ is measured beginning in the second trimester as one indicator of the progress of fetal growth. The _____ test determines whether the nipple is everted or inverted, by placing thumb and forefinger on the areola and pressing inward gently.

5. Assessment of fetal health status includes evaluating _____, _____, _____, and _____. The fetal _____ is estimated after determining the duration of pregnancy and the estimated date of birth.

6. Maternal and paternal adaptation during pregnancy includes mastery of certain _____ tasks that include _____, _____, _____, and _____.

7. As a pregnant woman establishes a relationship with her fetus and emotional attachment begins, she progresses through three phases. In phase one, she accepts the _____ and needs to be able to state _____. In phase two, the woman accepts the _____. She can now say _____. Finally, in phase three, the woman prepares realistically for the _____ and _____. She expresses the thought _____.

8. _____ refers to rapid unpredictable changes in mood related to profound _____ changes and concerns about _____ and _____. _____ refers to having conflicting feelings simultaneously about the pregnancy.

9. The _____ phase is the first, early period of paternal adaptation during which the father accepts the _____. During the second or _____ phase the father adjusts to the reality of the pregnancy. The developmental task is to _____. The father becomes actively involved in the pregnancy and the relationship with his child during the third or _____ phase. The developmental task is to _____ with his partner the role he is to play in _____ and to prepare for _____.

10. _____ refers to the rituals and taboos that a culture expects the male to follow when his partner is pregnant. _____ refers to the phenomenon of an expectant father's experiencing pregnancy-like symptoms such as emotional lability, ambivalence, nausea, fatigue, and other discomforts.

11. Certain cultural practices are expected by women of all cultures to ensure a good outcome to their pregnancy. Cultural _____ are practices that tell a woman what to do during pregnancy. Cultural _____ are practices that tell a woman what not to do during pregnancy; they establish _____.

12. The multiple marker or _____ blood test is used to screen for _____. It is done between _____ and _____ weeks' gestation and measures maternal serum levels of _____, _____, and _____.

13. CALCULATE the expected date of birth (EDB) for each of the following pregnant women using Nägele's rule.
    A. Diane's last menses began on May 5, 2003, and its last day occurred on May 10, 2003.

    B. Sara had intercourse on February 21, 2003. She has not had a menstrual period since the one that began on January 14, 2003 and ended 5 days later.

    C. Beth's last period began on September 4, 2003, and ended on September 10, 2003. Beth noted that her basal body temperature (BBT) began to rise on September 28, 2003.

14. Cultural beliefs and practices are important influencing factors during the prenatal period.
    A. DESCRIBE how cultural beliefs can affect a woman's participation in prenatal care as it is defined by the Western Biomedical Model of Care.

B. *IDENTIFY* one **prescription** and one **proscription** for each of the following areas:
Emotional responses

Clothing

Physical activity and rest

Sexual activity

Diet

15. *COMPLETE* the following table by identifying data to be collected for each component of maternal assessment during the initial visit and follow-up visits during pregnancy.

Component	Initial Visit	Follow-Up Visits
Health history interview		
Physical examination		
Laboratory and diagnostic testing		

16. Marie asks the nurse what can be done during a prenatal visit to make sure that her baby is healthy and doing well. *IDENTIFY and DESCRIBE* what the nurse could tell Marie about the components of fetal assessment that will determine her baby's health status.

17. Nurses responsible for the care management of pregnant women must be alert for warning signs of potential complications that women could develop as pregnancy progresses from trimester to trimester.

    A. *LIST* the signs of potential complications (warning signs) for each trimester of pregnancy. *INDICATE* possible cause(s) for each sign listed.

First Trimester	Second/Third Trimesters

    B. *DESCRIBE* the approach a nurse should take when discussing potential complications with a pregnant woman and her family.

TRUE OR FALSE: Circle "T" if true or "F" if false for each of the following statements. Correct the false statements.

T F 18. Women who are joggers should stop jogging and begin swimming for exercise as soon as they discover that they are pregnant.

T F 19. If a woman's pulse rises above 100 beats per minute during exercise, she should slow down until it reaches a maximum of 80 beats per minute.

T F 20. The use of a condom is necessary during pregnancy if the woman is at risk for acquiring or transmitting a sexually transmitted infection (STI).

T F 21. Intercourse is safe during a normal pregnancy as long as it is not uncomfortable.

T F 22. Exposure to second-hand smoke is associated with growth restriction and an increase in perinatal and infant morbidity and mortality.

T   F   23. It is not necessary to screen pregnant women for human immunodeficiency virus because there is no effective measure to reduce transmission to the fetus.

T   F   24. Women who are at low risk for complications should be scheduled for prenatal visits every 2 to 3 weeks throughout pregnancy.

T   F   25. A 1-hour, 50-g glucose tolerance test is performed on all pregnant women at 20 weeks' gestation to screen for the presence of gestational diabetes.

T   F   26. A rise in systolic blood pressure of 15 mm Hg or more and/or in diastolic blood pressure of 10 mm Hg or more above baseline should be viewed as an indicator of risk for pregnancy-induced hypertension.

T   F   27. From weeks 18 to 30 the height of the fundus in inches is approximately the same as the weeks' gestation if the woman's bladder is full.

T   F   28. Quickening usually occurs between weeks 16 and 20 of gestation.

T   F   29. A woman should avoid tub bathing and shower instead once she reaches the third trimester of her pregnancy to avoid injury from falling.

T   F   30. The side-lying position promotes uteroplacental perfusion and fetal oxygenation.

T   F   31. Once the uterus enlarges, the pregnant woman should use only the lap belt and avoid using a shoulder harness while in a car.

T   F   32. A woman with inverted nipples should perform nipple rolling and tugging exercises during the third trimester in order to break adhesions.

T   F   33. Hepatitis B vaccination can be safely administered during pregnancy.

T   F   34. A sign of preterm labor would be uterine contractions occurring every 10 minutes or more often (six or more per hour) for 1 hour.

T   F   35. Wearing breast shells for 1 to 2 hours each day during the third trimester can help inverted or flat nipples evert or become erect, thereby facilitating latch-on of the newborn once breastfeeding begins after birth.

T   F   36. Women who are positive for hepatitis B should not breastfeed.

T   F   37. Women often react to the confirmation of pregnancy with mixed feelings or ambivalence.

T   F   38. Emotional lability (mood swings) may be related to profound hormonal changes that are part of the maternal response to pregnancy.

T   F   39. Children typically respond to their mother's pregnancy in terms of their age and dependency needs.

T   F   40. Ambivalence expressed by a pregnant woman during the first trimester is an early sign that she is rejecting an unwanted pregnancy.

T   F   41. The reaction of a mother to her daughter's pregnancy can influence her daughter's self-confidence about her pregnancy.

T   F   42. Low birth weight and infant mortality have been associated with inadequate prenatal care.

T   F   43. Currently, 65% of pregnant women in the United States receive prenatal care.

T   F   44. Loss of calcium from teeth during pregnancy increases a woman's risk for dental caries and tooth loss.

T   F   45. No amount of alcohol is considered safe during pregnancy.

T   F   46. Morning sickness occurs in 50% to 75% of pregnant women.

47. *CREATE* a protocol for fundal measurement that will facilitate accuracy.

48. *IDENTIFY* four factors that can be used to estimate the gestational age of the fetus.

49. Prevention of injury is an important goal for nurses as they teach pregnant women about how to care for themselves during pregnancy.
    A. *DESCRIBE* three principles of body mechanics that a pregnant woman should be taught to prevent injury.

    B. *IDENTIFY* five safety guidelines that the nurse should include in a pamphlet entitled "Safety During Pregnancy" that will be distributed to pregnant women during a prenatal visit.

50. During the third trimester, parents often make a decision concerning the method they will use to feed their newborn. *LIST* the contraindications for breastfeeding.

51. Men experience pregnancy in many different ways. Three styles of involvement have been exhibited by men during their partners' first pregnancy (May, 1980, 1982). *DESCRIBE* the typical behaviors the nurse would expect to observe in fathers representing each of the following styles of involvement.
    Observer

    Expressive

MULTIPLE CHOICE: Circle the one correct option and state the rationale for the option chosen.

52. A nurse is assessing a pregnant woman during a prenatal visit. Several presumptive indicators of pregnancy are documented. Which one of the following is a presumptive indicator?
    A. Uterine enlargement
    B. Quickening
    C. Ballottement
    D. Palpation of fetal movement by the nurse

53. A woman's last menstrual period (LMP) began on November 9, 2003, and it ended on November 14, 2003. Using Nägele's rule, the estimated date of birth would be:
    A. February 2, 2004
    B. July 6, 2004
    C. August 16, 2004
    D. August 21, 2004

54. A woman at 30 weeks' gestation assumes a supine position for a fundal measurement and Leopold maneuvers. She begins to complain about feeling dizzy and nauseous. Her skin feels damp and cool. The nurse's first action would be to:
    A. Assess the woman's respiratory rate and effort
    B. Provide the woman with an emesis basin
    C. Elevate the woman's legs 20 degrees from her hips
    D. Turn the woman on her side

55. During an early bird prenatal class a nurse teaches a group of newly diagnosed pregnant women about their emotional reactions during pregnancy. Which of the following should the nurse discuss with the women?
    A. Sexual desire (libido) is decreased throughout pregnancy
    B. A referral for counseling should be sought if a woman experiences conflicting feelings about her pregnancy especially in the first trimester
    C. A quiet period of introspection is often experienced around the time a woman feels her baby move for the first time
    D. The need to seek safe passage and prepare for birth begins early in the second trimester

56. The nurse evaluates a pregnant woman's knowledge about prevention of urinary tract infections at the prenatal visit following a class on infection prevention that the woman attended. The nurse would recognize that the woman needs further instruction when she tells the nurse about which one of the following measures that she now uses to prevent urinary tract infections:
    A. "I drink about one quart of fluid a day."
    B. "I have stopped using bubble baths and bath oils."
    C. "I have started wearing panty hose and underpants with a cotton crotch."
    D. "I drink cranberry juice instead of orange juice and have yogurt for lunch."

CRITICAL THINKING EXERCISES

1. A health history interview of the pregnant woman by the nurse is included as part of the initial prenatal visit.
    A. *STATE* the purpose of the health history interview.

    B. *WRITE* two questions for each component that is included in the initial health history interview. Questions should be clear, concise, and understandable. Most of the questions should be open ended in order to elicit the most complete response from the client.

    C. *WRITE* four questions that should be included when doing an updating health history interview during follow-up visits.

2. *IMAGINE* that you are a nurse working in a prenatal clinic. You have been assigned to be the primary nurse for Martha, an 18-year-old, who has come to the clinic for confirmation of pregnancy. She tells you that she knows she is pregnant because she has already missed three periods and a home pregnancy test that she did last week was positive. Martha states that she has had very little contact with the health care system, and the only reason she came today is because her boyfriend insisted that she "make sure" she is really pregnant. *DESCRIBE* the approach that you would take regarding data collection and nursing intervention appropriate for this woman.

3. Terry is a primigravida in her first trimester of pregnancy. She is accompanied by her husband Tim to her second prenatal visit. *ANSWER* each of the following questions asked by Terry and Tim:
    A. "At the last visit I was told that my estimated date of birth is December 25, 2003!! Can I really count on my baby being born on Christmas Day?"

B. "Before I became pregnant my friend told be I should be doing Kegel exercises. I was too embarrassed to ask her about them. What are they and is it safe for me to do them while I am pregnant?"

C. "What effect will pregnancy have on our sex life? We are willing to abstain during pregnancy if we have to keep our baby safe."

D. "This morning sickness I am experiencing is driving my crazy. I become nauseous in the morning and again late in the afternoon. Occasionally I vomit or have the dry heaves. Will this last for my entire pregnancy? Is there anything I can do to feel better?"

4. Tara is 2 months' pregnant. She tells the nurse, at the prenatal clinic, that she is used to being active and exercises everyday. Now that she is pregnant she wonders if she should reduce or stop her exercise routine. *DISCUSS* the nurse's response to Tara.

5. *WRITE* one nursing diagnosis for each of the following situations. *STATE* one expected outcome, and *LIST* appropriate nursing measures for the nursing diagnosis you identified.
    A. Beth is 6 weeks' pregnant. During the health history interview, she tells you that she has limited her intake of fluids and tries to hold her urine as long as she can because "I just hate having to go to the bathroom so frequently."

Nursing Diagnosis	Expected Outcome	Nursing Measures

B. Doris, who is 23 weeks' pregnant, tells you that she is beginning to experience more frequent lower back pain. You note that when she walked into the examining room her posture exhibited a moderate degree of lordosis and neck flexion. She was wearing shoes with 2-inch narrow heels.

Nursing Diagnosis	Expected Outcome	Nursing Measures

C. Lisa, a primigravida at 32 weeks' gestation, comes for a prenatal visit accompanied by her partner, the father of the baby. They both express anxiety about the impending birth of the baby and how they will handle the experience of labor. Lisa is especially concerned about how she will survive the pain and her partner is primarily concerned about how he will help Lisa cope with labor and make sure she and the baby are safe.

Nursing Diagnosis	Expected Outcome	Nursing Measures

6. Jane is a primigravida in her second trimester of pregnancy. ANSWER each of the following questions asked by Jane during a prenatal visit.

A. "Why do you measure my abdomen every time I come in for a check-up?"

B. "How can you tell if my baby is doing okay?"

C. "I am going to start changing the way that I dress now that I am beginning to show. Do you have any suggestions I could follow, especially since I have a limited amount of money to spend?"

D. "What can I do about gas and constipation? I never had much of a problem before I was pregnant."

E. "Since yesterday I have started to feel itchy all over. Do you think I am coming down with some sort of infection?"

F. "I will be flying out to Chicago to visit my father in 1 month. Is airline travel safe for me when I am 5 months' pregnant?"

7. While a nurse is measuring a pregnant woman's fundus, the woman becomes pale and diaphoretic. The woman, who is at 23 weeks' gestation, states that she feels dizzy and lightheaded.
A. *STATE* the most likely explanation for the assessment findings exhibited by this woman.

B. *DESCRIBE* the nurse's immediate action.

8. Kelly is a primigravida in her third trimester of pregnancy. *ANSWER* each of the following questions asked by Kelly during a prenatal visit.
    A. "My husband and I have decided to breastfeed our baby but friends told me it is very difficult if my nipples do not come out. Is there any way I can tell now if my nipples are okay for breastfeeding?"

    B. "My ankles are swollen by the time I get home from work late in the afternoon (Kelly teaches second grade). I have been trying to drink about 3 liters of fluid every day. Should I reduce the amount of liquid I am drinking or ask my doctor for a water pill?"

    C. "I woke up last night with a terrible cramp in my leg. It finally went away but my husband and I just did not know what to do. What if this happens again tonight?"

9. Marge, a pregnant woman (2–0–0–1–0) beginning her third trimester, expresses concern about preterm birth. "I already had one miscarriage and my sister's baby died after being born too early. I am so worried that this will happen to me."
    A. *IDENTIFY* one nursing diagnosis with an expected outcome that reflects Marge's concern.

    B. *INDICATE* what the nurse can teach Marge about the signs of preterm labor.

    C. *DESCRIBE* the actions Marge should take if she experiences signs of preterm labor.

10. Carol is 4 months' pregnant and beginning to "show." She asks the nurse what she should expect as a reaction from her 13-year-old daughter and 3-year-old son. DESCRIBE the response the nurse would make.

11. Your neighbor, Jane Smith, is in her second month of pregnancy. Knowing that you are a nurse, her husband Tom confides in you that he just cannot "figure Jane out. One minute she is happy and the next minute she is crying for no reason at all! I do not know how I will be able to cope with this for seven more months."

    A. WRITE a nursing diagnosis and expected outcome that reflects Tom's concern.

    B. DISCUSS how you would respond to his concern.

12. Jim's partner Mary is 5 months' pregnant. He tells you that sometimes he feels "left out" of Mary's pregnancy and asks you if he is important to Mary as her partner and the father of the baby. SPECIFY how you would answer his question.

ONLINE LEARNING ACTIVITIES

Access the Lowdermilk, Perry **Evolve** website at **http://evolve.elsevier.com/Lowdermilk/MatWmnHlth/** and enter the **Student** portion through the **Learning Resources** section. Use Chapter 16 as a starting point of a search of the Internet for websites designed to help pregnant women cope effectively with the discomforts of pregnancy. Prepare a report that includes the following:

- List of at least three relevant sites
- Description of one site in terms of:
  - Sponsoring person(s), agency, organization
  - Clarity, accuracy, accessibility (ease of use), value, and depth of the information provided
  - Currency—frequency of site updates
  - Variety of links to other relevant sites
  - Ability of persons visiting the site to obtain additional information and individualized support through such services as e-mail and chat rooms
- Handout that will guide women in the use of these sites

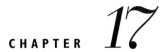

CHAPTER *17*

Childbirth and Perinatal Education

CHAPTER REVIEW ACTIVITIES

FILL IN THE BLANKS: Insert the term that corresponds to each of the following descriptions.

1. _____ is an important component of perinatal health care services that stresses risk management and healthy behaviors that promote the health of a woman, of a man, and their potential fetus. The period of greatest danger for the development of the fetus is between _____ and _____ days after fertilization.

2. The _____ method is the prepared childbirth method that is referred to as childbirth without fear. It is based on a theory that pain in childbirth is socially conditioned and caused by a _____ syndrome. _____ is an important component of this method.

3. The _____ method is the prepared childbirth method that is also referred to as the psychoprophylactic method. It combines _____ and _____ techniques.

4. The _____ method is the method known as partner (husband)-coached childbirth. It uses _____, _____, and _____. Environmental variables are emphasized such as _____, _____, and _____ to make childbirth a more natural experience.

5. Childbirth classes should focus on preparing families _____, _____, and _____ for childbirth and promoting _____ and improved _____ during the childbearing years.

6. A _____ is a tool used by parents to explore their childbirth options and choose those that are most important to them.

7. An _____ is a physician who specializes in the care of women during pregnancy.

8. A _____ is a registered nurse with added education and training in the care of women and their families during pregnancy.

9. _____, also known as _____, are caregivers trained through self-study, apprenticeship, midwifery schools or universities as a profession distinct from nursing.

10. A _____ is a labor attendant who is professionally trained to provide labor support including _____, _____, and _____ support to women and their partners during labor and birth.

11. _____ rooms are special units used for the labor, birth, and the first 1 to 2 hours afterwards, providing time for bonding with the newborn. The woman and her baby are then transferred to a postpartum unit.

12. _____ rooms are special units used for the total care of a woman from admission to labor until postpartum discharge. Women and their families may remain in these rooms for 6 to 48 hours.

13. A _____ center is built in a location separate from the hospital but usually located in close proximity to it in case transfer of a woman and/or her baby is required.

TRUE AND FALSE: Circle "T" if true or "F" if false for each of the following statements. Correct the false statements.

T   F   14. By the end of the 6th week after conception any major structural anomalies in the fetus are already present.

T   F   15. Preconception care is primarily directed toward women who have had a problem with a previous pregnancy and/or have a chronic illness.

T   F   16. An adequate maternal intake of folic acid before and after conception decreases the risk of having a child with a neural tube defect.

T   F   17. Approximately 50% of birth defects occur as a result of environmental factors that are amenable to educational awareness.

T   F   18. Nurse-midwives attend approximately 25% of births in the United States and Canada.

T   F   19. Certified nurse-midwives may practice independently with an arrangement for physician backup.

T   F   20. Most nurse-midwife births are managed in a home setting.

T   F   21. The doula does not become involved in clinical tasks required for the care of women in labor.

T   F   22. Six weeks after the birth, the doula-assisted woman is usually still breastfeeding and experiencing a higher level of self-esteem.

T   F   23. In North America, home births account for approximately 5% of births.

24. *OUTLINE* the role of the nurse in the preconception education and care of a couple considering pregnancy.

25. *EXPLAIN* the specific tension-reducing and pain relief measures advocated by each of the following childbirth education methods.
    Grantly Dick-Read method

    Lamaze method

    Bradley method

26. *IDENTIFY* the components of the philosophy of birth developed by Lamaze International and adopted by the Coalition to Improve Maternity Services (CIMS).

27. Women often fear the pain that will accompany childbirth. *DESCRIBE* how each of the following nonpharmacologic methods could be effective for pain relief during labor and birth.
    Relaxation

    Paced breathing

    Biofeedback

    Therapeutic touch

    Acupressure

    Music

28. In the United States, the rate of cesarean births is high and the rate of successful vaginal births after cesarean birth is low. *DISCUSS* the role that childbirth education could have in reversing this trend.

29. Which of the following methods of prepared childbirth advocate environmental modification?
    A. Psychoprophylactic method
    B. Lamaze method
    C. Grantly Dick-Read method
    D. Bradley method

30. The nurse is reviewing a pregnant couple's birth plan. The option that would require modification would be:
    A. Eight-year-old daughter will be present for the labor and birth
    B. Husband will cut the umbilical cord
    C. Woman will remain in bed for labor and birth as she did during her first labor
    D. A doula will be hired to provide labor support

31. Doulas are becoming important members of a laboring woman's health care team. Which of the following activities should be expected as part of the doula's role responsibilities?
    A. Monitor hydration of laboring woman including adjusting IV flow rates
    B. Interpret electronic fetal monitoring tracings to determine the well-being of the maternal-fetal unit
    C. Eliminate the need for the husband/partner to be present during labor and birth
    D. Provide continuous support throughout labor and birth including explanations of labor progress

32. The primary expected outcome of participation in childbirth preparation classes would be:
    A. Pain-free childbirth
    B. Family members present to observe the birth
    C. Enhanced ability to cope with pain and to remain in control
    D. No pharmacologic measures used for pain relief

CRITICAL THINKING EXERCISES

1. Mary Ann and her husband Sam have just been married. At her annual GYN check up, Mary Ann tells the nurse practitioner that she and Sam plan to get pregnant in about 1 year.
   A. *EXPLAIN* to Mary Ann and Sam why they should participate in preconception care before they become pregnant.

   B. *DESCRIBE* the process that the nurse should follow in providing Mary Ann and Sam with preconception care.

2. During a prenatal visit early in pregnancy, Tamara and Dan ask their nurse-midwife about developing a birth plan, stating "Our friends had one and they said it really helped them to have a satisfying birthing experience."

   A. *DESCRIBE* what the nurse should tell Tamara and Dan about the purpose of a birth plan.

   B. *STATE* the guidelines the nurse should follow when helping Tamara and Dan develop their plan.

   C. *OUTLINE* the topics for discussion and decision-making as the plan is created.

3. Jennifer (2–1–0–0–1) and her husband Dan are beginning their third trimester of a low risk pregnancy. As you work with them on their birth plan, they tell you that they are having trouble making a decision about their choice of a birth setting. They experienced a delivery room birth with their first child. Jennifer states, "My first pregnancy was perfectly normal just like this one, but the birth was disappointing, so medically focused with monitors, IVs, and staying in bed." They ask you for your advice about the different birth settings they have heard and read about, namely labor, delivery, recovery and postpartum (LDRP) rooms at their local hospital, the birthing center a few miles from their home, and even their own home. *DESCRIBE* the approach that you would take to guide Jennifer and Dan in their decision regarding a birth setting.

4. Nancy, a pregnant woman (3–2–0–0–2) at 26 weeks' gestation, asks the nurse about doulas. "My friend had a doula and she said that she was amazing. My first two birth experiences were difficult—my husband and I really needed someone to help us. Do you think a doula could be that person?"

   A. *EXPLAIN* the role of the doula so that Nancy will have the information she will need to make an informed decision.

B. Nancy decides to try a doula for her upcoming labor. *IDENTIFY* what you would tell Nancy about finding a doula.

C. *SPECIFY* questions that Nancy should ask when she is making a choice about the doula she will hire for her labor.

5. Tony and Andrea are considering the possibility of giving birth to their second baby at home. They have been receiving prenatal care from a certified nurse-midwife who has experience with home birth. Their 5-year-old son and both sets of grandparents want to be present for the birth.
   A. *DISCUSS* the decision-making process that Tony and Andrea should follow to ensure that they make an informed decision that is right for them and their family.

   B. Tony and Andrea decide that home birth is an ideal choice for them. *OUTLINE* the preparation measures you would recommend to Tony and Andrea to ensure a safe and positive experience for everyone.

6. During childbirth education classes couples often seek advice about how to care for their new baby and support their children through the sibling adjustment process. *DESCRIBE* the response you would give to the concerns expressed by the following couples.
   A. Anna and Rich express concern that their new baby will "cry all the time" just like their first baby. "When she cried we did everything, we fed her, changed her diaper, rocked her but nothing seemed to work. Our friends told us to be careful or we would spoil her if we went to her every time she cried."

   B. Anita and Joe are pregnant for the second time. They are excited about the pregnancy but are unsure about how to prepare their 4-year-old daughter for the new baby and the changes it will necessitate in her life. "We did not have to worry about this when we had our first baby!!"

ONLINE LEARNING ACTIVITIES

Access the Lowdermilk, Perry **Evolve** website at
http://evolve.elsevier.com/Lowdermilk/MatWmnHlth/ and enter the **Student** portion through the
Learning Resources section. Use Chapter 17 to begin a search for websites that will provide
expectant couples with information as they make decisions about birth setting options, childbirth
preparation methods, and the use of a doula. Prepare a handout for expectant couples that includes
the following:

- List of sites found in the search that provide the information they will require for decision making
- Summary of each site listed in terms of:
  - Sponsor of the site
  - Information provided
  - Services that will allow persons visiting the site to obtain further information such as links to
    other sites, e-mail, and chat rooms
- Guidelines related to using the site and for making a decision about the options they will choose
  for their childbirth experience

CHAPTER 18

Labor and Birth Processes

CHAPTER REVIEW ACTIVITIES

FILL IN THE BLANKS: Insert the term that corresponds to each of the following descriptions.

1. Five factors affecting the process of labor and birth are _____, _____, _____, _____, and _____.
2. Fontanels are _____ that are located where the _____ in the fetal/neonatal skull intersect.
3. Molding is the slight _____ of the _____ of the fetal _____ that occurs during childbirth.
4. Presentation refers to the _____ of the fetus that enters the pelvic _____ first. The three main types are _____ (head first), _____ (buttocks first), and _____.
5. The presenting part is the part of the fetal body _____ during a _____. The four types are _____, _____, _____, and _____.
6. The vertex presentation occurs when the fetal head is fully _____, making the _____ the fetal part first felt by the examining finger.
7. Fetal lie is the relationship of the fetal _____ to the maternal _____. There are two types: longitudinal (vertical) when the _____ and transverse (horizontal) when the _____.
8. Attitude is the relationship of the _____. The most common type is one of _____.
9. The biparietal diameter is the largest _____ diameter of the fetal skull. The suboccipitobregmatic diameter is the smallest _____ diameter of the fetal skull to enter the maternal pelvis when the fetal head is in complete _____.
10. Fetal position refers to the relationship of the _____ to the _____.
11. Engagement occurs when the _____ of the presenting part has passed through the _____, into the _____ reaching the level of the _____.
12. Station is the relationship of the _____ of the fetus to an imaginary line drawn between the _____. It is measured in _____ above or below the _____, thereby serving as a method of determining the progress of fetal _____.
13. Effacement refers to the _____ and _____ of the _____ during the _____ stage of labor. Degree of effacement is expressed in _____.

14. Dilation is the _____ or _____ of the _____ and the _____ that occurs once labor has begun. Degree of progress is expressed in _____ from less than _____ to _____.

15. Lightening occurs when the fetal _____ descends into the _____ approximately _____ before term in the primigravida and at the _____ in the multiparous woman.

16. The primary powers of labor are involuntary _____ and the secondary powers are the woman's _____ efforts or _____.

17. Bloody show is a _____ discharge representing the passage of the _____ as the cervix _____ in preparation for labor.

18. The mechanism of labor in a vertex presentation refers to the _____ and _____ of the _____, to facilitate passage through the maternal _____. Also known as the seven _____ of labor, they include _____, _____, _____, _____, _____, _____, and _____.

19. _____ maneuver is a pushing method during the second stage of labor whereby the woman holds her _____ and tightens her _____. It is not recommended because it increases _____, reduces _____, and increases _____. A temporary increase in maternal _____ and _____ occurs along with a slowing of the maternal _____. As a result, fetal _____ can occur.

20. _____ reflex or the maternal urge to _____ occurs when the presenting part of the fetus reaches the _____, stimulating stretch receptors and causing release of _____.

21. The first stage of labor begins with the onset of _____ and ends with full _____. It is divided into three phases, namely _____, _____, and _____.

22. The second stage of labor lasts from the time the _____ to the _____. Two phases of the second stage of labor are _____ and _____.

23. The third stage of labor lasts from the _____ until the _____.

24. The fourth stage of labor is the period of _____ when _____ is reestablished. It lasts approximately _____.

25. The four factors that affect fetal circulation during labor are maternal _____, _____, _____, and _____.

26. DESCRIBE how the five factors (the five P's) affect the process of labor and birth.

27. EXPLAIN how the cardinal movements of labor facilitate the birth of the fetus.

28. *LABEL* the following illustrations of the fetal skull and the maternal pelvis with the appropriate landmarks and diameters.

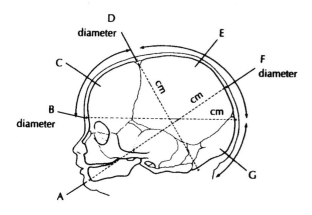
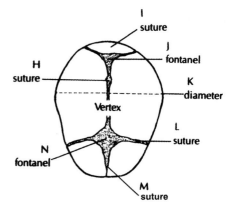

Fetal Skull

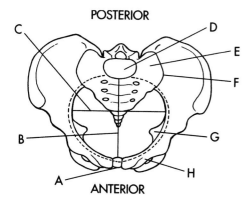

Pelvic Brim from Above

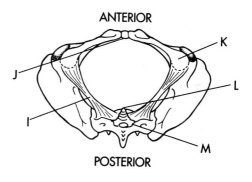

Pelvic Outlet from Above

Maternal Pelvis

29. *INDICATE* the presentation, presenting part, position, lie and attitude of the fetus, for each of the following illustrations.

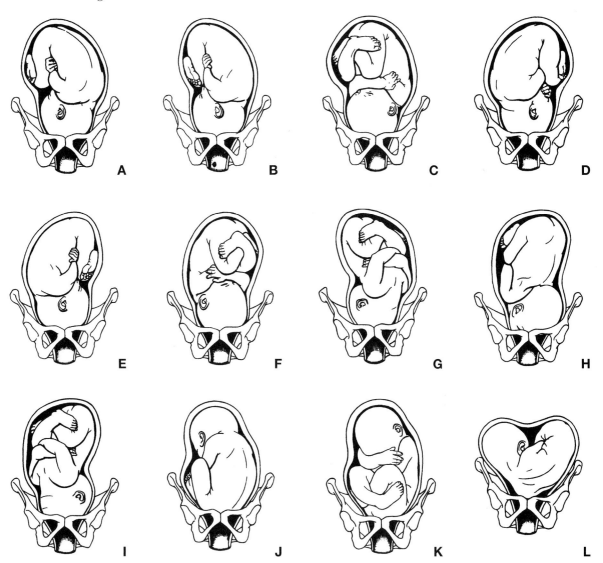

TRUE OR FALSE: Circle "T" if true or "F" if false for each of the following statements. Correct the false statements.

T   F   30. The most common fetal attitude is one of full extension of body parts.

T   F   31. A longitudinal lie results in either a cephalic or a breech presentation.

T   F   32. Fetal position is unlikely to change once labor begins.

T   F   33. A woman must have a gynecoid pelvis in order to experience a spontaneous vaginal birth.

T   F   34. Effacement usually precedes dilation for a nulliparous woman.

T   F   35. Women with a history of sexually transmitted infections may experience slowed or ineffective progress of cervical dilatation.

T   F   36. The hands and knees position is most helpful when the fetal presentation is breech.

T   F   37. Women often experience decreased dyspnea but increased urinary frequency after lightening occurs.

T   F   38. The expected range of the fetal heart rate of a full term fetus is 100 to 140 BPM.

T   F   39. An increase in fetal pO_2 and arterial pH and a decrease in pCO_2 prepares the fetus for initiating respirations immediately after its birth.

T   F   40. Because systolic blood pressure increases during a contraction assessment of maternal blood pressure *between* contractions provides more accurate data.

T   F   41. The maternal white blood cell count (WBC) increases in response to the stress, tissue trauma, and increased activity level associated with childbirth.

T   F   42. During labor, a woman should be encouraged to point her toes to reduce the incidence of leg cramps.

T   F   43. Endogenous endorphins secreted during labor raise a woman's pain threshold and produce sedation.

T   F   44. Fetal fibronectin is found in maternal plasma and cervicovaginal secretions of pregnant women before the onset of labor.

T   F   45. Effacement and dilation progress together during the first stage of labor for the multiparous woman.

T   F   46. The average duration of the second stage of labor is approximately 10 to 20 minutes.

T   F   47. Women are expected to experience an urge to bear down as soon as the second stage of labor begins.

MULTIPLE CHOICE: Circle the one correct option and state the rationale for the option chosen.

48. A vaginal examination during labor reveals the following information about the fetus: RMT—2. An accurate interpretation of these data would be:
   A. Attitude: flexed
   B. Station: above the ischial spines
   C. Presenting part: vertex
   D. Lie: transverse

49. Changes occur as a woman progresses through labor. Which of the following maternal adaptations would be expected during labor?
   A. Increase in both systolic and diastolic blood pressure during uterine contractions in the first stage of labor.
   B. Decrease in white blood cell count
   C. Slight increase in temperature, pulse, and respiration findings
   D. Increase in gastric motility leading to vomiting especially during the latent and active phases of the first stage of labor.

50. Duration of labor varies from woman to woman and is often influenced by a woman's obstetric history including parity. An expected duration for a nulliparous woman's stages of labor would be:
   A. First stage of labor: up to 20 hours for full dilatation to be achieved
   B. Second stage of labor: average of 20 minutes or less
   C. Third stage of labor: 45 to 60 minutes
   D. Fourth stage of labor: 6 to 8 hours

51. When instructing a group of primigravid women about the onset of labor, the nurse would tell them to be alert for:
   A. Urinary retention
   B. Weight gain of 2 kg
   C. Quickening
   D. Energy surge

CRITICAL THINKING EXERCISES

1. As part of their care of the laboring woman, nurses perform vaginal examinations and interpret the results. *STATE* the meaning of each of the following vaginal examination findings.

Exam I	Exam II	Exam III	Exam IV
ROP	RMA	LST	OA
−1	0	+1	+3
50%	25%	75%	100%
3 cm	2 cm	6 cm	10 cm

2. Brooke is a primigravida at 36 weeks' gestation. During a prenatal visit at 34 weeks' gestation, she asks you the following questions regarding her approaching labor. *DESCRIBE* how you would respond.
   A. "What gets labor to start?"

B. "Are there things I should watch for that would tell me my labor is getting closer to starting?"

C. "How long can I expect my labor to last once it gets started?"

D. "My friend just had a baby and she told me the nurses kept helping her to change her position and even encouraged her to walk! Isn't that dangerous for the baby and painful for the mom?"

ONLINE LEARNING ACTIVITIES

Access the Lowdermilk, Perry **Evolve** website at **http://evolve.elsevier.com/Lowdermilk/MatWmnHlth/** and enter the **Student** portion through the **Learning Resources** section. Use Chapter 18 as a starting point to search the Internet for websites designed to inform expectant parents about what to expect during each stage of labor and the effects their actions during labor can have on the process of labor including its duration. Prepare a report that includes:

- List of at least three sites
- Description of one site in terms of:
  - Sponsoring person(s), agency, organization
  - Clarity, accuracy, accessibility (ease of use), value, and depth of information provided
  - Currency—frequency of site updates
  - Variety of links to other relevant sites
  - Ability of persons visiting the site to obtain additional information through such services as e-mail and chat rooms
- Discussion about how a childbirth educator could use this information to enhance the prepared childbirth classes he or she conducts
- Handout that could be given to parents during a childbirth preparation class; the handout should include a brief description of each site and guidelines to use them effectively

CHAPTER 19

Management of Discomfort

CHAPTER REVIEW ACTIVITIES

MATCHING: Match the description in Column I with the appropriate pharmacologic method for discomfort management during childbirth in Column II.

COLUMN I

_____ 1. Abolition of pain perception by interrupting nerve impulses going to the brain. Loss of sensation (partial or complete) and sometimes loss of consciousness occurs.

_____ 2. Method used to repair a tear in the dura mater around the spinal cord as a result of spinal anesthesia; the goal is to treat postdural puncture headache (PDPH).

_____ 3. Single-injection, subarachnoid anesthesia useful for pain control during birth but not for labor.

_____ 4. Systemic analgesic that provides analgesia without causing maternal or neonatal respiratory depression.

_____ 5. Provides rapid perineal anesthesia for performing and repairing an episiotomy.

_____ 6. Injection of a dilute local anesthetic solution into the cervical mucosa to relieve pain from uterine contractions and cervical dilation. It has been associated with fetal bradycardia.

_____ 7. Medication such as a barbiturate that can be used in absence of pain to relieve anxiety and induce sleep in prodromal or early latent labor.

_____ 8. Co-drug used to potentiate the effect of an opioid agonist analgesic.

_____ 9. Drug that reverses the effects of opioid agonist analgesics including neonatal narcosis (CNS depression of the newborn).

_____ 10. Medication such as an opioid agonist analgesic that is usually administered intravenously for pain relief during labor.

COLUMN II

A. Opioid agonist-antagonist analgesic

B. Anesthesia

C. Analgesia

D. Ataractic

E. Epidural anesthesia/analgesia

F. Epidural blood patch

G. Local perineal infiltration anesthesia

H. Spinal anesthesia (block)

I. Opioid antagonist

J. Paracervical nerve block

K. Pudendal nerve block

L. Systemic analgesic

M. Sedative

_____ 11. Alleviation of pain sensation or raising of the pain threshold without loss of consciousness.

_____ 12. Relief from pain of uterine contractions and birth by injecting a local anesthetic and/or an opioid agonist analgesic into the peridural space.

_____ 13. Anesthetic that relieves pain in the lower vagina, vulva, and perineum, making it useful for episiotomy and forceps or vacuum-assisted birth.

FILL IN THE BLANKS: Insert the term that corresponds to each of the following descriptions.

14. _____ pain predominates during the first stage of labor. This type of pain results from _____ changes, distention of the _____, and uterine _____. It is located over the _____ of the abdomen.

15. _____ pain predominates during the second stage of labor. This type of pain results from stretching and distention of _____ and the _____ to allow passage of the fetus, from distention and traction on the _____-and _____ during contractions, and from _____.

16. _____ pain is felt in areas of the body other than the area of pain origin. During labor and birth, pain originating in the _____ radiates to the _____, _____, _____, _____, and down the _____.

17. The _____ theory of pain is based on the principle that certain nerve cell groupings within the spinal cord, brain stem, and cerebral cortex have the ability to modulate the pain impulse through a blocking mechanism. According to this theory, pain sensations travel along sensory nerve pathways to the brain, but only a limited number of sensations or messages can travel through these nerve pathways at one time. Pain relief techniques based on this theory include _____ or _____, _____, _____, and _____. _____ work involving concentration on _____ and _____ techniques are also based on this theory of pain.

18. _____ are endogenous opioids secreted by the pituitary gland that act on the central and peripheral nervous systems to reduce pain. It is thought that these opioid substances increase during pregnancy and birth in humans and may augment the ability of the woman in labor to tolerate acute pain.

19. Breathing techniques should be initiated when the laboring woman can no longer _____ or _____ through a contraction. _____ breathing is breathing at approximately _____ the woman's normal breathing rate. It is usually the first technique that is used in early labor.

20. As labor advances _____ breathing is used with techniques becoming _____ and increasing to about _____ the normal breathing rate.

21. A _____ should begin each breathing pattern and end each contraction exhaling to blow the contraction away.

22. A _____ breathing technique combining breaths and puffs in a ratio of 4:1, 6:1, or 8:1 is used to enhance concentration during the _____ phase of the first stage of labor. An undesirable effect of this type of breathing is _____ or rapid deep respirations, which can result in _____ as exhibited by the symptoms of _____, _____, _____, and _____. It can be eliminated by having the woman _____. This enables the woman to rebreathe _____ and replace the _____. Maintaining the breathing rate at no more than _____ the normal rate will decrease the occurrence of this breathing-related problem.

23. _____ or light stroking of the abdomen or other body part in rhythm with breathing during contractions and _____ or steady pressure against the sacrum using the _____ or _____ of the hand especially during back labor are two examples of nonpharmacologic methods to relieve discomfort that are based on the _____ theory of pain.

24. _____ (e.g., bathing, showering, whirlpool baths) uses the buoyancy of the warm water to provide support for tense muscles, relief from discomfort, and general body relaxation. It should not be initiated until the laboring woman is in the _____ phase of the first stage of labor.

25. _____ uses two pairs of electrodes placed on either side of the woman's _____ and _____ spine to provide continuous mild electrical currents that can be increased during a contraction. It may be effective because of a _____ effect that can stimulate the release of _____ in the woman's body and thereby alleviate discomfort.

26. _____ is a technique based on the application of pressure, heat, or cold on specific body points called tsubos.

27. _____ is a technique based on the premise that a person can learn to recognize her body's physical signals and use mental processes to control body responses and functions.

28. _____ uses essential oils from plants, flowers, herbs, and trees to promote health and well-being, enhance relaxation, and treat illness.

29. _____ is the injection of small amounts of sterile water using a fine needle into four locations on the lower back to relieve pain. Effectiveness of this method may be related to the mechanisms of _____, _____, or a rise in the level of _____.

30. *DESCRIBE* the factors that could influence the following nursing diagnosis identified for a woman in labor: Acute pain related to the processes involved in labor and birth.

31. *EXPLAIN* the theoretical basis for using such techniques as massage, stroking, music, and imagery in order to reduce the sensation of pain during childbirth.

32. *COMPLETE THE FOLLOWING TABLE* by listing the effects, criteria/timing for use, and nursing management for each of the following analgesic/anesthetic methods.

Anesthetic	Effects	Criteria/Timing	Management
Local perineal infiltration			
Pudendal nerve block			
Spinal anesthesia (block)			
Epidural anesthesia-analgesia (block)			
Nitrous oxide for analgesia			
General anesthesia			

33. Systemic analgesics cross the placenta and effect the fetus/newborn.
    A. *LIST* three factors that influence the effect systemic analgesics have on the fetus/newborn:

B. *IDENTIFY* the fetal/newborn effects of systemic analgesics.

34. *COMPLETE THE FOLLOWING TABLE* by giving one example for each of the following medication classifications and stating how each medication is administered and why it is used during the childbirth process.

Medication	Method of Administration	Purpose for Administration
Opioid agonist analgesic		
Opioid agonist-antagonist analgesic		
Ataractic		
Opioid antagonist		

35. *EXPLAIN* why the intravenous route is preferred to the intramuscular route for the administration of systemic analgesics during labor.

TRUE OR FALSE: Circle "T" if true or "F" if false for each of the following statements. Correct the false statements.

T   F   36. Somatic pain occurs as a result of perineal stretching and pressure exerted by the presenting part on the pelvic organs and structures.

T   F   37. Pain threshold is highly variable among individuals.

T   F   38. Pain perception is often affected by a person's gender and ethnicity.

T F 39. A woman's perception of her birth experience as "good" or "bad" is influenced by the degree to which she believes she met her personal goals related to coping effectively with pain.

T F 40. Water therapy can be used even if the laboring woman's membranes are ruptured.

T F 41. There is no limit on the time a laboring woman can spend in a whirlpool bath.

T F 42. Effectiveness of acupressure is based on the gate control theory of pain coupled with an increase in endorphin levels.

T F 43. Hyperventilation in labor can result in respiratory acidosis as the amount of carbon dioxide increases in the bloodstream.

T F 44. Sedatives given without an analgesic when a laboring woman is experiencing pain can increase apprehension and lead to hyperactivity and disorientation.

T F 45. Intramuscular administration of medications during labor offers more predictable onset of pain relief.

T F 46. Naloxone (Narcan) should be used cautiously if a woman is opioid dependent because it may precipitate abstinence syndrome in both mother and newborn.

T F 47. Before an epidural block is initiated, a woman should be adequately hydrated using an IV of 5% glucose in water.

T F 48. An epidural block is useful as a pain relief measure for both labor and birth.

T F 49. Keeping the woman in a flat position for at least 8 hours after birth is the most effective way to prevent headaches following a spinal block.

T F 50. Research findings indicate that women whose pain is managed with systemic analgesics are more satisfied with their pain management than those women who received epidural analgesia.

T F 51. Maternal hypotension is a major adverse reaction to both spinal and epidural blocks.

MULTIPLE CHOICE: Circle the one correct option and state the rationale for the option chosen.

52. In her birth plan, a woman requests that she be allowed to use the new whirlpool bath during labor. When implementing this woman's request the nurse would:
    A. Assist the woman to maintain a reclining position when in the tub
    B. Tell the woman she will need to leave the tub as soon as her membranes rupture
    C. Limit her to no longer than 1 hour in the tub
    D. Cool the water or have the woman step out of the tub if the fetal heart rate or maternal temperature increases

53. The use of ataractics can potentiate the action of analgesics. An ataractic the nurse could expect to give to a laboring woman would be:
    A. naloxone (Narcan)
    B. hydroxyzine (Vistaril)
    C. butorphanol tartrate (Stadol)
    D. fentanyl (Sublimaze)

54. The doctor has ordered meperidine (Demerol) 25 mg IV q 2–3 h prn for pain associated with labor. In fulfilling this order the nurse should know that:
    A. The onset of this analgesic's effect after IV administration would be approximately 10 minutes
    B. The dosage of the analgesic is too high for IV administration, necessitating a new order
    C. Respiratory depression of the woman or fetus is not a concern with this analgesic
    D. The newborn should be observed for respiratory depression if birth occurs within 4 hours of the dose

55. Following administration of fentanyl (Sublimaze) IV for labor pain, a woman's labor progresses more rapidly than expected. The physician orders that a stat dose of naloxone (Narcan) 0.1 mg be administered intravenously to the woman to reverse respiratory depression in the newborn after its birth. In fulfilling this order the nurse would:
    A. Question the route since this medication should be administered orally
    B. Recognize that the dose is too low
    C. Assess the woman's level of pain since it will return abruptly
    D. Observe maternal pulse for bradycardia

56. An anesthesiologist is preparing to begin a continuous epidural block using a combination local anesthetic and opioid agonist analgesic as a pain relief measure for a laboring woman. Nursing measures related to this type of nerve block would be:
    A. Assist the woman into a modified Sims position or upright position with back curved
    B. Keep the woman in a semirecumbent position after administration to ensure equal distribution of the pharmacologic agents
    C. Assess the woman for headaches especially after birth
    D. Assist the woman to urinate every 4 hours to prevent bladder distention

CRITICAL THINKING EXERCISES

1. A nurse working with a group of expectant fathers is asked if there really is "a physical reason for all the pain women say they feel when they are in labor." DESCRIBE the response that this nurse should give.

2. Nurses working on childbirth units must be sensitive to their clients' pain experiences.
    A. IDENTIFY physiologic effects, sensory and emotional responses, and affective expressions of pain that nurses could expect to observe when a client experiences pain.

B. *DESCRIBE* specific measures nurses could use to alter the laboring woman's perception of pain.

3. On admission to the labor unit in the latent phase of labor, Mr. and Mrs. Timins (2–0–0–1–0) tell you that they are so glad they took Lamaze classes and did so much reading about childbirth. "We will not need any medication now that we know what to do. But most importantly our baby will be safe!" *DESCRIBE* how you would respond if you were their primary nurse for childbirth.

4. *IMAGINE* you are the nurse manager of a labor and birth unit. Major renovations are being planned for your unit and your input is required. You and your staff nurses believe that water therapy including the use of showers and whirlpool baths is a beneficial nonpharmacologic method to relieve pain and discomfort and to enhance the progress of labor. *DISCUSS* the rationale you would use to convince planners that installation of a shower and a whirlpool bath into each birthing room is cost effective.

5. Tara has been in labor for 4 hours. Her blood pressure had been stable, averaging 130/80 when assessed between contractions and the FHR pattern consistently exhibited criteria of a reassuring pattern. A lumbar epidural block was initiated. Shortly afterwards during assessment of maternal vital signs and FHR, Tara's blood pressure decreased to 102/60 and the FHR pattern began to exhibit a decrease in rate and variability.
   A. *STATE* what Tara is experiencing. *SUPPORT* your answer and *EXPLAIN* the physiologic basis for what is happening to Tara.

   B. *WRITE* a nursing diagnosis that reflects this occurrence.

   C. *LIST* the immediate nursing actions.

6. Moira, a primigravida, has elected a continuous epidural block as her pharmacologic method of choice during childbirth.

   A. *IDENTIFY* the assessment procedures that should be used to determine Moira's readiness for the initiation of the epidural block.

   B. *DESCRIBE* the preparation methods that should be implemented.

   C. *DESCRIBE* two positions you could help Moira assume for the induction of the epidural block.

   D. *OUTLINE* the nursing care management interventions recommended while Moira is receiving the epidural block to ensure her well-being and that of her fetus.

ONLINE LEARNING ACTIVITIES

Access the Lowdermilk, Perry **Evolve** website at **http://evolve.elsevier.com/Lowdermilk/MatWmnHlth/** and enter the **Student** portion through the **Learning Resources** section to assist you in searching the medical literature for nursing research studies related to the effectiveness of nonpharmacologic pain relief measures.
- Create an annotated bibliography of at least five nursing research studies
- Choose one research study and complete a bibliography card that includes the following:
  - Hypothesis; research question
  - Summary of the methodology used and key findings
  - Reliability of the study and its findings
  - Recommendations for further research
- Discuss how you would use the findings from these research studies to provide pain relief measures to laboring women that are evidence based

CHAPTER 20

Fetal Assessment During Labor

CHAPTER REVIEW ACTIVITIES

MATCHING: Match the definition in Column I with the appropriate term related to FHR pattern from Column II.

COLUMN I

_____ 1. Average FHR range of 110–160 BPM at term as assessed during a 10-minute segment.

_____ 2. Absence of the expected irregular fluctuations in the baseline FHR.

_____ 3. Persistent (10 minutes or longer) baseline FHR below 110 BPM.

_____ 4. Visually apparent decrease in the FHR of 15 BPM or more below the baseline that lasts more than 2 minutes but less than 10 minutes.

_____ 5. Changes in FHR from the baseline that occur with uterine contractions.

_____ 6. Persistent (10 minutes or longer) baseline FHR above 160 BPM.

_____ 7. Expected irregular fluctuations of the baseline FHR of 2 or more cycles per minute as a result of the interaction of the sympathetic and parasympathetic nervous system.

_____ 8. FHR decrease starting before the peak of a contraction in response to fetal head compression.

_____ 9. FHR decrease after the peak of the contraction in response to uteroplacental insufficiency

_____ 10. FHR decrease any time during a contraction in response to umbilical cord compression.

_____ 11. Visually apparent abrupt increase in the FHR of 15 BPM or more above the baseline that lasts 15 seconds or more with return to baseline less than 2 minutes after onset.

_____ 12. Changes in FHR from the baseline that are not associated with uterine contraction.

COLUMN II

A. Acceleration
B. Early deceleration
C. Variability
D. Late deceleration
E. Variable deceleration
F. Tachycardia
G. Prolonged deceleration
H. Bradycardia
I. Baseline FHR
J. Undetected variability
K. Periodic changes
L. Episodic (nonperiodic) changes

FILL IN THE BLANKS: Insert the term that corresponds to each of the following descriptions related to fetal assessment.

13. The goals of intrapartum FHR monitoring are to identify and differentiate the _____ patterns from the _____ patterns that can be indicative of fetal _____. _____ is a deficiency of oxygen in the arterial blood, whereas _____ is an inadequate supply of oxygen at the cellular level.

14. One method to assess fetal status is intermittent _____ using a _____ or an _____ to listen to the FHR.

15. _____ is the method used for ongoing assessment of fetal oxygenation by analyzing fetal heart rate tracings for characteristic patterns signifying hypoxic and nonhypoxic events. Two modes can be used to accomplish this method of assessment. External monitoring uses an _____ to assess the FHR pattern and a _____ to monitor the frequency and duration of contractions. Internal monitoring uses a _____ applied to the fetal presenting part to assess the FHR pattern and an _____ to monitor the frequency, duration, and intensity of contractions.

16. _____ is an abnormally small amount or absence of amniotic fluid. It can lead to compression of the umbilical cord resulting in a _____ FHR pattern. _____ can be used to instill _____ or _____ solution into the uterine cavity via the intrauterine pressure catheter for the purpose of adding fluid around the umbilical cord and thus preventing its compression during uterine contractions.

17. _____ therapy can be used when fetal compromise is associated with increased uterine activity. _____ improves _____ through the _____ by inhibiting _____.

18. It is critical that a nurse working on a labor unit be knowledgeable concerning factors associated with a reduction in fetal oxygen supply, characteristics of a reassuring FHR pattern, and characteristics of normal uterine activity. *LIST* the required information for each of the following:

A. **Factors associated with a reduction in fetal oxygen supply**

B. **Characteristics of a reassuring FHR pattern**

C. **Characteristics of normal uterine activity**

19. *IDENTIFY* the characteristics of nonreassuring FHR patterns.

FILL IN THE BLANKS: In general, the recommended frequency of FHR assessment depends on the risk status of the mother and the stage of labor. Insert the appropriate time for each of the following assessment recommendations:

20. Obtain a _____ -minute strip by electronic fetal monitoring (EFM) on all women admitted to the labor unit.
21. Low risk client (risk factors are absent during labor): Auscultate FHR/assess tracing every _____ in the active phase of the first stage of labor and every _____ in the second stage of labor.
22. High risk client (risk factors are present during labor): Auscultate FHR/assess tracing every _____ in the active phase of the first stage of labor and every _____ in the second stage of labor.

23. Nurses caring for laboring women may need to use intermittent auscultation to assess fetal health and well-being during labor.
    A. *STATE* the advantages and disadvantages of intermittent auscultation as a method of fetal assessment during childbirth.

    B. *OUTLINE* the guidelines that should be followed when monitoring the fetus using the intermittent auscultation method.

24. *STATE* the legal responsibilities related to fetal monitoring for nurses who care for women during childbirth.

TRUE OR FALSE: Circle "T" if true or "F" if false for each of the following statements. Correct the false statements.

T   F   25. A nonreassuring FHR pattern indicates that the fetus is compromised and is experiencing some degree of hypoxemia, hypoxia, or both.
T   F   26. Auscultation should be performed during a uterine contraction and for at least 10 seconds after the end of the contraction to detect periodic changes in pattern.
T   F   27. FHR variability can temporarily decrease when the fetus is in a sleep state.

T F 28. When external monitoring is used the tocotransducer should be repositioned every 4 hours and reddened skin areas gently massaged.

T F 29. Maternal supine hypotensive syndrome reduces blood flow to the placenta resulting in fetal hypoxia as reflected in fetal bradycardia, decreased variability, and late deceleration patterns.

T F 30. Acceleration of the FHR associated with fetal movement is a reassuring sign.

T F 31. Decelerations of the FHR may be benign or nonreassuring in terms of fetal well-being.

T F 32. Late deceleration patterns are characterized by a **U** or **V** shape with acceleration shoulders before and after the deceleration.

T F 33. Early decelerations are nonreassuring patterns that typically occur when blood flow through the placenta is diminished.

T F 34. The average intrauterine (intraamniotic) pressure range during a uterine contraction is 50 to 85 mm Hg.

T F 35. The tocotransducer should be placed on the abdomen over the area of maximum intensity and clarity of fetal heart sounds.

T F 36. The intrauterine pressure catheter (IUPC) is able to assess uterine contraction frequency, duration, and intensity.

T F 37. Ritgen maneuver is used to determine the correct placement of the ultrasound transducer.

T F 38. Late deceleration patterns of any magnitude are considered to be nonreassuring FHR patterns.

T F 39. Periodic acceleration patterns are associated with breech presentations.

40. A nurse caring for a laboring woman in active labor notes a nonreassuring FHR pattern when evaluating the monitor tracing. *DESCRIBE* the action the nurse should take based on this finding.

41. *OUTLINE* the nursing interventions that should be implemented when caring for a woman who is being monitored using an external monitor.

MULTIPLE CHOICE: Circle the one correct option and state the rationale for the option chosen.

42. A laboring woman's uterine contractions are being internally monitored. When evaluating the monitor tracing, which of the following findings would be a source of concern and require further assessment?
   A. Frequency every 2½ to 3 minutes
   B. Duration of 80 to 85 seconds
   C. Intensity during a uterine contraction of 85 to 90 mm Hg
   D. Average resting pressure of 20 to 25 mm Hg

43. External electronic fetal monitoring will be used for a woman just admitted to the labor unit in active labor. A guideline the nurse should follow when implementing this form of monitoring would be:
    A. Use Leopold maneuvers to determine correct placement of the tocotransducer
    B. Apply contact gel to the ultrasound transducer prior to application over the point of maximum intensity
    C. Reposition the ultrasound transducer every hour and massage the site
    D. Apply a spiral electrode if nonreassuring FHR signs are noted

44. The nurse caring for women in labor should be aware of signs characterizing reassuring FHR patterns. A reassuring sign would be:
    A. Moderate baseline variability
    B. Average baseline FHR of 90 to 110 BPM
    C. Transient episodic deceleration with movement
    D. Late deceleration patterns approximately every three or four contractions

45. A laboring woman's temperature is elevated as a result of an upper respiratory infection. The FHR pattern that reflects maternal fever would be:
    A. Diminished variability
    B. Variable decelerations
    C. Tachycardia
    D. Early decelerations

46. A nulliparous woman is in the active phase of labor and her cervix has progressed to 6 cm dilatation. The nurse caring for this woman evaluates the external monitor tracing and notes the following: decrease in FHR shortly after onset of several uterine contractions returning to baseline rate by the end of the contraction; shape is uniform. Based on these findings the nurse should:
    A. Change the woman's position to her left side
    B. Document the finding on the woman's chart
    C. Notify the physician
    D. Perform a vaginal examination to check for cord prolapse

CRITICAL THINKING EXERCISES

1. Darlene, a primigravida in active labor, has just been admitted to the labor unit. She becomes very anxious when external electronic monitoring equipment is set up. She tells the nurse that her father had a heart attack 2 months ago. "He was so sick they had to put him on a monitor too. Does this mean that my baby has a heart problem just like my father?" DESCRIBE the nurse's expected response.

2. Terry is a primigravida at 43 weeks' gestation. Her labor is being stimulated with oxytocin administered IV. Her contractions have been increasing in intensity with a frequency of every 2 to 2½ minutes and a duration of 80 to 85 seconds. She is currently in a supine position with a 30-degree elevation of her head. On observation of the monitor tracing, you note that during the last two contractions the FHR decreased after the contraction peaked and did not return to baseline until about 10 seconds into the rest period. A slight decrease in variability and baseline rate was observed.

   A. *IDENTIFY* the pattern described and the possible factors responsible for it.

   B. *DESCRIBE* the actions you would take. *STATE* the rationale for each action.

3. *ANALYZE* each of the following monitor tracings and *DOCUMENT* your findings. *DESCRIBE* each FHR pattern depicted and the criteria used to determine if the pattern is reassuring or nonreassuring. *INDICATE* the possible causes, significance, and nursing actions required for each nonreassuring FHR pattern identified.

   A.
   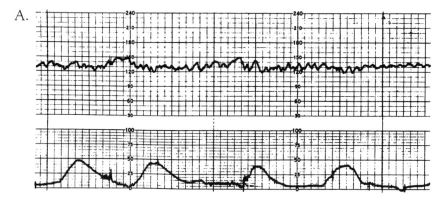

   B.
   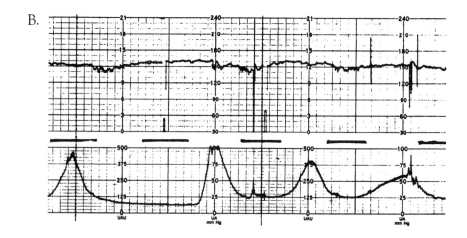

C.

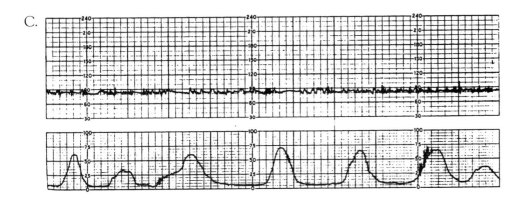

D.

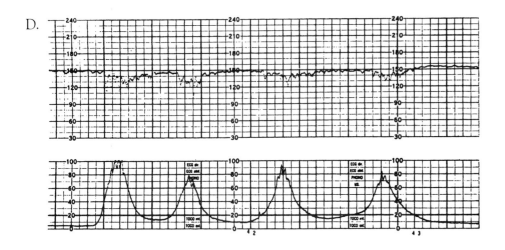

E.

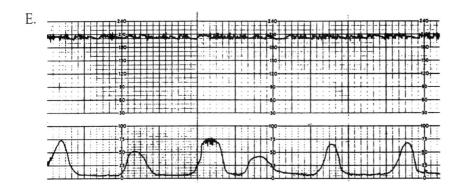

F.

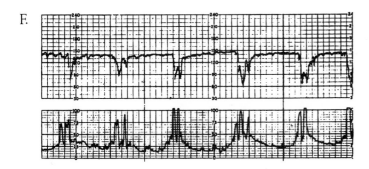

ONLINE LEARNING ACTIVITIES

Access the Lowdermilk, Perry **Evolve** website at
http://evolve.elsevier.com/Lowdermilk/MatWmnHlth/ and enter the **Student** portion through the
Learning Resources section to assist you in searching the medical literature for journal articles
related to assessment methods used to determine fetal responses to labor and effective measures to
prevent or treat nonreassuring FHR patterns.

- Create an annotated bibliography of at least five journal articles
- Choose one journal article and complete a bibliography card that includes the following:
  - Summary of the article's key points
  - Personal reaction to the ideas presented in the article
  - How the professional nurse can use the article's ideas to more effectively assess and care for the
    fetus's well being during labor

CHAPTER 21

Nursing Care During Labor

CHAPTER REVIEW ACTIVITIES

MATCHING: Match the description in Column I with the appropriate term from Column II.

COLUMN I

_____ 1. Prolonged breath holding while bearing down (closed glottis pushing)

_____ 2. Burning sensation of acute pain as vagina stretches and crowning occurs.

_____ 3. Artificial rupture of membranes (AROM, ARM).

_____ 4. Occurs when widest part of the head (biparietal diameter) distends the vulva just prior to birth.

_____ 5. Incision into perineum to enlarge the vaginal outlet.

_____ 6. Test to determine if membranes have ruptured by assessing pH of the fluid.

_____ 7. Technique used to control birth of fetal head and protect perineal musculature.

_____ 8. Expulsion of placenta with fetal side emerging first.

_____ 9. Cord encircles the fetal neck.

_____ 10. Method used to palpate fetus through abdomen.

_____ 11. Occurs when pressure of presenting part against pelvic floor stretch receptors results in a woman's perception of an urge to bear down.

_____ 12. Classification of medication that stimulates the uterus to contract.

_____ 13. Expulsion of placenta with maternal surface emerging first.

_____ 14. Protrusion of umbilical cord in advance of the presenting part.

COLUMN II

A. Ritgen maneuver
B. Episiotomy
C. Oxytocic
D. Ferguson reflex
E. Schultze mechanism
F. Valsalva maneuver
G. Ring of fire
H. Crowning
I. Duncan mechanism
J. Amniotomy
K. Nuchal cord
L. Prolapse of umbilical cord
M. Nitrazine test
N. Leopold maneuvers

EVALUATE each of the following assessment findings that are used to distinguish true labor from false labor. DESIGNATE whether the assessment finding is associated with TRUE LABOR (TL) or with FALSE LABOR (FL).

_____ 15. Contractions regular and progressive
_____ 16. Cervix soft and posterior
_____ 17. Contractions cease with ambulation
_____ 18. Cervix soft, 25%, 2 cm, mid position
_____ 19. Lightening occurs in multiparous woman
_____ 20. Discomfort present in abdomen above umbilicus
_____ 21. Contraction intensity increases with activity and ambulation
_____ 22. Presenting part is above ischial spines
_____ 23. Bloody show
_____ 24. Discomfort radiates from lower back to lower abdomen
_____ 25. Contractions continue even after a shower or back rub

FILL IN THE BLANKS: Insert the term that corresponds to each of the following descriptions related to the stages of labor.

26. The first stage of labor begins with the onset of _____ and ends with full _____ and _____ of the cervix. A blood-tinged mucous discharge (bloody show) usually indicates the passage of the _____.

27. During the latent phase of the first stage of labor, the cervix dilates from _____ to _____ cm in approximately _____ to _____ hours. Cervical dilation progresses from _____ to _____ cm in about _____ to _____ hours during the active phase of the first stage of labor. The duration of the transition phase is approximately _____ to _____ minutes and the cervix dilates from _____ to _____ cm.

28. The second stage of labor is the stage when the _____. It begins with full _____ and complete _____. It ends with the _____. Additional signs that the second stage of labor is beginning include _____, _____, _____, _____, _____, and _____. This stage consists of three phases: _____, _____, and _____. The duration of the second stage of labor is influenced by effectiveness of the _____, type and amount of _____ used, _____ condition, maternal _____ and _____ level, _____, _____ adequacy, _____ of the fetus, and the nature and source of _____ the woman receives.

29. The third stage of labor lasts from the time the _____ until the _____. Detachment of the placenta from the wall of the uterus or _____ is indicated by a _____, change from a _____ shape to a _____ shape, a sudden _____ from the introitus, apparent _____, and the finding of _____.

FILL IN THE BLANKS: Insert the term that corresponds to each of the following descriptions related to the characteristics of the powers of labor.

30. _____ The primary powers of labor that act involuntarily to expel the fetus and the placenta from the uterus.

31. _____ "Building up" phase of a contraction.
32. _____ The peak of a contraction.
33. _____ "Letting down" phase of a contraction.
34. _____ How often the contractions occur; the period of time from the beginning of one contraction to the beginning of the next or from the peak of one contraction to the peak of the next.
35. _____ The strength of the contraction at its peak.
36. _____ The period of time that elapses between the onset and end of a contraction.
37. _____ The tension of the uterine muscle between contractions.
38. _____ Period of rest between contractions.
39. _____ An involuntary urge to push in response to the Ferguson reflex.

40. Assessment of the characteristics and patterns of uterine contractions is an important nursing responsibility.

    A. *LABEL* the following illustration that depicts the characteristics of uterine contractions.

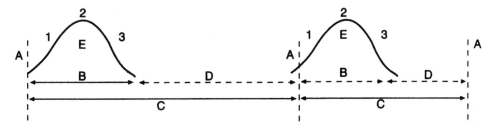

    B. *DESCRIBE* how you would assess each of these characteristics using the palpation method.

41. Laura (3–1–1–0–1) has just been admitted in the latent phase of the first stage of labor. As part of the admission procedure you review her prenatal record, and interview her regarding what she has observed regarding her labor and discuss her current health status.

    A. *LIST* the essential data you would need to obtain from her prenatal record in order to plan care that is appropriate for Laura.

    B. *IDENTIFY* the information required regarding the status of Laura's labor.

C. *STATE* the information required regarding Laura's current health status.

TRUE OR FALSE: Circle "T" if true or "F" if false for each of the following statements. Correct the false statements.

T   F   42. Amniotic fluid will turn Nitrazine test paper greenish-yellow.

T   F   43. A partogram is used to diagram the progress of uterine contractions.

T   F   44. A laboring woman should be encouraged to void at least every 2 hours during labor.

T   F   45. Ambulation should be encouraged only during the latent phase of the first stage of labor.

T   F   46. A hands and knees position is recommended during contractions to facilitate the internal rotation of an occiput posterior position to a more anterior position.

T   F   47. The nurse should perform a vaginal examination immediately, using strict sterile technique, if bright red, fresh vaginal bleeding is noted during active labor.

T   F   48. Amniotic fluid is alkaline as compared to urine which is usually acidic.

T   F   49. Leopold maneuvers can assist in the location of the point of maximum intensity (PMI) of the fetal heart beat.

T   F   50. Maternal body temperature should be monitored every 1 to 2 hours after the amniotic membranes rupture.

T   F   51. Increased sensitivity to touch or hyperesthesia, which develops as labor progress, can result in a woman's rejection of her partner's or the nurse's touch with comfort measures.

T   F   52. A woman should begin pushing as soon as the second stage of labor begins.

T   F   53. In order for childbirth to progress safely and in a timely fashion, a woman's bearing down efforts must be carefully regulated by the nurse and coach.

T   F   54. For pushing to be effective, the woman should maintain a push and hold her breath for at least 10 seconds.

T   F   55. The only certain objective sign of the onset of the second stage of labor is the woman's perception of an urge to bear down.

T   F   56. During the descent phase of the second stage of labor, pressure of the presenting part on the pelvic floor stimulates release of oxytocin from the pituitary gland thus intensifying uterine contractions.

T   F   57. During birth of the head, the woman must continue to fully bear down with uterine contractions to ensure prompt expulsion.

T   F   58. If stirrups are used during birth, it is important to place the legs into the stirrups one leg at a time.

T   F   59. The time of birth is recorded as the precise time when the newborn takes its first breath.

T   F   60. The priority goal for a newborn in the immediate post birth period is that the newborn's airway remains patent.

61. *COMPLETE THE FOLLOWING TABLE* by identifying the stressors that a woman and her partner/coach experience during childbirth and the nursing measures that can be supportive and reduce stress.

Woman and Partner/Coach	Stressors	Support Measures
Laboring woman		
Partner/coach		

62. A nurse caring for a laboring woman needs to be alert for signs of potential complications. *LIST* these signs.

63. *COMPLETE THE FOLLOWING TABLE* by identifying two advantages for each of the following labor positions.

Labor Position	Advantages
Semi-recumbent	
Upright	
Lateral	
Hands and knees	

64. *OUTLINE* the critical factors to be included in the physical assessment of the maternal-fetal unit during labor.

65. *INDICATE* the laboratory and diagnostic tests that are recommended during labor. *STATE* the purpose for each.

66. *COMPLETE THE FOLLOWING TABLE* by identifying two support measures you would use during each phase of the second stage of labor. Validate your response with events and behaviors typical of that phase.

Phase	Events/Behaviors	Support Measures
Latent		
Descent		
Transition		

67. *DESCRIBE* the maternal positions recommended to enhance the effectiveness of a woman's bearing down efforts during the second stage of labor. *STATE* the basis for each position's effectiveness in facilitating the descent and birth of the fetus.

MULTIPLE CHOICE: Circle the one correct option and state the rationale for the option chosen.

68. A primigravida calls the hospital and tells a nurse on the labor unit that she knows that she is in labor. The nurse's initial response would be:
    A. "Tell me why you know that you are in labor."
    B. "How far do you live from the hospital?"
    C. "How far along are you in your pregnancy?"
    D. "Have your membranes ruptured?"

69. A woman's amniotic membranes have apparently ruptured. The nurse assesses the fluid to determine its characteristics and confirm membrane rupture. An expected assessment finding would be:
    A. pH 5.5
    B. Absence of ferning
    C. Pale straw colored fluid with white flecks
    D. Strong odor

70. A vaginal examination is performed on a multiparous woman who is in labor. The results of the examination were documented as: 4 cm, 75%, +2, LOT. An accurate interpretation of this data would be:
    A. Woman is in the latent phase of the first stage of labor
    B. Station is 2 cm above the ischial spines
    C. Presentation is vertex
    D. Lie is transverse

71. A nulliparous woman is in active labor. She is considered to be at low risk for complications. Which of the following is a standard recommendation for assessment during this phase of labor?
    A. Maternal blood pressure, pulse, respirations—every hour
    B. FHR—every 15 to 30 minutes
    C. Temperature—twice per shift once membranes rupture
    D. Vaginal examination to determine progress of dilatation and effacement—every hour

72. A physical care measure for a laboring woman that has been identified as unlikely to be beneficial and may even be harmful would be:
    A. Allowing the laboring woman to drink fluids and eat light solids as tolerated
    B. Administering a Fleet enema at admission
    C. Ambulating periodically throughout labor as tolerated
    D. Using a whirlpool bath once active labor is established

CRITICAL THINKING EXERCISES

1. Alice, a primigravida, calls the labor unit. She tells the nurse that she thinks she is in labor. "I have had some pains for about 2 hours. Should my husband bring me to the hospital now?"
   A. *DESCRIBE* how the nurse should approach this situation.

   B. *WRITE* several questions the nurse could use to elicit the appropriate information required to determine the course of action required.

   C. Based on the data collected during the telephone interview, the nurse determines that Alice is in very early labor. Because she lives fairly close to the hospital she is instructed to stay home until her labor progresses. *OUTLINE* the instructions and recommendations for care Alice and her husband should be given.

2. *ANALYZE* the assessment findings documented for each of the following women.

   Denise
   > 5 cm
   > Moderate
   > q4min
   > 40-55 sec
   > 0

   Teresa
   > 9 cm
   > Very strong
   > q2-3min
   > 65-75 sec
   > +2

   Danielle
   > 2 cm
   > Mild
   > q6–8min
   > 30-35 sec
   > −1

A. *IDENTIFY* the phase of labor being experienced by each woman.

B. *DESCRIBE* the behavior and appearance you would expect to be exhibited by each woman.

C. *SPECIFY* the physical care and emotional support measures you would implement if you were caring for each of these women.

3. *DESCRIBE* the procedure that should be followed prior to auscultating the FHR or applying an ultrasound transducer to the abdomen of a laboring woman. *EXPLAIN* the rationale for using this procedure.

4. Tonya, a woman in active labor, begins to cry during a vaginal examination to assess her status. "Why not watch the monitor to see how I am progressing instead of doing these vaginal exams? They really hurt and they are embarrassing!!"

A. *DESCRIBE* the response the nurse should make to Tonya's concern.

B. *DISCUSS* the measures the nurse could use to meet Tonya's safety and comfort needs during a vaginal examination.

5. Tasha is 6 cm dilated. Her coach comes to tell you that her "water just broke with a gush!" *IDENTIFY* each action you would take in this situation, in order of priority. *STATE* the rationale for the actions you have identified.

6. Sara, a 17-year-old primigravida, is admitted in the latent phase of labor. Her boyfriend Dan is with her as her only support. They appear committed to each other. During the admission interview, Sara tells you that they did not go to any classes because she was embarrassed about not being married. Both Sara and Dan appear very nervous and assessment indicates they know little about what is happening, what to expect, and how to work together with the process of labor. *IDENTIFY* the nursing diagnosis reflected in this data. *STATE* one expected outcome and *LIST* nursing measures appropriate for the diagnosis you identified.

Nursing Diagnosis	Expected Outcome	Nursing Measures

7. Identifying a laboring couple's cultural and religious beliefs and practices regarding childbirth is a critical factor in providing culturally sensitive care that enhances the couple's sense of control and eventual satisfaction with their childbirth experience.
   A. *LIST* the questions you would ask when assessing a couple's cultural and religious preferences for childbirth.

   B. *DISCUSS* the problems that can occur if the nurse does not consider the couple's cultural and religious preferences when planning and implementing care.

8. Cori (4–3–0–0–3) is in latent labor. She and her husband are being oriented to the birthing room. Their last birth occurred in a delivery room 10 years ago. Both she and her husband are amazed by the birthing room and the birthing bed that will allow her to give birth in an upright position. They are also informed that changes in bearing down efforts now allow a woman to follow her own body feelings and even to vocalize with pushing. Both Cori and her husband state that with every other birth they put her legs in stirrups, she held her breath for as long as she could, and pushed quietly. "Everything turned out okay so why should we change?" DESCRIBE the response the primary nurse caring for this couple should make to their concerns.

9. A nurse living in a rural area is called to her neighbor's home to assist his wife who is in labor. "Everything is happening so fast. She says she is ready to deliver!!"

A. IDENTIFY the measures the nurse can use to reassure and comfort the woman.

B. Shortly after the nurse arrives crowning begins. STATE what the nurse should do.

C. DESCRIBE the action the nurse should take after the birth of the head.

D. LIST the measures the nurse should use to prevent excessive neonatal heat loss after its birth.

E. IDENTIFY the infection control measures that should be implemented during a home birth.

F. SPECIFY the measures the nurse should use to prevent excessive maternal blood loss or hemorrhage until the ambulance arrives.

G. *OUTLINE* the information the nurse should document regarding the childbirth.

10. Beth is in the descent phase of the second stage of labor. She is actively pushing/bearing down to facilitate birth. *INDICATE* the criteria a nurse would use to evaluate the correctness of Beth's technique.

11. Molly is entering the second stage of labor. She states that she is experiencing some perineal pressure but refuses to start pushing because as she states, "I am just not ready to push yet."

    A. *DISCUSS* the factors that might be inhibiting Molly's desire to bear down and give birth to her baby.

    B. *DESCRIBE* what the nurse could do to help Molly reach the point of readiness to give birth.

12. *IMAGINE* that you are participating in a panel discussion on childbirth practices. Your topic is "Episiotomy—is it needed to ensure the safety and well-being of the laboring woman and her fetus?" *OUTLINE* the information you would include in your presentation.

13. *IMAGINE* that you are a staff nurse on a childbirth unit. Your hospital is instituting a change in policy that would allow the participation of children in the labor and birth process of their mother. You are asked to be a part of the committee that will formulate the guidelines regarding sibling participation during childbirth. *DISCUSS* the suggestions you would make to help ensure a positive outcome for parents, children, and health care providers.

14. Annie is a primipara in the fourth stage of labor following a long and difficult labor and birth process. She seems disinterested in her baby. Annie looks him over quickly and then asks if you would take him back to the nursery.

A. *IDENTIFY* the factors that could be accounting for Annie's behavior.

B. *DISCUSS* the nursing measures you would use to encourage future maternal-newborn interactions and facilitate the attachment process.

ONLINE LEARNING ACTIVITIES

Access the website www.childbirth.org:
- Use the interactive section of the site to create your own birth plan. Identify some of the options you feel are critical to ensure that when the time comes you will have a childbirth that meets your expectations and goals
- Explain why creating a birth plan is a worthwhile activity for parents
- Develop guidelines for parents to follow as they create their own birth plan

CHAPTER 22

Postpartum Physiology

CHAPTER REVIEW ACTIVITIES

TRUE OR FALSE: Circle "T" if true or "F" if false for each of the following statements. Correct the false statements.

T F 1. Within 12 hours of birth the fundus of the uterus may be 1 cm above the umbilicus.

T F 2. The uterus is slightly smaller in size after every pregnancy.

T F 3. Regeneration of the entire endometrium, including the placental site, is completed approximately 4 weeks after birth.

T F 4. Subinvolution is the process of self-destruction of excess hypertrophied uterine tissue during the postpartum period.

T F 5. The external os of the cervix has a jagged, slit-like appearance in multiparous women.

T F 6. Until estrogen levels rise, the postpartum woman is likely to experience discomfort during intercourse (dyspareunia) associated with inadequate secretion of lubricating mucus.

T F 7. The appearance of colostrum is yellowish and thick compared with milk, which appears bluish-white and thin.

T F 8. For most nonlactating women (70%), menstruation resumes by 3 months after birth.

T F 9. During the first 24 hours after birth an elevated temperature of 38° C (100.4° F) is indicative of the onset of infection.

T F 10. It is to be expected that the hematocrit level will decrease by the seventh day postpartum.

T F 11. In the postpartum period a leukocytosis of 20,000/mm³ strongly suggests uterine or bladder infection.

T F 12. The process of autolysis results in a mild proteinuria of +1 for 1 to 2 days after birth.

T F 13. An elevated follicle-stimulating hormone (FHS) level in the postpartum period is responsible for the suppression of ovulation in lactating women.

T F 14. The presence of hematuria in the early postpartum period following vaginal birth is an expected finding.

T F 15. Lochia normally has a fleshy odor similar to menstrual flow.

T F 16. Women, who are diabetics, usually require more insulin for several days after they give birth.

T F 17. Most postpartum women will experience several anovulatory menstrual cycles before ovulation resumes.

T F 18. Saturation of a perineal pad in 1 hour or less with rubra lochia during the first 12 hours after birth would be considered an expected finding reflective of a moderate flow.

T F 19. Breastfeeding stimulates release of oxytocin, which enhances contraction and involution of the uterus.

T F 20. Postpartum women commonly experience faintness or dizziness upon rising from a supine position as a result of orthostatic hypotension.

21. When caring for a woman following vaginal birth, it is of critical importance for the nurse to assess the woman's bladder for distention.
    A. *EXPLAIN* why bladder distention is more likely to occur during the immediate postpartum period.

    B. *IDENTIFY* the problems that can occur if the bladder is allowed to become distended.

22. *CITE* the factors that can interfere with bowel elimination in the postpartum period.

23. *EXPLAIN* why hypovolemic shock is less likely to occur in the postpartum woman experiencing a normal or average blood loss.

24. *INDICATE* the factors that place a postpartum woman at increased risk for the development of thrombophlebitis.

25. *COMPARE and CONTRAST* the characteristics of lochial bleeding and nonlochial bleeding.

MULTIPLE CHOICE: Circle the one correct option and state the rationale for the option chosen.

26. A nurse has assessed a woman who gave birth vaginally 12 hours ago. Which of the following findings would require further assessment?
    A. Bright to dark red uterine discharge—¾ of pad saturated in 2 to 3 hours
    B. Midline episiotomy—approximated, moderate edema, slight erythema, absence of ecchymosis
    C. Protrusion of abdomen with sight separation of abdominal wall muscles
    D. Fundus firm at level of umbilicus and to the right of midline

27. A woman 24 hours after birth complains to the nurse that her sleep was interrupted the night before because of sweating and the need to have her gown and bed linen changed. The nurse's first action would be to:
    A. Assess this woman for additional clinical manifestations of infection
    B. Explain to the woman that the sweating represents her body's attempt to eliminate the fluid that was accumulated during pregnancy
    C. Notify her physician of the finding
    D. Document the finding as postpartum diaphoresis

28. Which of the following women at 24 hours following birth is least likely to experience afterpains?
    A. Primipara who is breastfeeding her twins that were born at 38 weeks' gestation
    B. Multipara who is breastfeeding her 10-pound full-term baby girl
    C. Multipara who is bottle feeding her 8-pound baby boy
    D. Primipara who is bottle feeding her 7-pound baby girl

CRITICAL THINKING EXERCISES

1. DESCRIBE how you would respond to each of the following typical questions/concerns of postpartum women.
    A. Mary is a primipara who is breastfeeding. "Why am I experiencing so many painful cramps in my uterus? I thought this happens only in women who have had babies before."

    B. Susan is being discharged after giving birth 20 hours ago. "For how many days should I be able to palpate my uterus to make sure it is firm?"

C. June is a primipara. "My friend, who had a baby last year, said she had a flow for 6 weeks. Isn't that a long time to bleed after having a baby?"

D. Jean is at 24 hours postpartum. "I cannot believe it—I look as if I am still pregnant!! How can this be?"

E. Marion is 1 day postpartum. "I perspired so much last night and I have such large amounts of urine when I go to the bathroom. I hope everything is okay and I can still go home!"

F. Joan is a primipara who is breastfeeding her baby. "My friend told me that I cannot get pregnant as long as I continue to breastfeed. This is great because I do not like to use birth control."

G. Alice, a multiparous woman who is bottle feeding her baby, is concerned. She states, "My doctor is not going to give me a drug to dry up my breasts like I had with my first baby. How will my breasts ever get back to normal now?"

H. Andrea, a primipara, is 1 day postpartum. While breastfeeding her baby she confides to the nurse that she does not know how long she will continue to breastfeed. "My husband and I have always had a satisfying sex life but my friend told me that as long as I breastfeed intercourse is painful."

ONLINE LEARNING ACTIVITIES

Access the Lowdermilk, Perry **Evolve** website at **http://evolve.elsevier.com/Lowdermilk/MatWmnHlth/** and enter the **Student** portion through the **Learning Resources** section. Use Chapter 22 to begin a search of the Internet for websites that are capable of informing postpartum women and their families about what to expect regarding the process of physical recovery following birth. Prepare a report that includes the following:

- List of the sites found
- Description of the site you found to be the most helpful in terms of:
  - Sponsoring person(s), agency, organization
  - Clarity, accuracy, accessibility (ease of use), depth, and value of the information provided
  - Currency—frequency of site updates
  - Variety of links to other relevant sites
  - Ability of persons visiting the site to obtain additional information through such services as e-mail and chat rooms
- Guidelines postpartum women should use when accessing these or other sites
- Assessment form, based on the information obtained in your search, that postpartum women can use after discharge to monitor the progress of their recovery in terms of expected findings and those findings that would indicate ineffective recovery and the need to notify their health care provider

Nursing Care of the Postpartum Woman

CHAPTER REVIEW ACTIVITIES

FILL IN THE BLANKS: Insert the term that corresponds to each of the following descriptions regarding the postpartum period.

1. _____ The first one to two hours after birth.
2. _____ Nursing care management approach where one nurse cares for both the mother and her infant. It is also called _____ care or _____ care.
3. _____ Term used for the decreasing length of hospital stays of mothers and their babies after low risk births. Other terms used are _____ and _____.
4. _____ Classification of medications that stimulate contraction of the uterine smooth muscle.
5. _____ Failure of the uterine muscle to contract firmly. It is the most frequent cause of _____ following childbirth.
6. _____ Perineal treatment that involves sitting in warm water for approximately 20 minutes in order to soothe and cleanse the site and to increase blood flow, thereby enhancing healing.
7. _____ Menstrual-like cramps experienced by many women as the uterus contracts after childbirth.
8. _____ Dilation of the blood vessels supplying the intestines as a result of the rapid decease in intraabdominal pressure after birth. It causes blood to pool in the viscera and thereby contributes to the development of _____ when the woman who has recently given birth stands up.
9. _____ Complaint of pain in calf muscles when dorsiflexion of the foot is forced. The presence of pain is associated with the presence of thrombophlebitis.
10. _____ Exercises that can assist women to regain muscle tone that is often lost when pelvic tissues are stretched and torn during pregnancy and birth.
11. _____ Swelling of breast tissue caused by increased blood and lymph supply to the breasts preceding lactation.
12. _____ Vaccine that can be given to postpartum women whose antibody titer is less than 1:8 or whose enzyme immunoassay (EIA) level is less than 0.8. It is used to prevent nonimmune women from contracting this TORCH infection during a subsequent pregnancy.

13. _____ is administered within 72 hours of birth to Rh-negative, antibody (Coombs test)-negative women who have Rh-positive newborns. The _____ test is performed if a large fetomaternal transfusion is suspected to more accurately determine the amount of fetal blood present in the maternal circulation so that the correct dosage of RhoGAM can be given.

14. *EXPLAIN* to a woman who has just given birth why breastfeeding her newborn during the fourth stage of labor is beneficial to her and to her baby.

15. A postpartum woman at 6 hours after a vaginal birth is having difficulty voiding. *LIST* the measures that you would try to help this woman to void spontaneously.

16. *IDENTIFY* the measures the nurse should teach a postpartum woman in an effort to prevent the development of thrombophlebitis.

17. During the fourth stage of labor, the nurse must assess a woman's recovery from anesthesia.
    A. *LIST* the components of the postanesthesia recovery (PAR) score.

    B. *STATE* the criteria the nurse should use to determine the progress of a woman's recovery from each of the following types of anesthesia:
    General anesthesia

    Epidural or spinal anesthesia

18. *IDENTIFY* the measures you would teach a bottle-feeding mother to suppress lactation naturally and to relieve discomfort during breast engorgement.

19. *STATE* the two most important interventions that can be used to prevent excessive bleeding in the early postpartum period. *INDICATE* the rationale for the effectiveness of each intervention you identified.

TRUE OR FALSE: Circle "T" if true or "F" if false for each of the following statements. Correct the false statements.

T F 20. The effectiveness of the rubella vaccine may be reduced if a postpartum woman receives both Rh immunoglobulin and a rubella vaccine.

T F 21. Before sitting down in a sitz bath, the woman should relax her gluteal muscles to reduce discomfort when entering the bath, then tighten them after she is sitting in the bath.

T F 22. Tucks can be used to soothe sore hemorrhoids.

T F 23. Medications such as estrogen and bromocriptine (Parlodel) are no longer used to suppress lactation for the bottle-feeding woman.

T F 24. For healthy women, the most dangerous potential complication of the fourth stage of labor is infection.

T F 25. Ice packs are most effective in minimizing perineal edema formation during the first 24 hours following birth.

T F 26. A good time to administer pain medication to a breastfeeding woman would be immediately after a feeding session.

T F 27. Rubella vaccine should not be given to a postpartum woman who is breastfeeding.

T F 28. A woman should be expected to void at least 250 ml of urine spontaneously within 2 hours following vaginal birth.

T F 29. RhoGAM should be administered intramuscularly into the deltoid or gluteal muscle.

T F 30. A Chinese woman is likely to use hormonal preparations as her primary method of contraception.

T F 31. Women who follow the cultural practice of balancing heat and cold will avoid bathing for a specified period of time after they have given birth.

T F 32. A critical nursing action at the time of discharge is to carefully check the mother's and baby's identification bands.

T F 33. A postpartum woman who is depressed and is experiencing thoughts of suicide or harming her child should call the warm line she learned about at discharge.

34. Tamara delivered vaginally 2 hours ago. She has a midline episiotomy.
    A. DESCRIBE the position that Tamara should assume in order to facilitate palpation of her fundus.

    B. IDENTIFY the characteristics of Tamara's fundus that should be assessed.

    C. DESCRIBE the position Tamara should assume in order to facilitate the examination of her episiotomy and perineum.

    D. IDENTIFY the characteristics that should be assessed to determine progress of healing and adequacy of Tamara's perineal self-care measures.

    E. STATE the characteristics of Tamara's uterine flow that should be assessed.

35. Imagine that you are the nurse who cared for a woman during her labor and birth and her recovery during the fourth stage of labor. OUTLINE the information that you would report to the mother-baby nurse when you transfer the new mother and her baby to her room on the postpartum unit.

36. Infection control measures should guide the practice of nurses working on a postpartum unit.
    A. DISCUSS the measures designed to prevent transmission of infection from person to person.

B. *DISCUSS* measures a postpartum woman should be taught to reduce her risk of infection.

37. *IDENTIFY* the signs of potential complications that may occur during the postpartum period.

MULTIPLE CHOICE: Circle the one correct option and state the rationale for the option chosen.

38. During the fourth stage of labor a woman experiences intense tremors that resemble shivers. Based on this finding the nurse would:
    A. Request an order for a sedative
    B. Assess the woman for signs of infection
    C. Check the woman's rectal temperature to determine if she is becoming hypothermic
    D. Wrap the woman in warm blankets and reassure her

39. The nurse is prepared to assess a postpartum woman's fundus. The nurse would tell the woman to:
    A. Elevate the head of the bed
    B. Place her hands under her head
    C. Flex her knees
    D. Lie flat with legs extended and toes pointed

40. The expected outcome for care when Methergine is administered to a postpartum woman during the fourth stage of labor would be: The woman will
    A. Demonstrate expected lochial characteristics
    B. Achieve relief of pain associated with uterine cramping
    C. Remain free from infection
    D. Void spontaneously within 4 hours of birth

41. A nurse is preparing to administer RhoGAM to a postpartum woman. Prior to implementing this care measure the nurse should:
    A. Ensure that medication is given within 24 hours of birth
    B. Verify that the Coombs' test results are negative
    C. Make sure that the newborn is Rh negative
    D. Cancel the administration of the RhoGAM if it was given to the woman during her pregnancy at 28 weeks' gestation

42. When teaching a postpartum woman with an episiotomy about using a sitz bath the nurse should emphasize
    A. Using sterile equipment
    B. Filling the sitz bath basin with hot water (at least 42° C)
    C. Taking a sitz bath once a day for 10 minutes
    D. Squeezing her buttocks together prior to sitting down then relaxing them

Chapter 23: Nursing Care of the Postpartum Woman   211

CRITICAL THINKING EXERCISES

1. Tara is a breastfeeding woman at 12 hours postpartum. She requests medication for pain. *DESCRIBE* the approach that you would take when fulfilling Tara's request.

2. When caring for a woman 4 hours after birth, the nurse notes an excessive rubra flow and early signs of hypovolemic shock.
   A. *STATE* the criteria that the nurse should have used to determine that the flow is rubra and excessive and that the early signs of hypovolemic shock are being exhibited.

   B. *IDENTIFY* the nurse's priority action in response to these assessment findings.

   C. *DESCRIBE* the nurse's legal responsibility in this clinical situation.

   D. *IDENTIFY* additional interventions that a nurse may need to implement to ensure this woman's safety and to prevent the development of further complications.

3. Carrie is a postpartum woman awaiting discharge. Because her rubella titre indicates that she is not immune, a rubella vaccination has been ordered before discharge. STATE what you would tell Carrie with regard to this vaccination.

4. The physician has written the following order for a postpartum woman: "Administer RhoGAM (Rh immunoglobulin) if indicated." *DESCRIBE* the actions the nurse should take in fulfilling this order.

5. Susan, a postpartum breastfeeding woman, confides to the nurse, "My partner and I have always had a very satisfying sex life even when I was pregnant. My sister told me that this will definitely change now that I have had a baby." DESCRIBE what the nurse should tell Susan regarding sexual changes and activity after birth.

6. IDENTIFY the priority nursing diagnosis as well as one expected outcome and appropriate nursing management for each of the following situations.

A. Tina is 2 days postpartum. During a home visit the nurse notes that Tina's episiotomy is edematous, slightly reddened, with approximated wound edges, and no drainage. A distinct odor is noted and there is a buildup of secretions and the Hurricaine gel Tina uses for discomfort. During the interview Tina reveals that she is afraid to wash the area, "I rinse with a little water in my peri bottle in the morning and again at night. I also apply plenty of my gel."

Nursing Diagnosis	Expected Outcome	Nursing Management

B. Erin, who gave birth 3 days ago, has not had a bowel movement since a day or two before labor. She tells the visiting nurse during the interview that she has been avoiding "fiber" foods for fear that the baby will get diarrhea. Her activity level is low. "My family is taking good care of me. I do not have to lift a finger! Besides I would prefer to wait until my episiotomy is less sore before trying to have a bowel movement."

Nursing Diagnosis	Expected Outcome	Nursing Management

Chapter 23: Nursing Care of the Postpartum Woman   213

C. Mary gave birth 24 hours ago. She complains of perineal discomfort. "My hemorrhoids and stitches are killing me but I do not want to take any medication because it will get into my breast milk and hurt my baby."

Nursing Diagnosis	Expected Outcome	Nursing Management

7. Dawn gave birth 8 hours ago. Upon palpation, her fundus was found to be 2 finger breadths above the umbilicus and deviated to the right of midline. It was also assessed to be less firm than previously noted.
A. *STATE* the most likely basis for these findings.

B. *DESCRIBE* the action that the nurse should take based on these assessment findings.

8. Jill gave birth 3 hours ago. During labor, epidural anesthesia was used for pain relief. Jill's primary health care provider has written the following order, "Out of bed and ambulating when able." *DISCUSS* the approach the nurse should take in safely fulfilling this order.

9. Andrea gave birth 1½ hours ago. She tells the nurse that she is ravenous. You check the chart, noting that Andrea's primary health care provider has ordered "diet as tolerated." *STATE* the criteria that should be met prior to fulfilling this order.

10. Dawn, a primiparous woman at 20 hours postpartum, is preparing for discharge within the next 4 hours. She is breastfeeding her new daughter.

A. *DESCRIBE* the nurse's legal responsibility in terms of early discharge.

B. *LIST* the criteria for discharge that Dawn and her newborn must meet prior to discharge from the hospital to home.

Maternal Criteria	Newborn Criteria	General Criteria

C. *OUTLINE* the essential content that must be taught before discharge. A home visit by a nurse is planned for Dawn's third postpartum day.

11. Cultural beliefs and practices must be considered when planning and implementing care in the postpartum period.

A. Discuss the importance of using a culturally sensitive approach when providing care to postpartum women and their families.

B. Kim, a Korean-American woman, has just given birth. Assessment reveals that she and her family are guided by beliefs and practices based on a balance of heat and cold. *DESCRIBE* how the nurse would adjust typical postpartum care in order to respect and accommodate Kim's cultural beliefs and practices.

C. A Muslim woman has been admitted to the postpartum unit following the birth of her second son. *DESCRIBE* the approach you would use in managing this woman's care in a culturally sensitive manner.

ONLINE LEARNING ACTIVITIES

Access the Lowdermilk, Perry **Evolve** website at **http://evolve.elsevier.com/Lowdermilk/MatWmnHlth/** and enter the **Student** portion through the **Learning Resources** section. Use Chapter 23 to search the Internet for websites that can provide postpartum women and their families with information regarding measures that they can use to facilitate physical recovery and provide them with support that will enhance their psychosocial adjustment to a new baby. Prepare a report that includes the following:

- List of sites
- Describe the site you found to be the most helpful in terms of the following:
  - Sponsoring person(s), agency, organization
  - Clarity, accuracy, accessibility (ease of use), value, and depth of information provided
  - Currency—frequency of site updates
  - Variety of links to other relevant sites
  - Nature of support offered to postpartum families including the ability to obtain additional information and individualized support through such services as e-mail and chat rooms.
- Handout that you could give to postpartum women and their families. It should include the following:
  - Outline of the most critical measures that should be implemented in order to facilitate physical recovery and psychosocial adjustment
  - List of relevant websites and guidelines for their use

CHAPTER 24

Transition to Parenthood

CHAPTER REVIEW ACTIVITIES

1. *COMPLETE THE FOLLOWING TABLE* by identifying the focus, characteristics (typical behaviors and concerns), and care requirements for postpartum women in each of the following phases of maternal adjustment and transition to parenthood.

Phase	Focus	Characteristics	Care Requirements
Dependent (taking-in)			
Dependent-independent (taking-hold)			
Interdependent (letting-go)			
Postpartum blues			

2. *COMPLETE THE FOLLOWING TABLE* by identifying the focus and characteristics (typical behaviors/concerns) and care requirements for fathers in each of the following stages of paternal adjustment and transition to the role of father.

Phase	Focus	Characteristics	Care Requirements
Stage 1: Expectations			
Stage 2: Reality			
Stage 3: Transition to Mastery			

3. Attachment of the newborn to parents and family is critical for optimum growth and development.
   A. *DEFINE* the process of attachment and bonding.

   B. *IDENTIFY* the critical attributes of the attachment process and *EXPLAIN* how each influences the developing parent-infant relationship.

   C. *LIST* conditions that must be present for the parent-newborn attachment process to begin favorably.

D. *DESCRIBE* the acquaintance process.

E. *DISCUSS* how you would assess the progress of attachment between parents and their new baby.

4. *IDENTIFY* the required parental tasks and responsibilities that are part of parental adjustment to a new baby.

5. *DISCUSS* how each of the following forms of parent-infant contact can facilitate attachment and promote the family as a focus of care.
Early contact

Extended contact

6. The parenting process is composed of two essential components. *DESCRIBE* each component and its importance for the optimum growth and development of children. *IDENTIFY* nursing strategies that can be effective in helping parents develop competency and self-confidence with regard to each component.

Skill and Knowledge Component	Affective Component

7. During the fourth trimester parents reorganize and modify their roles and relationships as they take on the role of parent to a new baby. *STATE* the focus for each period of the fourth trimester:
Early period (first 3 to 4 weeks)

Consolidation period

FILL IN THE BLANKS: Insert the appropriate term for each of the following descriptions regarding parent-infant interaction and parenting.

8. _____ is defined as a passage or process occurring over time involving development or movement from one state, condition, or place to another. Six conditions that influence this passage are _____, _____, _____, _____, _____, and _____ and _____. Indicators that the passage has been successful include _____, _____, and _____.

9. _____ is the term used to refer to the process by which a parent comes to love and accept a child and a child comes to love and accept a parent. The term _____ is often used to refer to this process; it is a sensitive period after birth when parents have close contact with their infant. The three critical attributes of this process are _____, _____, and _____.

10. _____ is the term used to refer to infant behaviors and characteristics that call forth a corresponding set of maternal behaviors and characteristics. Infant signaling behaviors include _____, _____, and _____. Infant executive behaviors include _____, _____, and _____ that maintain the contact.

11. An important part of attachment is _____, whereby parents use _____, _____ _____, and _____ to get to know their baby in the immediate postpartum period.

12. _____ or _____ is a position in which the parent's face and the infant's face are approximately 8 inches apart and are on the same plane. Nursing actions to encourage this interaction include _____, _____, and _____.

13. The _____ process is the identification of the new baby. The child is first identified in terms of _____ to other family members, then in terms of _____, and finally in terms of _____.

14. _____ is exhibited when newborns move in time with the structure of adult speech by _____, _____, and _____ seemingly _____ to a parent's voice.

15. One of the newborn's tasks is to establish a personal rhythm or _____. Parents can help in this process by giving consistent _____ and using their infant's _____ state to develop _____ behavior and thereby increase _____ and opportunities for _____.

16. _____ is a type of body movement or behavior that provides the observer with cues. The observer or receiver interprets those cues and responds to them. _____ refers to the "fit" between the infant's cues and the parents' response.

17. Infant-parent interactions can be facilitated by modulation of _____, modification of _____, and mutual _____.

18. To modulate _____, both parent and infant must be able to interact. Therefore the infant must be in the _____ state long enough for interactions to take place.

19. The infant and both parents have a _____ of behaviors they can use to facilitate interactions. For the infant these behaviors include _____, _____, and _____. For the parents these behaviors include various types of interactive behaviors such as constantly _____ at the infant and noting the infant's _____. Adults also _____ their speech to help the infant listen. _____ such as slow and exaggerated looks of surprise, happiness, and confusion are often used by parents to _____ these emotions to the infant.

20. Contingent responses or _____ are those that occur within a specific time and are similar in form to a stimulus behavior. The adult has the feeling of having an influence on the interaction. Infant behaviors such as _____, _____, and sustained _____, usually in the _____ position, are viewed as contingent responses.

21. _____ is a father's absorption, preoccupation, and interest in his infant. Characteristics of this absorption include _____ and _____.

22. COMPLETE THE FOLLOWING TABLE by identifying three infant and parent facilitating behaviors and three infant and parent inhibiting behaviors that can affect the process of attachment.

Infant/Parents	Facilitating Behaviors	Inhibiting Behaviors
Infant		
Parents		

23. *DESCRIBE* how each of the following factors influences the manner in which parents respond to the birth of their child. *STATE* two nursing implications/actions related to each factor.

Adolescent parents

Parental age older than 35 years of age

Social support

Culture

Socioeconomic conditions

Personal aspirations

Visual impairment

Hearing impairment

MULTIPLE CHOICE: Circle the one correct option and state the rationale for the option chosen.

24. During the final phase of the claiming process of a newborn, mother might say:
    A. "She has her grandfather's nose."
    B. "His ears lay nice and flat against his head not like mine and his sister's, which stick out."
    C. "She gave me nothing but trouble during pregnancy and now she is so stubborn she won't wake up to breastfeed."
    D. "He has such a sweet disposition and pleasant expression—I have never seen a baby quiet like him before."

25. Which of the following nursing actions would be least effective in facilitating parent attachment to their new infant?
    A. Referring the couple to a lactation consultant to ensure continuing success with breastfeeding
    B. Keeping the baby in the nursery as much as possible for the first 24 hours after birth so the mother can rest
    C. Extending visiting hours for the woman's partner or significant other as they desire
    D. Providing guidance and support as the parents care for their baby's nutrition and hygiene needs

26. A behavior that illustrates engrossment would be:
    A. Father is sitting in a rocking chair, holding his new baby boy, touching his toes, and making eye contact
    B. Mother tells her friends that her baby's eyes and nose are just like hers
    C. Mother picks up and cuddles her baby girl when she begins to cry
    D. Grandmother gazes into her new grandson's face, which she holds about 8 inches away from her own—she and the baby make eye-to-eye contact

27. A woman expresses a need to review her labor and birth experience with the nurse who cared for her while in labor. This behavior is most characteristic of which of the following phases of maternal postpartum adjustment?
    A. Taking hold (dependent-independent phase)
    B. Taking in (dependent phase)
    C. Letting go (interdependent)
    D. Postpartum blues (baby blues)

28. Prior to discharge, a postpartum woman and her partner ask the nurse about the baby blues. "Our friend said she felt so let down after she had her baby and we have heard that some women actually become very depressed. Is there anything we can do to prevent this from happening to us or at least coping with the blues if they occur?" The nurse could tell this couple:
    A. "Postpartum blues usually happens in pregnancies that are high risk or unplanned so there is no need for you to worry."
    B. "Try to become skillful in breastfeeding and caring for your baby as quickly as you can."
    C. "Get as much rest as you can, sleep when the baby sleeps, because fatigue can precipitate the blues or make them worse."
    D. "I will call your doctor before you leave to get you a prescription for an antidepressant to prevent the blues from happening."

CRITICAL THINKING EXERCISES

1. Jane and Andrew are parents of a newborn girl. *DESCRIBE* what you would teach them regarding the communication process as it relates to their newborn.
   A. Techniques they can use to communicate effectively with their newborn.

   B. The manner in which the baby is able to communicate with them.

2. Allison had a difficult labor that resulted in an emergency cesarean birth under general anesthesia. She did not see her baby until 12 hours after her birth. Allison tells the nurse who brings the baby to her room, "I am so disappointed. I had planned to breastfeed my baby and hold her close, skin to skin, right after her birth just like all the books say. I know that this is so important for our relationship." *DESCRIBE* how the nurse should respond to Allison's concern.

3. Angela is the mother of a 1-day-old boy and a 3-year-old girl. As you prepare Angela for discharge, she states, "My little girl just saw her brother. She says she loves him and cannot wait for him to come home. I am so glad that I do not have to worry about any of that sibling rivalry business!" *INDICATE* how you would respond to Angela's comments.

4. Sara and Ben have just experienced the birth of their first baby. They are very happy with their baby boy but appear very unsure of themselves and are obviously anxious about how to tell what their baby needs. Sara is trying very hard to breastfeed and is having some success but not as much as she had hoped. Both parents express self-doubt about their ability to succeed at the "most important role in our lives."
   A. *STATE* the nursing diagnosis that is most appropriate for this couple.

B. *DESCRIBE* what the nurse caring for this family can do to facilitate the attachment process.

5. Mary and Jim are the parents of three sons. They very much wanted to have a girl this time, but after a long and difficult birth they had another son who weighed 10 pounds. His appearance reflects the difficult birth process: occipital molding, caput succedaneum, and forceps marks on each cheek. Mary and Jim express their disappointment not only in the appearance of their son but also in the fact that they had another boy. "This was supposed to be our last child—now we just do not know what we will do." *DISCUSS* how you would facilitate Mary and Jim's attachment to their son and reconcile their fantasy ("dream") child with the reality of their actual child.

6. Dawn and Matthew have just given birth to their first baby. This is the first grandchild for both sets of grandparents. The grandmothers approach the nurse to ask how they can help the new family, stating, "We want to help Dawn and Matthew but at the same time not interfere with what they want to do." *DISCUSS* the role of the nurse in helping these grandparents to recognize their importance to the new family and to develop a mutually satisfying relationship with Dawn, Matthew, and the new baby.

7. Jane is 2 days postpartum. When the nurse makes a home visit, Jane is found crying. Jane states, "I have such a let-down feeling. I cannot understand why I feel this way when I should be so happy about the healthy outcome for myself and my baby." Jane's husband confirms her behavior and expresses confusion as well, stating, "I wish I knew what to do to help her." *IDENTIFY* the priority nursing diagnosis and one expected outcome for this situation. *DESCRIBE* the recommended nursing management for the nursing diagnosis you have identified.

Nursing Diagnosis	Expected Outcome	Nursing Management

ONLINE LEARNING ACTIVITIES

Access the Lowdermilk, Perry **Evolve** website at
http://evolve.elsevier.com/Lowdermilk/MatWmnHlth/ and enter the **Student** portion through the
Learning Resources section to search the medical literature for nursing research studies related to a
man's transition to fatherhood and the measures that have been effective in facilitating this process.
- Create an annotated bibliography of at least five nursing research studies
- Choose one study and complete a bibliography card that includes the following:
  - Hypothesis; research question
  - Summary of the methodology used and key findings
  - Reliability of the study and its findings
  - Recommendations for further research
- Write a description of how you would use the findings of these research studies to plan prenatal
  and postpartum classes for fathers that are evidence-based. Specify at least five content areas you
  would emphasize and strategies that you would use as you present these classes to prospective and
  new fathers.

CHAPTER 25

Physiologic and Behavioral Adaptations of the Newborn

CHAPTER REVIEW ACTIVITIES

MATCHING: Match the description in Column I with the appropriate newborn reflex from Column II.

COLUMN I

_____ 1. Apply pressure to soles of feet with fingers when the lower limbs are semiflexed—legs extend.

_____ 2. Place infant on flat surface and strike surface—symmetric abduction and extension of arms, fingers fan out, thumb and forefinger form a "C", slight tremor may occur.

_____ 3. Place finger in palm of hand or at base of toes—infant's fingers curl around examiner's finger, toes curl downward.

_____ 4. Place infant prone on flat surface, run finger down side of back 4 to 5 cm lateral to spine—body flexes and pelvis swings toward stimulated side.

_____ 5. Tap over forehead, bridge of nose, or maxilla when eyes are open—blinks for first four to five taps.

_____ 6. Use finger to stroke sole of foot beginning at heel, upward along lateral aspect of sole, then across ball of foot—all toes hyperextend, with dorsiflexion of big toe.

_____ 7. Clap hands sharply—arms abduct with flexion of elbows, hands stay clenched.

_____ 8. Touch infant's lip, cheek, or corner of mouth with nipple—turns head toward stimulus, opens mouth, takes hold, and sucks.

_____ 9. Place infant in a supine position, turn head quickly to one side as infant is falling asleep or is asleep—arm and leg extend on side to which head is turned while opposite arm and leg flex.

COLUMN II

A. Rooting
B. Grasp
C. Extrusion
D. Glabellar
E. Tonic neck
F. Moro
G. Stepping (walking)
H. Startle
I. Babinski
J. Trunk incurvation
K. Magnet

_____ 10. Hold infant vertically allowing one foot to touch table surface—infant alternates flexion and extension of its feet.

_____ 11. Touch or depress tip of tongue—tongue is forced outward.

Neonatal nurses are responsible for the assessment of the physiologic integrity of newborns. As part of this responsibility the nurse must be aware of the significance of data collected. *LABEL* each of the following assessment findings, if present, in a group of three full-term newborns who were born 12 hours ago, as "**N**" (reflective of normal adaptation or acceptable variation to extrauterine life) or "**P**" (reflective of potential problems with adaptation to extrauterine life).

Assessment Finding	Evaluation
12. Crackles upon auscultation of the lungs	_____
13. Respirations: 36, irregular, shallow	_____
14. Episodic apnea lasting 5 to 10 seconds	_____
15. Nasal flaring and sternal retractions	_____
16. Slight bluish discoloration of feet and hands	_____
17. Blood pressure 86/54	_____
18. Apical rate: 126 with murmurs	_____
19. Pink-tinged stains on diaper after first two urinations	_____
20. Small white cysts at gum margins and on palate	_____
21. Boggy, edematous swelling over occiput	_____
22. Overlapping of parietal bones	_____
23. White pimple-like spots on nose and chin	_____
24. Jaundice on face and chest	_____
25. Regurgitation of small amount of milk after feedings	_____
26. Liver palpated 1 cm below right costal margin	_____
27. Absence of bowel elimination since birth	_____
28. Spine straight with dimple at base	_____
29. Adhesion of prepuce—unable to fully retract	_____
30. Edema of scrotum and labia	_____
31. Flaring or hyperextension of toes when sole is stroked upward	_____
32. Hematocrit 36% and hemoglobin 12 g/dl	_____
33. White blood cell count (WBC) 20,000/mm^3	_____
34. Blood glucose 45 mg/dl	_____

35. The most critical adjustment that a newborn must make at birth is the establishment of respirations. *LIST* the factors that are responsible for the initiation of breathing after birth.

FILL IN THE BLANKS: Insert the term that corresponds to each of the following descriptions related to temperature regulation in the newborn.

36. _____ is the maintenance of balance between heat loss and heat production. _____ from excessive heat loss is a common and dangerous problem in neonates. Heat production is referred to as _____. Nonshivering thermogenesis is accomplished primarily by _____, which is unique to the newborn and secondarily by increased _____ in the brain, heart, and liver.

37. Major factors that affect a newborn's risk for thermogenic problems include _____ less than an adult's, _____ close to the skin surface, larger _____ ratio, and ability to maintain a _____ position.

38. When exposed to cold, the newborn may _____, become _____, increase _____ to generate heat, and increase _____ to stimulate muscle activity.

39. _____ is the flow of heat from the body surface to cooler ambient air. Two measures to reduce heat loss by this method would be to _____ infant and keep the ambient air temperature at _____.

40. _____ is the loss of heat from the body surface to a cooler, solid surface not in direct contact but in relative proximity. _____ and _____ are placed away from _____ to prevent this type of heat loss.

41. _____ is the loss of heat that occurs when a liquid is converted to vapor. This heat loss can be intensified by failure to _____ the newborn directly after birth or by _____ of the infant after a bath.

42. _____ is the loss of heat from the body surface to cooler surfaces in direct contact. When admitted to the nursery, the newborn is placed in a _____ to minimize heat loss.

43. *IDENTIFY* two nursing measures that can be used to limit the degree of physiologic hyperbilirubinemia. *STATE* the basis for the effectiveness of each measure identified.

FILL IN THE BLANKS: Insert the term that corresponds to each of the following descriptions of newborn behavioral adaptations and characteristics.

44. Variations in the state of consciousness of newborn infants are called the _____-_____ states.

45. The sleep states are _____ sleep and _____ sleep.

46. The wake states are _____, _____, _____, and _____. The optimum state of arousal is the _____ state, in which the infant can be observed smiling, responding to voices, watching faces, vocalizing, and moving in synchrony.

47. The newborn sleeps about _____ hours a day, with periods of wakefulness gradually _____.

48. _____ is a protective mechanism that allows the infant to become accustomed to environmental stimuli. It is a psychologic and physiologic phenomenon whereby the response to a constant or repetitive stimulus is decreased. The infant is able to _____ to and then _____ to discrete stimulus while asleep.

49. _____ refers to the quality of alert states and ability to attend to visual and auditory stimuli while alert.

50. *DESCRIBE* how each of the following factors can influence a newborn's behavior.
    Gestational age

    Time

    Stimuli

    Medication

51. During the first 6 to 8 hours after birth, newborns experience a transition period characterized by three phases of instability. *COMPLETE THE FOLLOWING TABLE* by identifying the timing/duration and typical behaviors for each phase of this transitional period.

Phase	Timing/Duration	Typical Behaviors
First period of reactivity		
Period of diminished response		
Second period of reactivity		

TRUE OR FALSE: Circle "T" if true or "F" if false for each of the following statements. Correct the false statements.

T F 52. The presence of phosphatidylglycerol (Pg) in amniotic fluid is more predictive of fetal lung maturity than is the L/S (lecithin/sphingomyelin) ratio.

T F 53. Crackles, audible grunting, nasal flaring, and retractions of the chest are often noted during the second period of reactivity.

T F 54. The white blood cell count will increase when the newborn develops an infection.

T F 55. Petechiae scattered over a newborn's body are a common finding during the first 24 hours following birth.

T F 56. Blood-tinged mucus on the diaper of the female newborn should be documented by the nurse as pseudomenstruation and recognized as an expected assessment finding related to the withdrawal of maternal estrogen.

T F 57. A newborn usually loses approximately 20% of its birth weight during the first 3 to 5 days of life as a result of fluid loss, limited fluid intake, and an increased metabolic rate.

T F 58. Jitteriness and tremors may indicate that the newborn is experiencing hypoglycemia.

T F 59. Physiologic jaundice in the full-term newborn disappears by the end of the first week of life.

T F 60. Kernicterus occurs when bilirubin invades the cells of the heart muscle, thereby weakening heart function.

T F 61. Abdominal movements are counted when determining the respiratory rate of newborns.

T F 62. Meconium stool often has a strong odor as a result of bacteria present in the fetal intestine during intrauterine life.

T F 63. The wink reflex can be used to test anal sphincter tone.

T F 64. Breast tissue in full-term male and female newborns may be swollen and secrete a thin milky-type discharge.

T F 65. Presence of a click and asymmetric movement during Ortolani's maneuver indicates hip dislocation or dysplasia.

T F 66. A cephalhematoma should be aspirated in order to prevent development of pathologic jaundice.

T F 67. In physiologic jaundice the level of unconjugated bilirubin often reaches 16 mg/dl in the full-term newborn.

T F 68. The newborn's white blood cell count will decrease rapidly after birth to stabilize at a level of 20,000/mm^3.

MULTIPLE CHOICE: Circle the one correct option and state the rationale for the option chosen.

69. A newborn, at 5 hours old, wakes from a sound sleep and becomes very active. He exhibits the following signs when assessed. Which one would require further assessment?
    A. Increased mucus production
    B. Passage of meconium
    C. Heart rate of 160 beats per minute
    D. Two apneic episodes of 16 and 20 seconds' duration

70. When assessing a newborn boy at 12 hours of age, the nurse notes a rash on his abdomen and thighs. The rash appears as irregular reddish blotches with pale centers. The nurse would:
   A. Document the finding as erythema toxicum
   B. Isolate the newborn and his mother until infection is ruled out
   C. Apply an antiseptic ointment to each lesion
   D. Request nonallergenic linen from the laundry

71. A newborn girl is 12 hours old and is being prepared for early discharge. Which of the following assessment findings if present could delay discharge?
   A. Dark green-black stool, tarry in consistency
   B. Yellowish tinge in sclera and on face
   C. Blood glucose level of 55 mg/dl
   D. Rust stain on diaper after urination

72. As part of a thorough assessment of a newborn the nurse should check for hip dislocation and dysplasia. The technique the nurse would most likely use would be:
   A. Measurement of each leg from hip to heel
   B. Stepping or walking reflex
   C. Magnet reflex
   D. Ortolani maneuver

73. When assessing a newborn after birth the nurse notes flat, irregular, pinkish marks on the bridge of the nose, nape of neck, and over the eyelids. The areas blanch when pressed with a finger. The nurse would document this finding as:
   A. Milia
   B. Nevus vasculosus
   C. Telangiectatic nevi
   D. Nevus flammeus

CRITICAL THINKING EXERCISES

1. Newborns are at risk for cold stress.
   A. *STATE* the dangers that cold stress poses for the newborn.

   B. *IDENTIFY* one nursing diagnosis and one expected outcome related to this danger.

C. *DESCRIBE* care measures the nurse should implement to prevent cold stress from occurring.

2. After a long and difficult labor, baby boy James was born with a caput succedaneum and significant molding over the occipital area. Low forceps were used for the birth, resulting in ecchymotic areas on both cheeks. *DESCRIBE* what you would tell the parents of James about these assessment findings.

3. Mary and Jim are concerned that their baby boy who weighed 8 lb 6 oz at birth now, at 2 days of age, "weighs only 7 lb 14 oz." *DESCRIBE* how you would respond to their concern.

4. Susan and Allen are first-time parents of a baby girl. They ask the nurse about their baby's ability to see and hear things around her and to interact with them.
   A. *SPECIFY* what the nurse should tell these parents about the sensory capabilities of their healthy full-term newborn.

   B. *NAME* four stimuli Susan and Allen could provide for their baby that would help to foster her development.

5. Tonya and Sam, an African-American couple, express concern that their new baby girl has several bruises on her back and buttocks. They ask if their baby was injured during birth or in the nursery. *DESCRIBE* the appropriate response of the nurse to Tonya and Sam's concern.

ONLINE LEARNING ACTIVITIES

Access the Lowdermilk, Perry **Evolve** website at
http://evolve.elsevier.com/Lowdermilk/MatWmnHlth/ and enter the **Student** portion through the
Learning Resources section. Use Chapter 25 as a starting point in a search of the Internet for
websites that are capable of informing parents about newborn biologic and behavioral characteristics.
Prepare a report that includes the following:

- List of relevant websites found
- Description of the website that you found to be the most helpful, in terms of:
  - Sponsoring person(s), agency, organization
  - Clarity, accuracy, accessibility (ease of use), value, and depth of information provided
  - Illustrations and photographs that depict newborn characteristics and behaviors
  - Currency—frequency of site updates
  - Variety of links to other relevant sites
  - Ability of persons visiting the site to obtain additional information through such services as e-mail and chat rooms
- Discussion regarding how these sites can be a tool used by nurses to help parents to accurately assess their newborns after discharge and distinguish between expected characteristics and behaviors and those that indicate illness and the need to contact the infant's health care provider
- Guidelines that could be given to new parents to assist them in fully accessing the sites and the information they have to provide

CHAPTER 26

Nursing Care of the Newborn

CHAPTER REVIEW ACTIVITIES

FILL IN THE BLANKS: Insert the term that corresponds to each of the following descriptions of newborns and their care.

1. _____ or _____ ointment is used to prevent ophthalmia neonatorum resulting from _____ or _____ infection. A _____ ribbon of ointment should be instilled into the _____ of each eye within _____ of birth.

2. _____ is administered intramuscularly to newborns to prevent hemorrhage. It is administered in a dose of _____ using a _____-gauge, _____-inch needle.

3. Gestational age assessment should be performed between _____ and _____ hours of age. When assessing gestational age, _____ and _____ maturity are determined using the New Ballard scale.

4. An infant born before completion of 37 weeks' gestation, regardless of birth weight, is referred to as _____ or _____.

5. An infant born between the beginning of week 38 and the end of week 42 of gestation is referred to as _____.

6. An infant who is born after the completion of week 42 of gestation is referred to as _____ or _____.

7. An infant born after 42 weeks of gestation and showing the effects of progressive placental insufficiency is referred to as _____.

8. An infant whose weight is above the 90th percentile (or two or more standard deviations above the norm) at any week is referred to as _____.

9. An infant whose weight falls between the 10th and the 90th percentiles for its gestational age is referred to as _____.

10. An infant whose weight is below the 10th percentile (or two or more standard deviations below the norm) at any week is referred to as _____.

11. _____ is the term applied to the fetus whose rate of growth does not meet expected norms.

12. An infant whose birth weight is 2500 g or less is described as being _____. These infants are considered to have had either _____ or a _____. _____ and _____ commonly occur together. An infant whose birth weight is 1500 g or less is described as being _____.

TRUE OR FALSE: Circle "T" if true or "F" if false for each of the following statements. Correct the false statements.

T   F   13. Placing a dressed newborn under a radiant warmer facilitates a faster stabilization of body temperature after birth.

T   F   14. The thermistor probe of a radiant heat panel should be taped to the right upper quadrant of the abdomen just below the intercostal margin.

T   F   15. The nurse should wear gloves, gown, and mask when handling a newborn until blood and amniotic fluid have been removed.

T   F   16. Wearing gloves when caring for the newborn is the single most important measure in the prevention of neonatal infection.

T   F   17. For the first 12 hours after birth, a newborn's temperature should be taken rectally.

T   F   18. The average axillary temperature for a newborn is 38.2°C.

T   F   19. A tympanic thermometer can be used once the newborn's ears have been cleared of vernix and fluid.

T   F   20. Acrocyanosis will disappear when the infant cries.

T   F   21. The clavicle is the bone most likely to be fractured during birth.

T   F   22. The recommended site for intramuscular injections in the newborn is the dorsogluteal muscle.

T   F   23. A major preventative measure for hyperbilirubinemia is early feeding of the newborn.

T   F   24. If bleeding is noted after a circumcision, the nurse should apply gentle pressure to the site of bleeding using a folded square of sterile gauze.

T   F   25. To facilitate obtaining a heel stick blood sample, the loose application of a warm wet washcloth around the foot for 5–10 minutes is sufficient to dilate the blood vessels in the heel.

T   F   26. An alcohol swab should be used to apply pressure to the heel after a blood sample is obtained.

T   F   27. Pressure should be applied over an arterial or femoral vein puncture for at least 3–5 minutes to prevent bleeding from the site.

T   F   28. Before application of a U–Bag, the genitalia, perineum, and surrounding skin should be sprinkled with talcum powder to prevent irritation of the skin.

T   F   29. Universal hearing screening should be performed when the infant is at least 1 month of age.

T   F   30. The ointment used for eye prophylaxis should be flushed out of the eyes with normal saline 5 minutes after instillation.

T   F   31. A blood glucose level of less than 35 mg/dl during the early newborn period is indicative of hypoglycemia.

T   F   32. Hepatitis B vaccine should only be administered to newborns exposed to the hepatitis B virus.

T   F   33. When using a bulb syringe, the nose should be suctioned before the mouth.

34. *OUTLINE* the specific measures nurses should use when caring for newborns to ensure a safe and protective environment.

35. Nurses caring for newborns as they recover following their birth must be alert for signs of hypoglycemia and hypocalcemia. COMPLETE the following table related to the signs, risk factors, and care management of hypoglycemia and hypocalcemia.

Imbalance	Signs	Risk Factors	Care Management
Hypoglycemia			
Hypocalcemia			

36. SPECIFY the guidelines a nurse should follow to ensure accuracy of the findings and safety of the newborn when measuring the newborn. INDICATE the expected range for the term newborn.
Weight

Head circumference

Chest circumference

Abdominal circumference

Length

37. Maintaining a patent airway and supporting respirations to ensure an adequate oxygen supply in the newborn are essential focuses of nursing care management of the newborn especially in the early postbirth period.

   A. *STATE* the four conditions that are essential for maintaining an adequate oxygen supply in the newborn.

   B. *LIST* four signs that the nurse who is assessing a newborn would recognize as indicative of abnormal breathing.

   C. *DESCRIBE* three methods of relieving airway obstruction in an infant.

MULTIPLE CHOICE: Circle the one correct option and state the rationale for the option chosen.

38. A newborn male is estimated to be 40 weeks' gestation following an assessment using the New Ballard scale. A Ballard scale finding consistent with this newborn's full-term status would be:
   A. Apical pulse rate of 120 beats per minute, regular, and strong
   B. Popliteal angle of 160 degrees
   C. Weight of 3200 g placing him at the 50th percentile
   D. Thinning of lanugo with some bald areas

39. The nurse evaluates the laboratory test results of a 1-day-old, term newborn. Which of the following results would require notification of the pediatrician?
   A. Hemoglobin 22 g/dl
   B. Hematocrit 54%
   C. Glucose 45 mg/dl
   D. Total bilirubin 10 mg/dl

40. A newborn male has been designated as large for gestational age. His mother was diagnosed with gestational diabetes late in her pregnancy. The nurse should be alert for signs of hypoglycemia. Which of the following assessment findings would be consistent with a diagnosis of hypoglycemia?
   A. Unstable body temperature
   B. Cyanosis
   C. Edema of the extremities
   D. Abdominal distention

41. A radiant warmer will be used to help a newborn girl to stabilize her temperature. The nurse implementing this care measure should:
    A. Undress and dry the infant before placing her under the warmer
    B. Set the control panel between 35° to 38° C
    C. Place the thermistor probe on the left side of her chest just below her nipple
    D. Assess her rectal temperature every hour until her temperature stabilizes

42. A newborn male has been scheduled for a circumcision. Essential nursing care measures as part of this surgical procedure would include which one of the following?
    A. Feed the bottle-fed infant just prior to the procedure to help him remain relaxed and quiet
    B. Apply petrolatum to the site with every diaper change for the first 24 hours
    C. Check the penis for bleeding every 2 hours for the first 24 hours
    D. Teach the parents to remove the yellowish exudate that forms over the glans using a diaper wipe

CRITICAL THINKING EXERCISES

1. Apgar scoring is a method of newborn assessment used in the immediate postbirth period, at 1 and 5 minutes. *INDICATE* the Apgar score for each of the following newborns.

    Baby boy at 1 minute after birth:
       Heart rate—160 beats per minute
       Respiratory effort—good, crying vigorously
       Muscle tone—active movement, well flexed
       Reflex irritability—cries with stimulus to soles of feet
       Color—body pink, feet and hands cyanotic

    SCORE:
    INTERPRETATION:
    Baby girl at 5 minutes after birth:
       Heart rate—102 beats per minute
       Respiratory effort—slow, irregular with weak cry
       Muscle tone—some flexion of extremities
       Reflex irritability—grimace with stimulus to soles of feet
       Color—pale

    SCORE:
    INTERPRETATION:

2. Baby girl June was just born.
    A. *OUTLINE* the protocol that the nurse should follow when assessing June's physical status during the 2 hours after her birth.

B. *STATE* the nurse's legal responsibility regarding identification of June and her mother after birth.

C. *CITE* two priority nursing diagnoses appropriate for June during the first 2 hours after birth.

D. *IDENTIFY* the priority nursing care measures that the nurse must implement to ensure June's well-being and safety during the first 2 hours after birth.

3. Baby boy Tim is 24 hours old. The nurse is preparing to perform a physical examination of this newborn prior to his discharge.
   A. *LIST* the actions the nurse should take in order to ensure safety and accuracy. *INCLUDE* the rationale for the actions identified.

   B. *IDENTIFY* the major points that should be assessed as part of this physical examination.

   C. *SUPPORT* the premise that Tim's parents should be present during this examination.

4. Baby girl Susan has an accumulation of mucus in her nasal passages and mouth making breathing difficult.
   A. *STATE* the nursing diagnosis represented by the assessment findings.

B. *LIST* the steps that the nurse should follow when clearing Susan's airway using a bulb syringe.

C. If mucus accumulation continues and breathing is compromised, use of a nasopharyngeal catheter with mechanical suction may be required. *LIST* the guidelines a nurse should follow when using this method to clear the newborn's airway.

5. Susan and James are taking their newly circumcised (6 hours postprocedure) baby home. This is their first baby and they express anxiety concerning care of the circumcision.
   A. *STATE* one nursing diagnosis related to this situation.

   B. *STATE* one expected outcome related to the nursing diagnosis identified.

   C. *SPECIFY* the instructions that the nurse should give to Susan and James regarding the assessment and care measures required to facilitate healing of the circumcision site.

6. Andrew and Marion are parents of a newborn, 30 hours old, who has developed hyper-bilirubinemia. They are very concerned about the color of their baby and the need to put the baby under special lights. "A relative was yellow just like our baby and later died of liver cancer!!"
   A. *DESCRIBE* how the nurse should respond to Andrew and Marion's concern.

   B. *DESCRIBE* the blanch test as a method of assessment for jaundice.

C. *IDENTIFY* the expected assessment findings and physiologic effects related to hyperbilirubinemia.

D. *LIST* the precautions and care measures required by the newborn undergoing phototherapy in order to prevent injury to the newborn yet maintain the effectiveness of the treatment. *STATE* the rationale for each action identified.

7. A newborn is scheduled for a circumcision. The nurse caring for this newborn is aware that he will experience pain as a result of this procedure.
    A. *DESCRIBE* the most common behavioral responses to pain.

    B. *INDICATE* how a newborn's vital signs and integument will change when he experiences pain.

    C. *EXPLAIN* how the CRIES assessment can be used to monitor a newborn's pain during circumcision.

    D. *STATE* the nursing diagnosis reflective of this pain experience.

    E. *OUTLINE* the nonpharmacologic and pharmacologic measures the nurse could use or suggest be used to minimize the pain experience and its effects and maximize the newborn's ability to cope with the pain and recover.

ONLINE LEARNING ACTIVITIES

A couple is expecting their baby's birth in approximately 2 weeks. A sonogram has revealed that they are going to have a baby boy. They are unsure about having their baby circumcised. Describe how you would help this couple search the Internet for information that will help them to make an informed decision. Identify several sites that they could use.

CHAPTER 27

Newborn Nutrition and Feeding

CHAPTER REVIEW ACTIVITIES

1. It is critical that infants ingest an appropriate amount of calories and fluid each day to support their rapid growth and development.

A. *FILL IN THE BLANKS:* The daily energy requirements for the first 3 months of life is _____ kcal/kg; for 3 to 6 months of life, the daily requirement is _____ kcal/kg; for 6 to 9 months it is _____ kcal/kg; and it is _____ kcal/kg from 9 months to 1 year. Human milk provides _____ kcal/100 ml or _____ kcal/oz. Infants require _____ ml/kg of water/fluid in a 24-hour period. Formula or breast milk easily meets this requirement.

B. *CALCULATE* the daily energy (kcal) requirement for each of the following newborns.

Infant	Calories (kcal)
Jim: 1 month 4 kg	
Sue: 4 months 6 kg	
Sam: 7 months 7.5 kg	
Jean: 10 months 10.5 kg	

2. Development and function of lactation structures within the breast are critical to the success of lactogenesis.
   A. *LABEL* the following illustration as indicated:

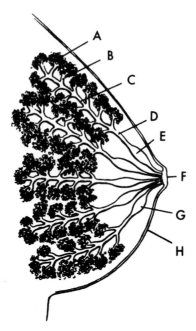

Lactation Structures of the Female Breast

B. *FILL IN THE BLANKS:* Insert the lactation structure that corresponds to the following descriptions:

   1) _____ Structures in the breast that are composed of alveoli, milk ductules, and myoepithelial cells. There are 15 to 20 in each female breast.
   2) _____ Milk-producing cells.
   3) _____ Breast structure that connects several alveoli.
   4) _____ Breast structure that connects a duct to the lactiferous sinus.
   5) _____ Milk collection structures that narrow to form many openings or pores in the nipple. They are compressed with infant sucking and the milk is ejected.
   6) _____ Cells surrounding alveoli; these cells contract in response to oxytocin, resulting in the milk ejection reflex or let-down.
   7) _____ Rounded, pigmented section of tissue surrounding the nipple.

3. A nurse has been asked to participate in a women's health seminar for women of childbearing age in the community. Her topic will be "Breastfeeding—The Goals for Healthy People 2010 and Beyond." *OUTLINE* the points that this nurse should emphasize in order to help women to appreciate the benefits of breastfeeding and to seriously consider breastfeeding when they have a baby.

4. It is important that a breastfeeding woman alter the position she uses for breastfeeding as one means of preserving nipple and areolar integrity. *DESCRIBE* four breastfeeding positions the nurse should demonstrate to a woman who is breastfeeding her newborn.

5. Infants exhibit feeding readiness cues as they recognize and express their hunger.
   A. *IDENTIFY* feeding readiness cues of the infant.

   B. *STATE* why the new mother should be guided by these cues when determining the timing of feeding sessions.

6. *INDICATE* the difference between foremilk and hindmilk.

7. *LABEL* each of the following illustrations depicting the maternal breastfeeding reflexes.

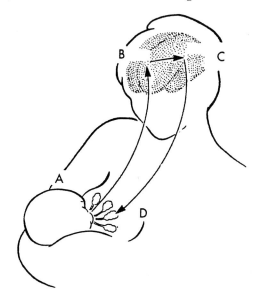

Milk Production Reflex

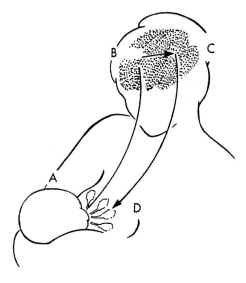

Let-Down Reflex

8. There are three stages of lactogenesis. *STATE* expected time of occurrence for each stage and *DESCRIBE* the events typical of each stage.

Stage I

Stage II

Stage III

9. Proper latch-on is essential for effective breastfeeding and preservation of nipple and areolar tissue integrity.

A. *INDICATE* the steps the nurse should teach a breastfeeding woman to follow to ensure a proper latch-on.

B. When observing a woman breastfeeding, it is essential that the nurse determine the effectiveness of the latch-on. *STATE* the signs a nurse should look for that would indicate a proper latch-on.

C. *DESCRIBE* the way a woman should remove her baby from her breast after feeding is completed.

10. A breastfeeding woman has been having difficulty calming down her fussy baby daughter in order to feed her. *IDENTIFY* several techniques that the nurse could teach this woman to calm her baby in preparation for feeding.

11. *COMPLETE THE FOLLOWING TABLE* by identifying the factors that should be assessed before and during breastfeeding and the factors for ongoing assessment as related to the infant and the breastfeeding mother.

Infant/Mother	Assessment Before and During Breastfeeding	Ongoing Assessment
Infant		
Mother		

FILL IN THE BLANKS: Insert the term that corresponds to each of the following descriptions associated with the breastfeeding process.

12. _____ is an infection of the breast which may be manifested by a swollen, tender breast and sudden onset of flu-like symptoms.
13. _____ is manual application of gentle but deep pressure to the breasts in order to trigger the let-down reflex and facilitate expression of milk.
14. The process of milk production is termed _____ or _____.
15. Exposing the newborn to both breast and bottle nipples can lead to nipple _____, a difficulty in knowing how to latch on to the breast after having taken a bottle.
16. A _____ is a professional who specializes in breastfeeding and may be available to assist a new mother with breastfeeding while in the hospital or after discharge.
17. _____ occurs 3 to 5 days after birth, when an increased volume of milk fills the breasts, which then become tender, swollen, hot and hard, and even shiny and red.
18. _____ are newborn behaviors that indicate hunger and a desire to eat.
19. Process whereby the infant is gradually introduced to drinking from a cup and eating solid food while breastfeeding is reduced by gradually decreasing the number of feedings is termed _____.
20. An _____ nipple becomes hard, erect, and protrudes upon stimulation, thereby facilitating latch-on. An _____ nipple remains flat and soft and does not protrude even when stimulated. A breast _____ is a plastic device that can be placed over the nipple and areola to keep clothing off the nipple and put pressure around the base of the nipple to promote protrusion of the nipple. The _____ reflex occurs when the infant cries, suckles, or rubs up against the breast and as a result the nipple becomes erect. This reflex is an integral part of lactation.
21. _____ is a very concentrated, high-protein, immunoglobulin-rich substance present in the breasts before the formation of milk.

22. Pituitary hormones play an essential role in lactation. _____, the lactogenic hormone, is secreted by the anterior pituitary gland in response to the infant's suck and emptying of the breast. _____ is the posterior pituitary hormone that triggers the let-down reflex.

23. _____ is a late sign of hunger in infants. Some infants will _____ or go into a deep sleep if their hunger needs are not met promptly.

24. _____ refers to a period lasting about 24 to 48 hours when the infant will be fussy and desires to eat more often than usual. Milk production will increase in response to demand.

25. _____ is an infection that is caused by a fungus or yeast. It causes thrush in the newborn's mouth. Both of the mother's nipples and the baby's mouth must be treated simultaneously.

26. For the _____ position, the mother holds the baby's head and shoulders in her hand with the baby's back and body tucked under the arm. For this _____ position, the baby's head is positioned in the crook of the arm and the mother and baby are "tummy to tummy."

27. The _____ reflex, also known as the _____ reflex, is triggered by the contraction of myoepithelial cells. Colostrum and later milk are ejected toward the nipple.

28. The _____ reflex is stimulated when a hungry baby's mouth or lips are touched. The baby opens its mouth and begins to suck. A newborn will automatically push solid food out of its mouth when it is placed on its tongue as a result of the _____ reflex.

29. _____ occurs when the baby is positioned onto the breast with its mouth open wide and tongue down. The nipple and some of the areola should be in the baby's mouth.

TRUE OR FALSE: Circle "T" if true or "F" if false for each of the following statements. Correct the false statements.

T F 30. Approximately 75% of infants in the United States are breastfed till they are 6 months of age.

T F 31. The most significant increase in breastfeeding is among well-educated, upper-income, Caucasian women.

T F 32. A newborn should lose no more than 10% of its birth weight.

T F 33. The birth weight of a full-term newborn is usually regained within 10 to 14 days of life.

T F 34. In order to prevent fat-related cardiovascular problems later in life, bottle-fed infants should be given low-fat or skim milk after the first 6 months of life.

T F 35. Infants who are entirely breastfed should receive iron supplementation in the form of iron-containing foods such as cereals after the first 6 months of life.

T F 36. Women who have large breasts will produce more milk than women who have small breasts.

T F 37. Milk production primarily depends on prolactin secretion.

T F 38. Women from some cultures do not give colostrum to their babies and breastfeed only when the milk comes.

T F 39. Early and frequent feeding facilitates the elimination of bilirubin in feces, thereby reducing the incidence or severity of hyperbilirubinemia.

T F 40. Diabetic women should avoid breastfeeding because insulin requirements are increased.

T F 41. Colostrum acts a laxative to remove meconium from the newborn's intestine.

T F 42. Breastfed babies require vitamin C supplementation.

T   F   43. Smoking can inhibit milk production.

T   F   44. When a newborn is breastfed, pacifiers should be avoided until breastfeeding is well established.

T   F   45. Uterine cramping during and after breastfeeding for the first 3 to 5 days indicates that oxytocin is being secreted during breastfeeding.

T   F   46. Fluoride supplementation should begin at 2 months for breastfed and bottle-fed babies not receiving fluoridated water.

T   F   47. A woman with mastitis should stop breastfeeding temporarily as soon as the diagnosis of infection is made.

MULTIPLE CHOICE: Circle the one correct option and state the rationale for the option chosen.

48. During a home visit, the mother of a 1-week-old infant son tells the nurse that she is very concerned about whether her baby is getting enough breast milk. The nurse would tell this mother that at 1 week of age a well-nourished newborn should exhibit
   A. Weight gain sufficient to reach his birth weight
   B. A minimum of three bowel movements each day
   C. Approximately 10 to 12 wet diapers each day
   D. Breastfeeding at a frequency of every 4 hours or about 6 times each day

49. A woman is trying to calm her fussy baby daughter in preparation for feeding. She would exhibit a need for further instruction if she:
   A. Removes all clothing from infant except the diaper
   B. Dims lights in the room and turns off the television
   C. Gently rocks the baby and talks to her in a low voice
   D. Allows the baby to suck on her finger

50. The nurse should teach breastfeeding mothers about breast care measures to preserve the integrity of the nipples and areola. Which of the following should the nurse include in these instructions?
   A. Cleanse nipples and areola twice a day with mild soap and water
   B. Apply vitamin E cream to nipples and areola before each feeding
   C. Insert plastic-lined pads into the bra to absorb leakage and protect clothing
   D. Apply modified lanolin to both dry and sore nipples

51. A breastfeeding woman asks the nurse about birth control that she should use during the postpartum period. Which is the best recommendation for a safe, yet effective method during the first 6 weeks after birth?
   A. Combination oral contraceptive that she used before she was pregnant
   B. Barrier method using a combination of a condom and spermicide foam
   C. Progestin-only contraceptive such as Norplant or Depo-Provera
   D. Complete breastfeeding—baby only receives breast milk for nourishment

52. A woman has determined that bottle feeding is the best feeding method for her. Instructions the woman should receive regarding this feeding method should include
    A. Place baby in a prone position after a feeding to facilitate passage of air bubbles
    B. Sterilize water by boiling, then cool and mix with formula powder or concentrate
    C. Expect a 1-week-old newborn to drink approximately 30 to 60 ml of formula at each feeding
    D. Microwave refrigerated formula prior to feeding the newborn

CRITICAL THINKING EXERCISES

1. *EVALUATE* each of the following actions of Janet, a breastfeeding mother. *DETERMINE* if the action indicates competency (+) or a need for further instruction (−). *INDICATE* what information you would give Janet to correct actions that require further instruction.

    _____ A. Washes her breasts thoroughly with soap and water twice a day.

    _____ B. Expresses a small amount of breast milk into her nipple and areola before initiating latch-on.

    _____ C. Lines her bra with a thick plastic-lined pad to absorb leakage.

    _____ D. Positions baby supporting back and shoulders securely and then brings her breast toward the baby, putting the nipple in its mouth.

    _____ E. Alternates breastfeeding positions among football, cradle, and modified cradle holds.

    _____ F. Limits breastfeeding at the first breast to a maximum of 10 minutes, then switches to the second breast.

    _____ G. Supports her breast with four fingers underneath the breast and thumb on the top at the back edge of the areola.

    _____ H. Inserts her finger into the corner of her baby's mouth between the gums to break the suction, before removing him from the breast.

    _____ I. Awakens the baby every 2–3 hours day and night to feed.

    _____ J. Increases her fluid intake to 3 L/day by drinking water, coffee, juice, milk, cola, wine, and beer.

    _____ K. Increases her caloric intake by 500 calories each day with a gradual weight loss noted.

    _____ L. Plans to use the "pill" for birth control beginning at 3 weeks postpartum.

2. Tonya is bottle feeding her baby. She expresses concern to the nurse at the well-baby clinic about heart disease and cholesterol levels as they relate to her 2-month-old baby. She tells the nurse that her family has a history of cardiac disease and hypertension and she has already changed her diet and wants to do the same for her baby. Tonya asks, "When should I start giving my baby skim milk instead of the prepared formula that I am using, which seems to contain quite a bit of fat?" *DISCUSS* how the nurse should respond to Tonya's question.

3. Elise and her husband Mark are experiencing their first pregnancy. During one of their prenatal visits, they tell the nurse that they are as yet unsure about the method they want to use for feeding their baby. "Everyone has an opinion—some say breastfeeding is best, yet others tell us that bottle feeding is more convenient especially because the father can help. What should we do?"

A. *IDENTIFY* one nursing diagnosis and one expected outcome appropriate for this situation.

B. *DISCUSS* why is it important for the pregnant couple to make this decision together.

C. *INDICATE* why is it preferable to make this decision during the prenatal period rather than waiting until the baby is born.

D. *DESCRIBE* how the nurse could use the decision-making process to assist Elise and Mark to choose the method that is best for them.

4. Mary, as a first time breastfeeding mother, has many questions. *DESCRIBE* how you would respond to the following questions and comments.

A. "I am so afraid that I will not make enough milk for my baby. My breasts are not as large as some of my friends who breastfeed."

B. "Everyone keeps talking about this let-down that is supposed to happen. What is it and how will I know I have it?"

C. "How can I possibly know if breastfeeding is going well and my baby is getting enough if I cannot tell how many ounces he gets with each feeding?"

D. "It is only the first day that I am breastfeeding and my nipples already feel sore. What can I do to relieve this soreness and prevent it from getting worse?"

E. "My friends all told me to watch out for the fourth day and engorgement. What can I do to keep it from happening or at least take care of myself when it does?"

F. "Every time I breastfeed, I get cramps and my flow seems to get heavier. Is there something wrong with me?"

G. "I am so glad I do not have to worry about getting pregnant again as long as I am breastfeeding. I hate using birth control and my friend told me I do not have to as long as I am breastfeeding!!"

H. "What should I do when I am ready to stop feeding my baby?"

5. Before discharge with her healthy, full-term baby boy, Jane, a primiparous woman, asks the nurse about when she should start solid foods such as cereals "so that the baby will sleep through the night?" *DESCRIBE* how the nurse should respond to Jane's request for information.

6. Susan is 2 days old. She last fed 5 hours ago. Her mother tells the nurse that Susan is so sleepy that she just does not have the heart to wake her.
   A. *IDENTIFY* one nursing diagnosis and one expected outcome appropriate for this newborn.

   B. *DISCUSS* the approach the nurse should take with regard to this situation.

7. Alice has decided that for personal and professional reasons, bottle feeding with a commercially prepared formula is the feeding method that is best for her. She tells the nurse that she hopes she made a good decision for her baby. "I hope she will be well nourished and feel that I love her even though I am bottle feeding."
   A. *DESCRIBE* how the nurse should respond to Alice's concern.

   B. *STATE* three guidelines for bottle-feeding technique that the nurse should teach Alice to ensure the safety and health of her baby.

ONLINE LEARNING ACTIVITIES

Access the Lowdermilk, Perry **Evolve** website at **http://evolve.elsevier.com/Lowdermilk/MatWmnHlth/** and enter the **Student** portion through the **Learning Resources** section. Use Chapter 27 as a starting point to search the Internet for websites that are designed to inform and support breastfeeding women. Prepare a report that includes the following:
- List of at least three relevant sites
- Description of the site that you found to be the most helpful, in terms of:
  - Sponsoring person(s), agency, organization
  - Clarity, accuracy, accessibility (ease of use), depth, and value of the information provided
  - Nature of the support provided
  - Currency—frequency of site updates
  - Variety of links to other relevant sites
  - Ability of persons visiting the site to obtain additional information and individualized support through such services as e-mail and chat rooms

- Discussion regarding how you would use these sites and the services they provide to assist women who are breastfeeding. Prepare a handout that you could give to women in a prenatal or postpartum breastfeeding class about the sites that you found and guidelines that the women could follow in using these or other relevant sites

CHAPTER **28**

Care of the Newborn at Home

CHAPTER REVIEW ACTIVITIES

TRUE OR FALSE: Circle "T" if true or "F" if false for each of the following statements. Correct the false statements.

T F 1. Helping to bring the baby home from the hospital is a good way to facilitate sibling adjustment to the changes the newborn will bring to their lives.

T F 2. The infant's crib should be placed on an inner wall to prevent cold stress as a result of heat loss by radiation.

T F 3. Parents should apply alcohol to their newborn's umbilical cord at every diaper change.

T F 4. The cord will fall off about 7 days after birth.

T F 5. When caring for their circumcised newborn, parents should apply petrolatum to the glans with each diaper change.

T F 6. Infants should be placed in a rear-facing car seat that is secured in the back seat of the car until they are at least 20 pounds and 1 year of age.

T F 7. Nonnutritive sucking with a pacifier or finger should be discouraged in the infant because it leads to malformation of the jaw and to dependency.

T F 8. The posterior fontanel closes by 1 month of age.

T F 9. An infant usually develops the ability to smile in response to various stimuli by 2 months of age.

T F 10. Infant massage can be used to reduce discomfort associated with colic.

T F 11. The first DPT (diphtheria, tetanus, pertussis) immunization should be given when the infant is 4 months of age.

T F 12. Breastfeeding provides a form of passive immunity as a result of antibodies present in colostrum and breast milk.

T F 13. Parents should report diarrhea as soon as their infant has four consecutive green, watery stools.

T F 14. An infant temperature above 36° C is considered fever.

T F 15. By 3 weeks of age, many newborns develop a regular end-of-the-day fussy period.

T F 16. Four back blows between the infant's shoulder blades using the heel of the hand is a recommended technique for the relief of airway obstruction in the newborn.

T F 17. CPR for infants recommends 10 cycles of 5 compressions and 1 ventilation (a 5:1 ratio) should be performed followed by a check of the brachial artery for pulsation.

T F 18. Five chest compressions should be completed in 10 seconds or less.

Chapter 28: Care of the Newborn at Home   257

19. *STATE* the factors parents should consider when creating a protective environment at home for their newborn.

20. *EXPLAIN* how parents can help their 2-month-old infant to learn.

21. Massage offers an excellent opportunity for parents and infants to interact with one another. *IDENTIFY* three infant benefits and three parental benefits for each of the following domains.
    Psychosocial domain

    Physiologic/physical domain

22. *DESCRIBE* the four recommended maneuvers that parents should be taught for relieving an airway obstruction in their infant.

MULTIPLE CHOICE: Circle the one correct option and state the rationale for the option chosen.

23. When caring for their newborn's circumcision, parents should:
    A. Check the circumcision site for bleeding every 4 hours until their newborn is 2 days old
    B. Apply firm pressure using an alcohol swab if bleeding occurs
    C. Wash area gently with warm water and apply petrolatum at every diaper change
    D. Remove the yellowish exudate that forms to prevent infection

24. Parents would require additional instruction regarding bathing their newborn baby boy if they:
    A. Adjust the temperature of the room where they will bathe their baby to 24° C (75° F)
    B. Cleanse the eyes from inner to outer canthus using separate parts of the washcloth for each eye
    C. Retract the foreskin of their newborn's uncircumcised penis, wash and rinse glans, then replace foreskin
    D. Sprinkle baby powder on their newborn's skin after it is dried thoroughly

25. Which of the following actions will help keep the infant safe within his or her home environment?
    A. Place infant in its carrier on the floor rather than on an elevated surface (e.g., table, counter, sofa)
    B. Ensure shade or blind is down at night if the infant's crib is placed under a window
    C. Tie a pacifier loosely around the infant's neck using a soft ribbon
    D. Purchase a crib with slats that are approximately 3 inches apart

26. Parents should be informed regarding the recommended schedule for immunizations. Which of the following reflects the current recommendations?
    A. DTP (diphtheria, tetanus, pertussis)—second dose at 6 months
    B. MMR (measles, mumps, rubella)—first dose at 15 months if no community outbreak
    C. HIBTITER (*Haemophilus influenzae* b conjugate)—third dose at 8 months of age
    D. HBV (hepatitis B)—first dose at 6 months of age

27. A 3-day-old newborn is receiving home phototherapy for hyperbilirubinemia. Which of the following signs, if noted in their newborn, should parents report immediately to their health care provider?
    A. Regurgitation after one or two feedings.
    B. Loose greenish stools
    C. Four voidings in the past 24 hours
    D. Axillary temperature of 37.2° C (99° F)

CRITICAL THINKING EXERCISES

1. Jane and Matthew are first-time parents of a baby girl. You are preparing them for discharge tomorrow morning. *EXPLAIN* what you should tell them about each of the following concerns in order to ease the stress they may experience during the first week at home with their baby.
   Activities of daily living

   Visitors

   Activity and rest

Sexuality

2. Prior to discharge, Mary, a primiparous mother, asks questions about basic care measures for her new son. *EXPLAIN* how you would respond to each of Mary's questions.

   A. How should I take care of my baby's umbilical cord? My grandmother told me I should always keep it covered but that does not sound right to me.

   B. My friends gave me a wonderful basket filled with special lotions, powders, and soaps. When should I start to use them because I love that "fresh baby smell"?

   C. How should I keep my baby clean? One of my friends told me I did not need to give my baby a bath every day but my mother said I should wash my baby in the tub she gave me every morning so my baby develops a routine.

   D. My son was just circumcised. What should I do to take care of him properly and make sure he stays comfortable and infection free?

   E. I know babies can get cold very quickly. What should I do to keep my baby nice and warm?

3. Mary Beth and Tim are the parents of a 3-week-old baby girl. They call the *warm line* to express their concern that their baby seems to sleep well during the day and stays awake more at night. In addition, they tell you that she has started to get very irritable late in the afternoon. *EXPLAIN* how you would respond to the concerns these parents have expressed.

4. Andrew and Marion are parents of a newborn, 36 hours old, who has developed jaundice. They are very concerned about the color of their baby. Following a serum bilirubin determination, their primary health care provider explains to Andrew and Marion that their baby needs phototherapy treatment.

   A. Andrew and Marion ask if their baby can be treated at home rather than being hospitalized. *STATE* three criteria that their infant should meet in order to be considered as a candidate for home phototherapy.

   B. *STATE* the criteria that should be met by Marion and Andrew and their home environment.

   C. *IDENTIFY* the behaviors that Marion and Andrew should report, if they note them in their baby.

5. Angela, the mother of a newborn, tells the nurse, "I know that I should get my baby immunized, but I have heard that each shot is so expensive and there are so many. Since I am breastfeeding, my baby is protected from infection anyway. Do you think it would be all right to wait until the baby's first birthday? Then he will need fewer shots." *DESCRIBE* how the nurse should reply to Angela.

ONLINE LEARNING ACTIVITIES

Access the Lowdermilk, Perry **Evolve** website at
http://evolve.elsevier.com/Lowdermilk/MatWmnHlth/ and enter the **Student** portion through the **Learning Resources** section. Use Chapter 28 as a starting point in a search of the Internet for websites designed to inform and support first-time parents as they assume the responsibilities of caring for their new baby. Prepare a report that includes the following:
- List of relevant websites
- Description of the site that you found to be the most appealing and useful, in terms of the following:
  - Sponsoring person(s), agency, organization
  - Clarity, accuracy, accessibility (ease of use), value, and depth of information provided

- List of topics covered related to newborn care measures such as feeding, bathing, safety, fostering development, etc.
- Currency—frequency of site updates
- Links to other relevant sites
- Ability of persons visiting the site to obtain additional information and advice and individualized support through such services as e-mail and chat rooms
- Discuss how nurses who teach parenting classes could use these sites to extend the support available to new parents into their homes

Assessment for Risk Factors

CHAPTER REVIEW ACTIVITIES

FILL IN THE BLANKS: Insert the term that corresponds to each of the following descriptions.

1. A _____ is a pregnancy in which the life or health of the mother or her fetus is jeopardized by a disorder coincidental with or unique to pregnancy.

2. The major expected outcome of antepartum testing is the detection of potential _____ ideally before intrauterine _____ of the fetus occurs so that the health care provider can take measures to _____ or _____ adverse perinatal outcomes.

3. _____ or "_____" is the assessment of fetal activity by the mother. It is a simple yet valuable method for monitoring the condition of the fetus. The fetal alarm signal refers to the cessation of fetal movements entirely for _____. A count of less than _____ warrants further evaluation by _____, _____, _____, or a combination of these. Fetal movements are usually not present during the fetal _____; they may be temporarily reduced if the woman is taking _____, drinking _____, or _____; they do not _____ as the woman nears term.

4. _____ is the use of sound having a frequency higher than that detectable by humans to examine structures inside the body. It can be done _____ or _____ during pregnancy. _____ is more useful after the first trimester when the pregnant uterus rises out of the pelvis. _____, in which the probe is inserted into the _____, allows _____ anatomy to be evaluated in greater detail and _____ to be diagnosed earlier. It is optimally used in the first trimester to detect _____ pregnancies, monitor the developing _____, help identify _____, and help to establish _____.

5. _____ is the noninvasive study of blood flow in the fetus and placenta. It is a helpful adjunct in the management of pregnancies at risk because of _____, _____, _____, _____, or _____.

6. _____ is a noninvasive dynamic assessment of the fetus and its environment by _____ and external _____. This test includes assessment of five variables, namely fetal _____, fetal _____, fetal _____, fetal _____ by means of a _____, and _____ volume. The presence of normal fetal _____ activities indicates that the _____ is functional and the fetus is therefore not _____.

7. _____ is a noninvasive radiologic technique used for obstetric and gynecologic diagnosis. It provides excellent pictures of soft tissue without _____.

8. _____ is performed to obtain amniotic fluid, which contains fetal cells. A needle is inserted _____ into the uterus, _____ is withdrawn, and various assessments are performed. Indications for this procedure are prenatal diagnosis of _____, assessment of _____, and diagnosis of _____.

9. Direct access to the fetal circulation during the second and third trimesters is possible through _____ or _____, which is the most widely used method for fetal _____ and _____. It involves the insertion of a needle directly into a fetal _____ under ultrasound guidance.

10. _____ is a procedure that involves the removal of a small tissue specimen from the fetal portion of the placenta. Because this tissue originates form the zygote it reflects the _____ of the fetus. It is performed between _____ and _____ weeks of gestation.

11. Determination of the _____ level is used as a screening tool for neural tube defects in pregnancy. The test is ideally performed between _____ and _____ weeks of gestation.

12. The _____ is a screening test for Down syndrome. It is performed between _____ and _____ weeks of gestation. The levels of three markers namely _____, _____, and _____, in combination with maternal _____ are used to determine risk.

13. A _____ test is based on the fact that the heart rate of a healthy fetus with an intact central nervous system will _____ in response to fetal movement.

14. The purpose of a _____ test is to identify the jeopardized fetus that is stable at rest but shows evidence of compromise when exposed to the stress of uterine contractions. If the resultant hypoxia of the fetus is sufficient, a _____ of the FHR will result. Two methods used for this test are the _____ test and the _____ test.

15. *IDENTIFY* factors that would place the pregnant woman and fetus/neonate at risk, for each of the following categories.
Biophysical

Psychosocial

Sociodemographic

Environmental

16. *DISCUSS* the role of the nurse when caring for high risk pregnant women who are required to undergo antepartal assessment testing to determine fetal well-being.

17. Annie is a primigravida who is at 10 weeks' gestation. Her prenatal history reveals that she was treated for pelvic inflammatory disease 2 years ago. She describes irregular menstrual cycles and is therefore unsure about the first day of her last menstrual period. Annie is scheduled for a transvaginal ultrasound.
    A. *CITE* the likely reasons for the performance of this test.

    B. *DESCRIBE* how the nurse should prepare Annie for this test.

18. Ally, a pregnant woman at 20 weeks' gestation, is scheduled for a series of transabdominal ultrasound tests to monitor the growth of her fetus. *DESCRIBE* the nursing role as it applies to Ally and ultrasound examinations.

19. *STATE* two risk factors for each of the following pregnancy problems.
    Preterm labor

    Polyhydramnios

    Oligohydramnios

Intrauterine growth restriction

Postterm pregnancy

Chromosomal abnormalities

TRUE OR FALSE: Circle "T" if true or "F" if false for each of the following statements. Correct the false statements.

T F 20. Over one million births that occur in the United States each year are categorized as high risk.

T F 21. In 2000, the infant mortality rate in the United States was 6.9 per 1000 live births.

T F 22. The United States has one of the lowest infant mortality rates in the world.

T F 23. During the 1990s, the maternal mortality rate in the United States ranged between 7 and 8 per 100,000 live births.

T F 24. Currently, the three major causes for maternal mortality are hypertensive disorders (e.g., preeclampsia), pulmonary embolism, and hemorrhage.

T F 25. Maternal mortality remains a significant problem because a high proportion of deaths are preventable.

T F 26. African-American women have a maternal mortality rate that is twice as high as that of Caucasian women.

T F 27. Antepartum fetal deaths account for approximately 75% of all perinatal mortality.

T F 28. Respiratory distress syndrome continues as the leading cause of neonatal mortality.

T F 29. The major expected outcome of all antepartum testing is the detection of potential fetal compromise.

T F 30. Serial measurement of the fetal biparietal diameter, limb length, and abdominal circumference by means of ultrasonography can differentiate between size discrepancy resulting from inaccurate dates, true intrauterine growth restriction (IUGR), and macrosomia.

T F 31. Oligohydramnios or a decrease in amniotic fluid amount has been associated with neural tube defects.

T F 32. The presence of meconium in amniotic fluid antepartally is usually associated with adverse fetal outcome.

T F 33. After amniocentesis or chorionic villi sampling (CVS), an Rh-negative woman should receive RhoGAM.

T F 34. The major disadvantage of a nonstress test relates to its high rate of false-negative results.

T   F   35. A lower than normal alpha-fetoprotein level in the maternal serum and in the amniotic fluid has been associated with Down syndrome.

T   F   36. In order to accurately assess results of a contraction stress test, four uterine contractions in a 15-minute period are required.

T   F   37. Higher than normal levels of alpha-fetoprotein in maternal serum are diagnostic of a fetal neural tube defect.

T   F   38. A hyperstimulation result on a contraction stress test refers to late deceleration fetal heart rate (FHR) patterns occurring as a result of excessive uterine activity or a persistent increase in uterine tone.

T   F   39. When performing a daily fetal movement count, a pregnant woman should call her health care provider if she notes five or fewer fetal movements in 1 hour.

MULTIPLE CHOICE: Circle the one correct option and state the rationale for the option chosen.

40. A 34-year-old woman at 36 weeks' gestation has been scheduled for a biophysical profile. She asks the nurse why the test needs to be performed. The nurse would tell her that the test:
    A. Determines how well her baby will breathe after it is born
    B. Evaluates the response of her baby's heart to uterine contractions
    C. Measures her baby's head and length
    D. Observes her baby's activities to ensure that her baby is getting enough oxygen

41. As part of preparing a 24-year-old woman at 42 weeks' gestation for a nonstress test, the nurse would:
    A. Tell the woman to fast for 8 hours prior to the test
    B. Explain that the test will evaluate how well her baby is moving inside her uterus
    C. Show her how to indicate when her baby moves
    D. Attach a spiral electrode to the presenting part to determine FHR patterns

42. A 40-year-old woman at 18 weeks' gestation is having a Triple Marker test performed. She is obese and her health history reveals that she is Rh negative. The primary purpose of this test is to screen for:
    A. Spina bifida
    B. Down syndrome
    C. Gestational diabetes
    D. Rh antibodies

43. During a contraction stress test, four contractions lasting 45 to 55 seconds were recorded in a 10-minute period. A late deceleration was noted during the third contraction. The nurse conducting the test would document which of the following results?
    A. Negative
    B. Positive
    C. Suspicious
    D. Unsatisfactory

44. A pregnant woman is scheduled for a transvaginal ultrasound test to establish gestational age. In preparing this woman for the test the nurse would:
    A. Place the woman in a supine position with her hips elevated on a folded pillow
    B. Instruct her to come for the test with a full bladder
    C. Administer an analgesic 30 minutes before the test
    D. Lubricate the vaginal probe with transmission gel

CRITICAL THINKING EXERCISES

1. Mary is at 42 weeks' gestation. Her physician has ordered a biophysical profile (BPP). She is very upset and tells the nurse, "All my doctor told me is that this test will see if my baby is okay. I do not know what is going to happen and if it will be painful to me or harmful for my baby."
   A. *STATE* a nursing diagnosis that reflects this situation.

   B. *DESCRIBE* how the nurse should respond to Mary's concerns.

   C. Mary receives a score of 8 for the BPP. *LIST* the factors that were evaluated to obtain this score and *SPECIFY* the meaning of Mary's test result of 8.

2. Jan, age 42, is 18 weeks' pregnant. Because of her age, Jan's fetus is at risk for genetic anomalies. Jan's blood type is A negative and her partner's, the father of her baby, is B positive. Her primary health care provider has suggested an amniocentesis. *DESCRIBE* the nurse's role in terms of each of the following:
   A. **Preparing Jan for the amniocentesis**

   B. **Supporting Jan during the procedure**

C. **Providing Jan with postprocedure care and instructions**

3. Susan, who has diabetes and is in week 36 of pregnancy, has been scheduled for a nonstress test.
   A. *DISCUSS* what you would tell Susan about the purpose of this test and what will be learned about her baby's well-being.

   B. *DESCRIBE* how you would prepare Susan for this test.

   C. *INDICATE* how you would conduct the test.

   D. *ANALYZE* the following tracings. *DESIGNATE* the result each represents and *INDICATE* the criteria you used to determine the result.

   1)

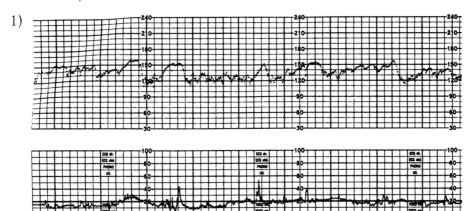

2)

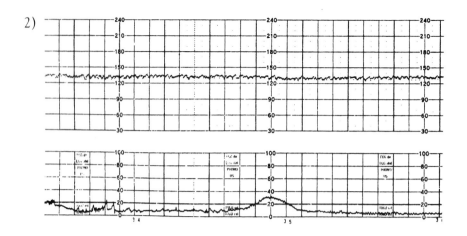

4. Beth is scheduled for a contraction stress test following a nonreactive result on a nonstress test. Nipple stimulation will be used to stimulate the required contractions.

A. *DISCUSS* what you would tell Beth about the purpose of this test and what will be learned about her baby's well-being.

B. *DESCRIBE* how you would prepare Beth for the test.

C. *INDICATE* how you would conduct the test.

D. *STATE* how you would conduct the test differently if exogenous Pitocin is used instead of nipple stimulation.

E. *ANALYZE* the following tracings. *DESIGNATE* the result each represents and *INDICATE* the criteria you used to determine the results.

1)

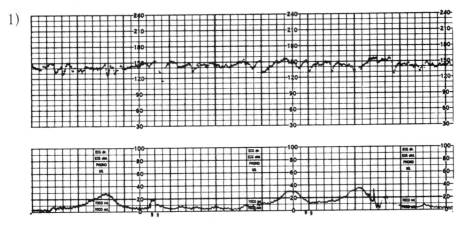

2)

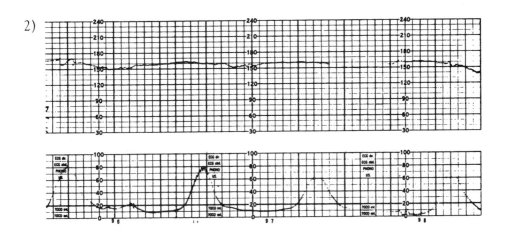

ONLINE LEARNING ACTIVITIES

1. Access the Lowdermilk, Perry **Evolve** website at **http://evolve.elsevier.com/Lowdermilk/MatWmnHlth/** and enter the **Student** portion through the **Learning Resources** section to assist you in searching the medical literature for nursing research studies related to the psychosocial impact of a high risk pregnancy on a woman and her family and the nursing measures found to be effective in providing support.
   - Create an annotated bibliography of at least five studies
   - Choose one study and complete a bibliography that includes the following:
     - Hypothesis; research question
     - Summary of the methodology used and key findings
     - Reliability of the study and its findings
     - Recommendations for further research
   - How you would use the information in these studies to improve the quality of supportive care to high risk pregnant women and their families?

Chapter 29: Assessment for Risk Factors   271

2. Use Chapter 29 of Evolve as a starting point for an Internet search to gather information about the antepartal assessment procedures discussed in this chapter. Prepare a report that includes the following:
   - List of sites that provide information about antepartal assessment methods
   - Summary of the information gathered about each test
   - Comparison of findings with the information provided in the chapter
   - Description of how you would use these sites and the information they provide to help high risk pregnant women and their families gain an understanding of the tests they are about to experience—what to expect and their role in the process

CHAPTER 30

Hypertensive Disorders in Pregnancy

CHAPTER REVIEW ACTIVITIES

MATCHING: Match the client description in Column I with the appropriate diagnosis from Column II.

COLUMN I

_____ 1. At 30 weeks' gestation, Angela's MAP was 108 mm Hg; her urinalysis indicated a protein level of +2; her weight increased 2 kg in 1 week; she exhibited dependent and upper body edema.

_____ 2. At 24 weeks' gestation, Mary's BP rose to 150/92 from a prepregnant baseline of 120/70. No other problematic signs and symptoms were noted.

_____ 3. Susan, a 34-year-old pregnant woman, has had a consistently high BP ranging from 148/92 to 160/98 since she was 28 years old. Her weight gain has followed normal patterns and urinalysis remains normal as well.

_____ 4. At 32 weeks' gestation, Maria, with hypertension since 28 weeks, generalized edema, and proteinuria of +4, has a convulsion.

_____ 5. Dawn has been hypertensive since her 24th week of pregnancy. Urinalysis indicates a protein content of +4. Further testing reveals a platelet count of 95,000 and elevated AST and ALT levels; in addition, her hematocrit is decreased and burr cells appear on a peripheral smear.

COLUMN II

A. Eclampsia
B. Chronic hypertension
C. Gestational hypertension
D. HELLP syndrome
E. Preeclampsia

FILL IN THE BLANKS: Insert the term that corresponds to each of the following descriptions of hypertensive disorders during pregnancy.

6. _____ is the onset of hypertension without proteinuria after the 20th week of pregnancy. _____ is hypertension that is present and observable before pregnancy or that is diagnosed before the 20th week of pregnancy.

7. _____, a pregnancy-specific syndrome in which hypertension usually develops after _____ of gestation in a previously normotensive woman, is a multisystem, vasospastic disease process characterized by the presence of _____ and _____. It is usually categorized as _____ or _____ in terms of management. An elevated blood pressure is often the first sign to develop.

8. _____ is defined as a systolic blood pressure greater than _____ or a diastolic blood pressure greater than _____ or mean arterial pressure of greater than _____. The elevated values must be present on _____ occasions at least _____ hours apart.

9. _____ is defined as a protein concentration of _____ g/L (_____ on dipstick measurement) or more in at least _____ random urine samples collected at least _____ apart with no evidence of urinary tract infection.

10. _____ is clinically evident, generalized accumulation of fluid in the face, hands, or abdomen that is not responsive to _____ hours of bed rest. It may also be manifested as a rapid weight gain of more than _____ in one week.

11. _____ is the presence of any one of the following in women diagnosed with preeclampsia: systolic blood pressure of at least _____ or a diastolic blood pressure of at least _____; protein concentration in the urine greater than _____ on dipstick measurement; _____, less than 400 to 500 ml of urine output over 24 hours; _____ or _____ disturbances; _____ involvement; _____ with a platelet count less than _____; _____ or _____ involvement; increased serum _____; or severe fetal _____.

12. _____ is the onset of seizure activity or coma in the woman diagnosed with preeclampsia, with no history of preexisting pathology that can result in seizure activity.

13. _____ syndrome is a laboratory diagnosis for a variant of severe preeclampsia that involves _____ dysfunction, characterized by _____, elevated _____, and low _____.

14. _____ diminishes the diameter of blood vessels, which impedes blood flow to all organs and raises blood pressure. Impaired _____ leads to degenerative aging of the placenta and possible _____ of the fetus. Reduced kidney perfusion leads to degenerative _____ changes and _____.

15. COMPLETE THE FOLLOWING TABLE by contrasting the expected physiologic adaptations of pregnancy with the ineffective responses to pregnancy characteristic of preeclampsia and eclampsia.

Expected Physiologic Adaptations	Ineffective Responses

16. *STATE* the principles you would follow to ensure the accuracy of blood pressure measurement during pregnancy.

TRUE OR FALSE: Circle "T" if true or "F" if false for each of the following statements. Correct the false statements.

T   F   17. Preeclampsia complicates 25% of all pregnancies that progress beyond the first trimester.

T   F   18. The rate for pregnancy-related hypertension has risen steadily since 1990.

T   F   19. The major maternal hazard of preeclampsia is liver failure.

T   F   20. A genetic predisposition may be partly responsible for the development of preeclampsia in some women.

T   F   21. HELLP syndrome occurs in approximately 2% to 12% of women with severe preeclampsia.

T   F   22. HELLP syndrome occurs most often in young, nulliparous African-American women.

T   F   23. Calcium gluconate is the antidote for magnesium sulfate toxicity.

T   F   24. The therapeutic serum magnesium level for the treatment of severe preeclampsia would be 10 to 12 mg/dl.

T   F   25. Pregnant women with chronic renal disease are at increased risk for developing preeclampsia.

T   F   26. Research studies have confirmed that a daily dose of low-dose aspirin is effective in preventing preeclampsia.

T   F   27. The increased incidence of preeclampsia or eclampsia in primigravidas and women pregnant by a new partner may be a result of an adverse response of the immunologic system to pregnancy.

T   F   28. When on bed rest, the woman with preeclampsia should maintain a dorsal recumbent position.

T   F   29. Sodium should be restricted to a minimal level when a woman has preeclampsia.

T   F   30. Administration of magnesium sulfate to a woman with severe preeclampsia may precipitate labor by stimulating the uterus to contract.

T   F   31. An expected outcome for the use of magnesium sulfate is the prevention of progress from preeclampsia to eclampsia.

T   F   32. Hydralazine (Apresoline) may be used to lower the blood pressure of a woman with preeclampsia.

T   F   33. Severe epigastric pain is one of the premonitory signs of eclampsia.

T   F   34. Protein restriction in the diet of a woman with preeclampsia can reduce blood pressure and edema.

T   F   35. Prompt treatment of a woman using appropriate medications, bed rest, and diet can cure preeclampsia.

T   F   36. Methergine is the oxytocic of choice to prevent or treat postpartum hemorrhage for women with preeclampsia.

37. Preeclampsia is a serious complication of pregnancy. *STATE* the risk factors associated with preeclampsia for which the nurse should be alert when doing the health history interview at the first prenatal visit.

38. *DESCRIBE* the assessment technique used to determine if the following findings are present in women with preeclampsia. (Note: You may wish to review this information in a physical assessment textbook for a complete explanation of each technique.)
Hyperreflexia

Ankle clonus

Proteinuria

Pitting edema

39. Preeclampsia and eclampsia affect both maternal and fetal well-being.
    A. *DESCRIBE* how preeclampsia and eclampsia can adversely affect the health and well-being of the fetus.

    B. *INDICATE* the fetal surveillance measures recommended for women experiencing preeclampsia.

MULTIPLE CHOICE: Circle the one correct option and state the rationale for the option chosen.

40. When measuring the blood pressure to ensure consistency and to facilitate early detection of blood pressure changes consistent with preeclampsia, the nurse should:
    A. Place the woman in a seated or a left lateral position
    B. Allow the woman to rest for 15 minutes after positioning before measuring her blood pressure
    C. Use the woman's right arm if she is lying on her left side.
    D. Use a proper sized cuff that covers at least 50% of her upper arm

41. When caring for a woman with mild preeclampsia, it is critical that during assessment the nurse is alert for signs of progress to severe preeclampsia. Progress to severe preeclampsia would be indicated by which one of the following assessment findings?
    A. Proteinuria greater than 4+, in two specimens collected 6 hours apart
    B. Dependent edema in the ankles and feet at bedtime
    C. Deep tendon reflexes 2+, ankle clonus is absent
    D. Blood pressure of 154/94 and 156/100, 6 hours apart

42. A woman's preeclampsia has advanced to the severe stage. She is admitted to the hospital and her primary health care provider has ordered an infusion of magnesium sulfate be started. In implementing this order the nurse would:
    A. Prepare a solution of 20 g of magnesium sulfate in 100 cc of 5% glucose in water
    B. Monitor maternal vital signs, FHR patterns, and uterine contractions every hour
    C. Expect the maintenance dose to be approximately 4 g/hour
    D. Report a respiratory rate of 12 breaths or less per minute to the primary health care provider immediately

43. The primary expected outcome for care associated with the administration of magnesium sulfate would be met if the woman:
    A. Exhibits a decrease in both systolic and diastolic blood pressure
    B. Experiences no seizures
    C. States that she feels more relaxed and calm
    D. Urinates more frequently resulting in a decrease in pathologic edema

44. A woman has been diagnosed with mild preeclampsia and will be treated at home. The nurse, in teaching this woman about her treatment regimen for mild preeclampsia, would tell her to:
    A. Weigh herself daily after dinner or just before going to bed
    B. Place a dipstick into her urine stream as she begins to urinate to check for protein in the urine
    C. Reduce her fluid intake to four to five 8-ounce glasses each day
    D. Do gentle exercises such as hand and feet circles and gently tensing and relaxing of arm and leg muscles

CRITICAL THINKING EXERCISES

1. Jean (2–1–0–0–1) is at 30 weeks' gestation and has been diagnosed with mild preeclampsia. The treatment plan includes home care with limited activity consisting of bed rest with bathroom privileges and out of bed twice a day for meals, appropriate nutrition, and stress reduction. She and her husband are very anxious about the diagnosis and are also concerned about how they will manage the care of their active 3-year-old daughter Anne.

   A. *INDICATE* the clinical manifestations that would have been present to indicate this diagnosis.

   B. *LIST* three priority nursing diagnoses for Jean and her family.

   C. *DESCRIBE* how you would help this couple to organize their home care routine.

   D. *SPECIFY* what you would teach them with regard to assessment of Jean's status in terms of each of the following:
   Blood pressure

   Weight

   Protein in urine

   Fetal well-being

Signs of a worsening condition

E. *DESCRIBE* the instructions you would give Jean regarding her nutrient and fluid intake.

F. *DISCUSS* the measures Jean can use to cope with the boredom and alteration in circulation and muscle tone that accompany bed rest.

G. Limited activity can lead to a nursing diagnosis of Risk for constipation related to changes in bowel function associated with pregnancy and limited activity. *CITE* two measures that Jean can use to enhance bowel elimination and prevent constipation.

2. Ellen, a pregnant woman at 37 weeks' gestation, is admitted to the hospital with a diagnosis of severe preeclampsia.
A. *INDICATE* the signs and symptoms that would have been present to indicate this diagnosis.

B. *LIST* three priority nursing diagnoses for Ellen.

C. *SPECIFY* the precautionary measures that should be taken to protect Ellen and her fetus from injury.

D. Ellen's physician orders magnesium sulfate to be infused at 4 g in 20 minutes as a loading dose, then a maintenance intravenous infusion of 2 g/hr.

   1) *IDENTIFY* the guidelines that must be followed when administering the magnesium sulfate infusion.

   2) *WRITE* one nursing diagnosis related to the treatment with magnesium sulfate.

   3) *EXPLAIN* the expected therapeutic effect of magnesium sulfate to Ellen and her family.

   4) *LIST* the maternal-fetal assessments that should be accomplished on a regular basis during the infusion of magnesium sulfate.

   5) *IDENTIFY* the progressive signs of magnesium sulfate toxicity.

   6) *STATE* the interventions that must be instituted immediately if magnesium sulfate toxicity occurs.

E. Despite all prevention efforts, Ellen has a convulsion.

   1) *SPECIFY* the nursing measures that should be implemented at the onset of the convulsion and immediately afterwards.

   2) *LIST* the problems that can occur as a result of the convulsion that Ellen experienced.

F.   Ellen successfully gave birth vaginally despite her high risk status. *DESCRIBE* Ellen's care management during the first 48 hours of her postpartum recovery period.

ONLINE LEARNING ACTIVITIES

Access the Centers for Disease Control and Prevention (CDC) and the National Center for Health Statistics (NCHS) websites to gather statistical information regarding the scope of the problem of hypertensive disorders in pregnancy. Create a chart that includes the following:
- Incidence of each of the types of pregnancy-related hypertensive disorders in your state and in the nation as a whole
- Characteristics of women who develop these disorders
- Impact of pregnancy-related hypertensive disorders on maternal and fetal/newborn morbidity and mortality
- Types of treatment modalities used (e.g., home care, hospital care, magnesium sulfate infusion, antihypertensive therapy)

CHAPTER 31

Antepartal Hemorrhagic Disorders

CHAPTER REVIEW ACTIVITIES

FILL IN THE BLANKS: Insert the appropriate term for each description of antepartal bleeding.

1. Early in pregnancy _____, _____, _____, or _____ are the most common causes for excessive bleeding.

2. Late in pregnancy _____, _____, or variations in the _____ and the _____ may cause hemorrhage.

3. _____ is defined as the termination of pregnancy that occurs before the fetus is able to _____. This period is before _____ weeks of gestation. A fetal weight of less than _____ may also be used to define this type of pregnancy loss. A _____, commonly called a miscarriage results from natural causes. There are five types of miscarriage: _____, _____, _____, _____, and _____.

4. Evaluation of the serum level of the placental hormone _____ and assessment of the viability of the _____ using _____ are two diagnostic tests that can be used when a pregnant woman is exhibiting signs of miscarriage.

5. Incompetent cervix or _____ is a cause of late miscarriage. Current research contends that cervical incompetence is _____ and exists as a continuum that is determined in part by cervical _____. Other factors include _____ of the cervical tissue and the individual circumstances associated with the pregnancy in terms of maternal _____ and _____. _____ and _____ of the pregnancy at progressively earlier gestational ages are characteristics of this cervical disorder. A cervical _____ may be performed at _____ weeks of gestation in an attempt to maintain the pregnancy. Conservative management may include _____, _____, and _____.

6. _____ is one in which the _____ is implanted outside the uterine cavity, usually in the _____ of the uterine _____. An ecchymotic blueness around the umbilicus called _____ indicates _____ as a result of an undiagnosed intraabdominal pregnancy.

7. _____ or _____ is a gestational trophoblastic disease. There are two distinct types: _____ resulting from fertilization of an egg whose nucleus has been lost or inactivated and _____ resulting from two sperm fertilizing an apparently normal ovum.

8. _____ is the implantation of the placenta in the lower uterine segment near or over the _____. It is described as total or complete if the _____ is _____ covered by the placenta when the cervix is fully dilated. It is described as partial when there is _____ coverage of the _____. It is described as marginal when only an _____ of the placenta extends to the _____ but may extend into the _____ when the cervix _____ during labor. The term _____ is used when the placenta is implanted in the lower uterine segment but does not reach the _____. Risk for postpartum hemorrhage is increased because the _____ is unable to _____ around the open blood vessels of the placental site. The most important risks factors for this placental disorder are previous _____, previous _____, and _____. The risk also increases with _____ gestation, _____ pregnancies, advanced _____, _____, or _____ ethnicity, _____, and _____ use.

9. _____ or abruptio placentae is the _____ of _____ or _____ of the placenta from its _____ site. A woman who experienced abruptio placentae is at higher risk for postpartum hemorrhage as a result of _____, _____, or both. Risks for abruptio placentae include maternal _____, _____ use, _____ trauma, maternal _____, and _____.

10. _____ is a placental anomaly where the cord vessels begin to branch at the membranes and then course into the placenta. With _____, the cord blood vessels are not surrounded by Wharton's jelly or supportive tissue, thereby increasing the risk for fetal hemorrhage with _____ or _____. _____ is the term used for a marginal insertion of the cord into the placenta, which also increases the risk for fetal hemorrhage. _____ refers to a condition where the placenta is divided into two or more separate lobes.

11. _____ is a pathologic form of clotting that is diffuse and consumes large amounts of clotting factors, causing widespread _____, _____, or both.

TRUE OR FALSE: Circle "T" if true or "F" if false for each of the following statements. Correct the false statements.

T F 12. Miscarriages (spontaneous abortions) are often related to maternal behavior.
T F 13. There is little that nurses can do to reduce the incidence of miscarriages.
T F 14. A missed miscarriage refers to a pregnancy in which the fetus has died but miscarriage does not occur.
T F 15. Approximately 20% of all clinically recognized pregnancies end in miscarriage.
T F 16. A late miscarriage is one that occurs between 12 and 20 weeks of gestation.
T F 17. A woman should be advised to wait approximately 6 months after a miscarriage before attempting another pregnancy.
T F 18. An etiologic factor for incompetent cervix is the woman's mother's use of diethylstilbestrol during pregnancy with the woman.
T F 19. Ectopic pregnancy accounts for 30% of all maternal deaths.
T F 20. Ectopic pregnancy is the leading pregnancy-related cause of first-trimester maternal mortality.
T F 21. Ectopic pregnancy is a leading cause of infertility.

T F 22. The incidence of ectopic pregnancy is decreasing as a result of more effective treatment for pelvic inflammatory disease.

T F 23. Following treatment of ectopic pregnancy with methotrexate, women must return for follow-up laboratory studies until estrogen and progesterone levels decrease.

T F 24. Women who smoke are at higher risk for development of hydatidiform mole.

T F 25. Complete molar pregnancies contain embryonic or fetal parts and an amniotic sac.

T F 26. There is a lower rate of malignant transformation with an incomplete molar pregnancy.

T F 27. Multiple gestation and closely spaced pregnancies increase the risk for placenta previa.

T F 28. A woman should avoid pregnancy for at least 1 year following treatment for molar pregnancy.

T F 29. The standard for the diagnosis of placenta previa is transabdominal ultrasonic examination.

T F 30. The greatest fetal risk related to placenta previa is malpresentation.

T F 31. Maternal mortality is approximately 10% with placenta previa.

T F 32. A vaginal examination performed when a woman is exhibiting signs of placenta previa can result in profound hemorrhage.

T F 33. Premature separation of the placenta accounts for about 15% of all perinatal deaths.

T F 34. About 50% of the perinatal deaths associated with abruptio placentae occurs as a result of preterm birth.

T F 35. Abdominal trauma is the major risk factor for abruptio placentae.

T F 36. Use of cocaine can precipitate a premature separation of the placenta partly because of cocaine-induced hypertension.

T F 37. It is safe to manage a woman with a grade I premature separation of the placenta at home.

T F 38. The urinary output of women diagnosed with disseminated intravascular coagulation should be carefully monitored because renal failure is a potential complication.

39. Clotting disorders in pregnancy can result from a number of obstetric problems.
    A. *IDENTIFY* three predisposing conditions for clotting problems during pregnancy.

    B. *DESCRIBE* the pathophysiology that leads to disseminated intravascular coagulation (DIC).

    C. *INDICATE* the clinical manifestations of DIC that would be noted during physical examination and with laboratory testing.

D. *DESCRIBE* four priority nursing measures that should be used when caring for a woman experiencing DIC.

40. *EXPLAIN* the positive effects of the maternal hypervolemic state that occurs during pregnancy.

MULTIPLE CHOICE: Circle the one correct option and state the rationale for the option chosen.

41. A primigravida at 10 weeks' gestation reports mild uterine cramping and slight vaginal spotting without passage of tissue. When she is examined, no cervical dilation is noted. The nurse caring for this woman would:
    A Anticipate that the woman will be sent home and placed on bed rest with instructions to avoid stress or orgasm
    B. Prepare the woman for a dilation and curettage
    C. Notify a grief counselor to assist the woman with the imminent loss of her fetus
    D. Tell the woman that the doctor will most likely perform a cerclage to help her maintain her pregnancy

42. A woman is admitted through the emergency room with a medical diagnosis of ruptured ectopic pregnancy. The primary nursing diagnosis at this time would be:
    A. Acute pain related to irritation of the peritoneum with blood
    B. Risk for infection related to tissue trauma
    C. Deficient fluid volume related to blood loss associated with rupture of the uterine tube
    D. Anticipatory grieving related to unexpected pregnancy outcome

43. A woman diagnosed with an ectopic pregnancy is given an intramuscular injection of methotrexate. The nurse would tell the woman that:
    A. Methotrexate is an analgesic that will relieve the dull abdominal pain she is experiencing
    B. She should avoid alcohol until her primary care provider tells her the treatment is complete
    C. Follow-up blood tests will be required for at least 6 months after the injection of the methotrexate
    D. She should continue to take her prenatal vitamin to enhance healing

44. A pregnant woman at 32 weeks' gestation comes to the emergency room because she has begun to experience bright red vaginal bleeding. She reports that she is experiencing no pain. The admission nurse suspects:
    A. Abruptio placentae
    B. Disseminated intravascular coagulation
    C. Placenta previa
    D. Preterm labor

45. A pregnant woman at 38 weeks' gestation diagnosed with marginal placenta previa has just given birth to a healthy newborn male. The nurse recognizes that the immediate focus for the care of this woman would be:
   A. Preventing hemorrhage
   B. Relieving acute pain
   C. Preventing infection
   D. Fostering attachment of the woman with her new son

CRITICAL THINKING EXERCISES

1. Andrea is admitted to the hospital where a diagnosis of acute ruptured ectopic pregnancy in her fallopian tube is made.
   A. *STATE* the risk factors associated with ectopic pregnancy.

   B. *DESCRIBE* the findings that were most likely experienced and exhibited by Andrea as her ectopic pregnancy progressed and then ruptured.

   C. *IDENTIFY* the other health care problems that share the same or similar clinical manifestations as ectopic pregnancy.

   D. *STATE* the major care management problem at this time. *SUPPORT* your answer.

   E. *IDENTIFY* two priority nursing diagnoses appropriate for Andrea.

   F. *OUTLINE* the nursing measures Andrea will require during the preoperative and postoperative period.

2. Janet is 10 weeks' pregnant. She comes to the clinic and states that she has been experiencing slight bleeding with mild cramping for about 4 hours. No tissue has been passed and pelvic examination reveals that the cervical os is closed.
    A. *INDICATE* the most likely basis for Janet's signs and symptoms.

    B. *OUTLINE* the expected care management of Janet's problem.

3. Denise, a primigravida, calls the clinic. She is crying while she tells the nurse that she has noted "a lot of bleeding" and that she is sure she is losing her baby.
    A. *WRITE* several questions the nurse should ask Denise in order to obtain a more definitive picture of the bleeding she is experiencing.

    B. Based on the data collected Denise is admitted to the hospital for further evaluation. A medical diagnosis of incomplete miscarriage is made. *DESCRIBE* the assessment findings that would indicate the diagnosis of incomplete miscarriage.

    C. *STATE* the nursing diagnosis that would take priority at this time.

    D. *OUTLINE* the nursing measures that would be appropriate for the priority nursing diagnosis you identified and for the expected medical management of Denise's health problem.

    E. *SPECIFY* the instructions that Denise should receive prior to her discharge from the hospital.

F. *LIST* the nursing measures appropriate for the nursing diagnosis: Anticipatory grieving related to unexpected outcome of pregnancy.

4. Marsha (5–0–1–4–0) is a pregnant woman at 12 weeks of gestation. She has a history of early and recurring pregnancy loss. In an attempt to maintain the current pregnancy to term, a prophylactic cerclage has been performed. *OUTLINE* the discharge care and instructions the nurse should give Marsha to ensure her safe recovery at home.

5. Mary has been diagnosed with hydatidiform mole (complete).
   A. *IDENTIFY* the typical signs and symptoms Mary would most likely exhibit to establish this diagnosis.

   B. *SPECIFY* the posttreatment care and instructions that the nurse should include in a follow-up management plan with Mary and her family.

   C. A major concern, associated with hydatidiform mole, is the development of _____ which is indicated by a rising _____ titer and enlarging _____.

6. Two pregnant women are admitted to the labor unit with vaginal bleeding. Sara is at 29 weeks' gestation and is diagnosed with marginal placenta previa. Jane is at 34 weeks' gestation and is diagnosed with a moderate (grade II) premature separation of the placenta (abruptio placentae).

   A. *COMPARE* the clinical picture each of these women is likely to exhibit during assessment.

Sara	Jane

B. *IDENTIFY* two priority nursing diagnoses for both Sara and Jane.

Sara	Jane

C. *CONTRAST* the care management approach required by each of the women as it relates to their diagnosis and the typical medical management.

Sara	Jane

D. *INDICATE* the considerations that must be given top priority following birth for each of these women.

Sara	Jane

ONLINE LEARNING ACTIVITIES

Access the Lowdermilk, Perry **Evolve** website at
http://evolve.elsevier.com/Lowdermilk/MatWmnHlth/ and enter the **Student** portion through the
Learning Resources section to assist you in searching the medical literature for nursing research
studies related to a woman's reaction to early pregnancy loss as a result of miscarriage or ectopic
pregnancy.

- Create an annotated bibliography of at least four nursing research studies
- Choose one study and complete a bibliography card that includes the following:
  - Hypothesis; research question
  - Summary of the methodology used and key findings
  - Reliability of the study and its findings
  - Recommendations for further research
- Describe how you would use the findings from these research studies to provide evidenced-based
  emotional support to women who have experienced early pregnancy loss and their families
- Compare the reactions of women experiencing early pregnancy loss with those experiencing loss
  later in pregnancy

CHAPTER 32

Endocrine and Metabolic Disorders

CHAPTER REVIEW ACTIVITIES

1. *EXPLAIN* the interrelationship of each of the following clinical manifestations associated with diabetes mellitus.

   Hyperglycemia

   Polyuria

   Glycosuria

   Polydipsia

   Weight loss

   Polyphagia

FILL IN THE BLANKS: Insert the term that corresponds to each of the following descriptions.

2. Diabetes mellitus is a group of metabolic diseases characterized by _____ resulting from defects in _____, _____, or both.

3. _____ refers to excretion of large volumes of urine. _____ refers to excessive thirst and _____ refers to excessive eating. Excretion of unusable glucose results in _____.

4. _____ is the label given to type 1 or type 2 diabetes that existed before pregnancy. _____ is any degree of glucose intolerance with onset or first recognition occurring during pregnancy.

5. The key to optimal outcome of a diabetic pregnancy is strict maternal _____ before _____ and throughout the _____ period.

6. During the first trimester, the insulin dosage for the client with well-controlled diabetes may need to be reduced to avoid _____. There is an increased incidence of _____ episodes in women with type 1 diabetes during early pregnancy because _____, _____, and food _____ typical of early pregnancy result in dietary fluctuations that influence maternal _____ levels and necessitate a reduction in insulin dosage.

7. During the second and third trimester the dosage of insulin must be increased to avoid _____ and _____. _____ resistance begins as early in the second trimester of pregnancy.

8. For the pregnancy complicated by diabetes, fetal lung maturation is better predicted by the presence of _____ in the amniotic fluid rather than by the _____ / _____ ratio.

9. Glycemic control over the previous 4 to 6 weeks can be evaluated based on the determination of the level of _____ in the blood. Acceptable fasting blood glucose levels should be greater than _____ but less than _____. The 1-hour postprandial glucose should be less than _____ and the 2-hour postprandial should be less than _____. The goal of treatment is to maintain a state of _____ or normal blood glucose within a range of _____ and _____. Hypoglycemia is a blood glucose level less than _____. Hyperglycemia is a blood glucose level greater than _____.

10. Dietary management during a diabetic pregnancy must be based upon _____ levels. Energy needs are usually estimated based on _____ calories/kg of ideal body weight. _____ of total calories should be from carbohydrates. _____ carbohydrates should be limited and _____ carbohydrates that are high in fiber content should be emphasized when food choices are made. _____ of total calories should be from protein and _____ should be from fat with no more than _____ from saturated fat. Weight gain should be approximately _____ during pregnancy.

11. Blood glucose levels are measured throughout each day: before _____, _____, and _____, at _____, and in the _____. _____ measurements, 2 hours after meals may also be done. More frequent testing may be done during the _____ and _____ trimesters when insulin needs are _____. In addition, glucose levels should be checked at any sign of _____ or _____; when there is a readjustment of _____ or _____; and if _____, _____, or _____ occurs or if any _____ is present.

12. Typically _____ of the daily insulin dose is given in the morning _____
    using a combination of _____ and _____ insulin. The remaining
    _____ may be administered in the evening _____. To reduce the risk of
    _____ during the night often separate injections are given with _____
    insulin given _____ followed by _____ insulin at _____.
    Another insulin regimen would be to administer _____ insulin before each meal and
    _____ insulin at bedtime.
13. A diagnosis of _____ is made when vomiting becomes excessive enough to cause
    weight loss of at least _____ of prepregnancy weight and is accompanied by
    _____, _____, _____, and _____. Women with this
    disorder tend to be younger than _____, _____, and _____.
    They are also more likely to have _____ or _____ pregnancies.

14. COMPLETE THE FOLLOWING TABLE by identifying the major maternal and fetal/neonatal
    risks and complications associated with diabetic pregnancies.

Maternal Risks/Complications	Fetal and Neonatal Risks

15. COMPLETE THE FOLLOWING TABLE by identifying the metabolic changes that occur
    during pregnancy and indicating how these changes affect the woman with pregestational
    diabetes during the first trimester, the second and third trimesters, and the postpartum period.

Stage of Pregnancy	Metabolic Changes of Pregnancy	Impact on Diabetes
First trimester		
Second/third trimesters		
Postpartum period		

16. *EXPLAIN* the current recommendations for screening for and diagnosing gestational diabetes mellitus.

17. *STATE* how hyperthyroidism and hypothyroidism can affect reproductive well-being and pregnancy.

TRUE OR FALSE: Circle "T" if true or "F" if false for each of the following statements. Correct the false statements.

T F 18. Preconception counseling is a critical factor in the care management of the pregnancy of a woman with pregestational diabetes mellitus.

T F 19. Insulin requirements increase during the second and third trimesters.

T F 20. Women with type 2 diabetes can continue to use tolbutamide to maintain glycemic control during pregnancy.

T F 21. Strict metabolic control before conception and in the early weeks of pregnancy is an essential factor in reducing the risk of congenital anomalies.

T F 22. Even mild to moderate hypoglycemic episodes can have significant harmful effects on the fetus.

T F 23. The major cause of perinatal deaths in diabetic pregnancy is intrauterine growth restriction.

T F 24. Fasting blood glucose (FBS) levels should fall between 40 and 75 mg/dl.

T F 25. Multiple injections of insulin daily are usually required to maintain glucose control for the pregestational diabetic woman especially during the second half of pregnancy.

T F 26. Ketoacidosis occurring at any time during pregnancy can lead to intrauterine fetal death.

T F 27. Cardiac defects are the most common congenital anomalies associated with pregestational diabetes.

T F 28. A glycosylated hemoglobin level of 13% to 20% indicates good glycemic control.

T F 29. Women with diabetes should not have bedtime snacks when they are pregnant.

T F 30. It is recommended that the 2-hour postmeal (postprandial) blood glucose level be less than 120 mg/dl.

T F 31. During labor a woman's blood glucose level should be maintained between 70 and 90 mg/dl to prevent neonatal hypoglycemia.

T F 32. Insulin requirements increase substantially during the postpartum period as a result of the stress of childbirth.

T F 33. About 20% of women diagnosed with gestational diabetes will require insulin at some point during their pregnancy to maintain glycemic control.

T F 34. Women with gestational diabetes often convert to type 2 diabetes mellitus within 1 year after pregnancy.

T F 35. Gestational diabetes is primarily a condition complicating the pregnancies of young Caucasian women.

T   F   36. The incidence of congenital anomalies among infants of gestational diabetic mothers is nearly the same as for the general population.

T   F   37. A 1-hour 50-g glucose tolerance test result that is greater than 140 mg/dl confirms the diagnosis of gestational diabetes.

T   F   38. To avoid the risk of fetal intrauterine death, labor should be induced for the diabetic woman as soon as the fetal lungs are mature (usually at approximately 36 weeks' gestation).

T   F   39. The initial goal for the care management of a woman diagnosed with hyperemesis gravidarum would be restoration of her ability to retain oral fluids.

T   F   40. The primary treatment of hyperthyroidism during pregnancy is drug therapy with propylthiouracil (PTU).

T   F   41. Effectiveness of treatment for hyperthyroidism involves the monitoring of free T_3 levels on a weekly basis.

T   F   42. Infants of women with hypothyroidism often exhibit thyroid dysfunction for several months after birth.

T   F   43. Phenylketonuria (PKU) is an inborn error of metabolism that causes mental retardation if left untreated.

MULTIPLE CHOICE: Circle the one correct option and state the rationale for the option chosen.

44. A pregestational diabetic woman at 20 weeks' gestation exhibits the following: thirst, nausea and vomiting, abdominal pain, drowsiness, and increased urination. Her skin is flushed and dry and her breathing is rapid with a fruity odor. A priority nursing action when caring for this woman would be to:
    A. Provide the woman with a simple carbohydrate immediately
    B. Request an order for an antiemetic
    C. Assist the woman into a lateral position to rest
    D. Administer insulin according to the woman's blood glucose level

45. During her pregnancy, a woman with pregestational diabetes has been monitoring her blood glucose level several times a day. Which of the following levels would require further assessment?
    A. 85 mg/dl—prior to breakfast
    B. 90 mg/dl—prior to lunch
    C. 135 mg/dl—two hours after supper
    D. 100 mg/dl—at bedtime

46. Specific guidelines should be followed when planning a diet with a pregestational diabetic woman to ensure a euglycemic state. An appropriate diet would reflect:
    A. 40 calories per kg of prepregnancy weight daily
    B. A caloric distribution among three meals and at least two snacks
    C. A minimum of 350 mg of carbohydrate daily
    D. A protein intake of at least 30% of the total kcal in a day

47. An obese pregnant woman with gestational diabetes is learning self-injection of insulin. While evaluating the woman's technique for self-injection, the nurse would recognize that the woman understood the instructions when she:
    A. Washes her hands and puts on a pair of clean gloves
    B. Shakes the NPH insulin vial vigorously to fully mix the insulin
    C. Draws the NPH insulin into her syringe first
    D. Spreads her skin taut and punctures the skin at a 90-degree angle

48. A woman has just been admitted with a diagnosis of hyperemesis gravidarum. She has been unable to retain any oral intake and as a result has lost weight and is exhibiting signs of dehydration with electrolyte imbalance and acetonuria. The care management of this woman would include:
    A. Administering diphenhydramine (Benadryl) to control nausea and vomiting
    B. Keeping the woman on nothing-by-mouth status (NPO) for a maximum of 24 hours after intravenous fluids are started
    C. Avoiding oral hygiene until the woman is able to tolerate oral fluids
    D. Providing small frequent meals of bland foods and warm fluids once the woman begins to respond to treatment

CRITICAL THINKING EXERCISES

1. Mary is a 24-year-old diabetic woman. When Mary informed her gynecologist that she and her husband were trying to get pregnant, she was referred to an endocrinologist for preconception counseling. Mary tells the nurse that she just cannot understand why this is necessary. "I have been a diabetic since I was 12 years old and I have not had many problems. All I want to do is get pregnant!" DISCUSS how the nurse should respond to Mary's comments.

2. Luann is a 25-year-old nulliparous woman in her first trimester of pregnancy (sixth week of gestation). She has had type 1 diabetes since she was 15 years old. Recently, she has been experiencing some nausea and is eating less as a result. She took her usual dose of regular and NPH insulin prior to eating a very light breakfast of tea and a piece of toast. Just before her midmorning snack at work she began to experience nervousness and weakness. She felt dizzy and became diaphoretic and pale.
    A. IDENTIFY the problem that Luann is experiencing. INDICATE the basis for her symptoms.

    B. STATE the action that Luann should take.

C. *LIST* several "glucose boosters" that Luann should have on hand should this problem occur again.

3. Judy's pregnancy has just been confirmed. She also has type 1 diabetes.

A. As a result of her high risk status a variety of additional assessment measures are emphasized during her prenatal period to evaluate the status of her fetus. *IDENTIFY* these additional assessment measures and their relevance in a diabetic pregnancy.

B. *DISCUSS* the stressors that might confront Judy and her family as a result of her status as a diabetic woman who is pregnant.

C. *WRITE* two nursing diagnoses that reflect Judy's current health status.

D. *INDICATE* the activity and exercise recommendations that Judy should be given.

E. *COMPLETE THE FOLLOWING TABLE* by describing the focus, nursing interventions, and health teaching for the major components of health care required at each stage of Judy's pregnancy.

Care Component	Antepartum	Intrapartum	Postpartum
Diet			
Glucose monitoring			
Insulin requirements			

F. After birth, Judy, who will be bottle feeding, asks the nurse about birth control. *DISCUSS* the birth control options that would be best for Judy and her partner.

4. Elena (2–1–0–0–1) is a 32-year-old Hispanic-American woman in week 28 of her pregnancy. She is obese. Her mother, who is 59, was recently diagnosed with type 2 diabetes. Elena's first pregnancy resulted in the birth of a 10-pound 6-ounce daughter who is now 2 years old. A 1-hour, 50-g glucose tolerance test last week revealed a glucose level of 152 mg/dl. A 3-hour glucose tolerance test was done yesterday with the following results: Fasting—110 mg/dl, 1 hr—192 mg/dl, 2 hr—166 mg/dl, 3 hr—142 mg/dl.

A. *IDENTIFY* the complication of pregnancy Elena is exhibiting. *STATE* the rationale for your answer.

B. *LIST* the risk factors for this health problem that are present in Elena's assessment data.

C. *DESCRIBE* the pathophysiology involved in creating Elena's problem.

D. *IDENTIFY* the maternal and fetal/neonatal risks and complications that are possible in this situation.

E. *OUTLINE* the ongoing assessment measures necessitated by Elena's health problem.

F. *STATE* two nursing diagnoses for Elena and her fetus.

G. *STATE* the dietary changes Elena will have to make to maintain glycemic control during the rest of her pregnancy.

H. Before discharge after the birth of her second daughter, Elena asks the nurse if the health problem she experienced during this pregnancy will continue now that she has had her baby. She also wonders if it will happen with her next pregnancy because she wants to get pregnant again soon so she can "try for a son." *DISCUSS* the response the nurse should give to Elena's concerns.

5. Jennifer's pregnancy has just been confirmed. She has type 2 diabetes and is told that she now must learn how to give herself insulin. Jennifer becomes very upset and states, "I cannot possibly give myself a shot. Why not let me continue to take my pills since they have been working fine so far?" *DESCRIBE* how you would respond to Jennifer.

6. Marie, an 18-year-old obese primigravida, is diagnosed with hyperemesis gravidarum. She is unmarried and lives at home with her parents. Marie is admitted to the high-risk antepartal unit.
   A. *IDENTIFY* the etiologic factors that may have contributed to Marie's current health problem.

   B. *LIST* the physiologic and psychologic factors that the nurse should be alert for when assessing Marie upon her admission.

   C. *STATE* two nursing diagnoses related to Marie's current health status.

   D. *OUTLINE* the nursing care measures appropriate for Marie while hospitalized.

E. Once stabilized, Marie is discharged to home care. She is able to tolerate oral food and fluid intake. *EXPLAIN* the important care measures that the nurse should discuss with Marie and her family before she goes home.

ONLINE LEARNING ACTIVITIES

Access the website for the American Diabetes Association (ADA). Explore the site and prepare a report that includes the following:

- Summary of the information available regarding diabetes and pregnancy including both pregestational and gestational diabetes
- Types of services provided for health care professionals and services provided for pregnant women with diabetes and their families
- Discussion about how professional nurses working with women with diabetes could use the ADA site and its services to enhance the care they provide to women before they become pregnant and once they are pregnant, including the woman who is diagnosed with gestational diabetes

CHAPTER **33**

Medical-Surgical Problems in Pregnancy

CHAPTER REVIEW ACTIVITIES

FILL IN THE BLANKS: Insert the term that corresponds to each of the following descriptions.

1. _____ is the inability of the heart to maintain a sufficient cardiac output. Physiologic stress on the heart is greatest between the _____ and _____ weeks' gestation because the cardiac output is at its peak. Risk for this complication is also higher during _____ and the first _____ to _____ hours after birth.

2. _____ is a classification system for cardiovascular disorders developed by the New York Heart Association. Class I implies: _____. Class II implies: _____. Class III implies _____. Class IV implies: _____.

3. _____ is congestive heart failure with cardiomyopathy found in the last month of pregnancy or within the first 5 months postpartum, lack of another cause for heart failure, and absence of heart disease prior to the last month of pregnancy.

4. _____ refers to the damage of the heart valves and the chordae tendineae cordis as a result of an infection originating from an inadequately treated group A β-hemolytic streptococcal infection of the throat.

5. _____ is a narrowing of the opening of the valve between the left atrium and the left ventricle of the heart by stiffening of the valve leaflets, which obstructs blood flow from the atrium to the ventricles. It is the characteristic lesion resulting from _____.

6. _____ is an inflammation of the innermost lining of the heart caused by invasion of microorganisms.

7. _____ is a right-to-left or bidirectional shunting at either the atrial or ventricular level, combined with elevated pulmonary vascular resistance.

8. _____ is a common, usually benign cardiac condition that involves the protrusion of the leaflets of the mitral valve back into the left atrium during ventricular systole allowing some backflow of blood.

9. _____ is an autosomal dominant genetic disorder characterized by generalized weakness of the connective tissue, resulting in joint deformities, ocular lens dislocation, and weakness of the aortic wall and root.

10. _____ is a disorder characterized by constriction of the arteriolar vessels in the lungs leading to an increase in the pulmonary artery pressure.

11. _____ is a disease caused by the presence of abnormal hemoglobin in the blood. It is a recessive, hereditary, familial hemolytic _____ that affects those of _____ or _____ ancestry.

12. _____ is a relatively common anemia in which an insufficient amount of hemoglobin is produced to fill red blood cells.

13. _____ is an acute respiratory illness caused by allergens, marked change in ambient temperature, or emotional tension. In response to stimuli, there is widespread but reversible narrowing of the _____, making it difficult to _____. The clinical manifestations are expiratory _____, productive _____, thick _____, and/or _____.

14. _____ or shock lung occurs when the lungs are unable to maintain levels of oxygen and carbon dioxide within normal limits. In pregnancy it can be precipitated by inhalation of _____ during anesthesia, _____, _____ disorders, _____, _____ syndrome, or _____.

15. _____ is a common autosomal recessive genetic disorder in which exocrine glands produce excessive viscous secretions, which cause problems with both respiratory and digestive functions.

16. _____ is a disorder of the brain causing recurrent seizures; it is the most common neurologic disorder accompanying pregnancy.

17. _____ is a chronic, multisystem, inflammatory disease characterized by autoimmune antibody production that affects the skin, joints, kidneys, lungs, central nervous system, liver, and other body organs.

18. _____ refers to presence of gallstones in the gallbladder.

19. _____ refers to inflammation of the gallbladder.

20. _____ is the most common acute surgical condition seen in pregnancy.

21. _____ is idiopathic facial paralysis.

22. IDENTIFY the maternal and fetal complications that are more common among pregnant women who have cardiac problems.

23. At times pregnant women require abdominal surgery.
    A. IDENTIFY the factors that can complicate diagnosis of and surgical treatment for abdominal problems during pregnancy.

    B. CITE the major fear expressed by pregnant women undergoing surgery.

C. Preoperative care for a pregnant woman differs from that for a nonpregnant woman in one significant aspect, namely the presence of the _____. General preoperative observations and ongoing care are the same as for any surgery, with the addition of continuous _____ and _____ monitoring if the fetus is considered to be viable. Intrapartally fetal oxygenation is improved by placing the woman on an operating table with a _____ to avoid maternal _____. Continuous _____ and _____ must take place during the surgical procedures and in the postoperative period if intrauterine pregnancy continues. There is an increase for the onset of _____. _____ may be required to suppress uterine contractions.

D. *IDENTIFY* the nursing considerations and topics for teaching related to the discharge planning process of the pregnant woman who experienced abdominal surgery.

24. *EXPLAIN* the modifications that should be made in the protocol used for cardiopulmonary resuscitation (CPR) and the Heimlich maneuver when a woman is pregnant.

TRUE OR FALSE: Circle "T" if true or "F" if false for each of the following statements. Correct the false statements.

T F 25. A pregnant woman with a cardiac problem may be experiencing cardiovascular decompensation if she notices a sudden limitation of her ability to perform her usual activities.

T F 26. Pregnant women with cardiac problems require a diet low in both salt and potassium.

T F 27. Pregnancy is contraindicated for a woman who has had a heart transplant.

T F 28. Women using heparin during pregnancy should increase their intake of foods high in vitamin K to enhance the anticoagulant effects of the drug.

T F 29. Epidural anesthesia is generally a more effective method of pain relief than are narcotics for the labor of a woman with cardiac problems.

T F 30. Beta-adrenergic agents should be avoided if a pregnant woman with heart disease requires tocolysis.

T F 31. Anemia is the most common medical disorder of pregnancy.

T F 32. Folic acid deficiency anemia is the most common type of anemia in pregnancy.

T F 33. The pregnant woman is considered anemic when her hemoglobin level is less than 11 g/dl or her hematocrit is less than 33%.

T F 34. Iron deficiency anemia increases the incidence of cleft lip and cleft palate.

T F 35. A well-balanced diet alone is unable to prevent iron deficiency anemia in pregnancy.

T F 36. During pregnancy a woman requires a daily intake of 600 mcg of folic acid.

T F 37. Exacerbations of sickle cell crises are diminished during pregnancy if the woman has sickle cell anemia.

T F 38. Preeclampsia is more common in pregnancies complicated by thalassemia major.

T F 39. Approximately 50% of pregnant women with asthma will improve during pregnancy.

T F 40. Fentanyl should be avoided for laboring women with asthma because it may precipitate an asthmatic attack.

T F 41. In pregnancy, adult respiratory distress syndrome (ARDS) may be precipitated by severe preeclampsia.

T F 42. In the management of care for a laboring woman with cystic fibrosis, close monitoring of serum sodium and fluid balance is critical.

T F 43. The pregnant woman is more vulnerable to cholelithiasis than the nonpregnant woman.

T F 44. The incidence of Bell palsy peaks during the third trimester of pregnancy and the puerperium.

T F 45. Risk for preeclampsia and the HELLP syndrome is increased among pregnant women with systemic lupus erythematosus (SLE).

T F 46. Therapeutic abortion is recommended when a woman has multiple sclerosis because pregnancy can cause irreversible worsening of the condition.

MULTIPLE CHOICE: Circle the one correct option and state the rationale for the option chosen.

47. When assessing a pregnant woman at 28 weeks' gestation who is diagnosed with rheumatic heart disease, it is important that the nurse be alert for signs indicating cardiac decompensation. A sign of cardiac decompensation would be:
    A. Dry, hacking cough
    B. Supine hypotension
    C. Wheezing with inspiration and expiration
    D. Rapid pulse that is irregular and weak

48. A woman at 30 weeks' gestation with a class II cardiac disorder calls her primary health care provider's office and speaks to the nurse practitioner. She tells the nurse that she has been experiencing a frequent, moist cough for the past few days. In addition, she has been feeling more tired and is having difficulty completing her routine activities as a result of some difficulty with breathing. The nurse's best response would be:
    A. "Have someone bring you to the office so we can assess your cardiac status."
    B. "Try to get more rest during the day because this is a difficult time for your heart."
    C. "Take an extra diuretic tonight before you go to bed because you may be developing some fluid in your lungs."
    D. "Ask your family to come over and do your housework for the next few days so you can rest."

49. A pregnant woman with a cardiac disorder will begin anticoagulant therapy to prevent clot formation. In preparing this woman for this treatment measure the nurse would expect to teach the woman about self-administration of which of the following medications?
    A. Furosemide
    B. Propranolol
    C. Heparin
    D. Warfarin

50. At a previous antepartal visit, the nurse taught a pregnant woman diagnosed with a class II cardiac disorder about measures to use to lower her risk for cardiac decompensation. This woman would demonstrate need for further instruction if she:
    A. Increases roughage in her diet
    B. Remains on bed rest only getting out of bed to go to the bathroom
    C. Sleeps 10 hours every night and rests after meals
    D. States she will call the nurse immediately if she experiences any pain or swelling in her legs

51. A pregnant woman has been diagnosed with cholelithiasis. An important component of her treatment regimen will be dietary modification. The nurse would help this woman to plan a diet that:
    A. Reduces dietary fat to approximately 60 g per day
    B. Limits protein to 30% of total calories
    C. Chooses foods so that most calories come from carbohydrates
    D. Avoids spicy foods

CRITICAL THINKING EXERCISES

1. Linda, age 26, had rheumatic fever as a child and subsequently developed mitral valve stenosis. She is presently 6 weeks' pregnant. She is classified as class II according to the New York Heart Association functional classification of organic heart disease. This is the first pregnancy for Linda and her husband Sam.

   A. *IDENTIFY* two nursing diagnoses appropriate for Linda related to her cardiac status and her anticipated care management. *STATE* an expected outcome for each nursing diagnosis identified.

   B. *DISCUSS* a recommended therapeutic plan for Linda that will reduce her risk for cardiac decompensation in terms of each of the following:
   Rest/sleep/activity patterns

   Prevention of infection

   Nutrition

C. *IDENTIFY* physiologic and psychosocial factors that could increase the stress placed on Linda's heart during her pregnancy.

Physiologic factors

Psychosocial factors

D. *LIST* the subjective symptoms that the nurse should teach Linda and her family to look for as indicators of possible cardiac decompensation.

E. *LIST* the objective signs that could indicate that Linda is experiencing signs of cardiac decompensation and heart failure.

F. Linda is admitted to the labor unit. Her cardiac condition is still classified as class II. *OUTLINE* the nursing measures designed to assess Linda and promote optimum cardiac function during labor and birth.

G. Linda should be observed carefully during the postpartum period because cardiac risk continues. *INDICATE* the physiologic events after birth that place Linda at risk for cardiac decompensation.

H. *IDENTIFY* two nursing diagnoses that would be appropriate for the first 24 to 48 hours of Linda's postpartum period.

I. *DISCUSS* the measures the nurse can use to reduce the stress placed on the Linda's heart during the postpartum period.

J. Linda indicates that she wishes to breastfeed her infant. *DESCRIBE* the nurse's response.

K. *IDENTIFY* the important factors to be considered when preparing Linda's discharge plan.

2. Allison is a pregnant woman with a cardiac disorder. As part of her medical regimen, her primary health care provider substituted subcutaneous heparin for the oral warfarin sodium (Coumadin) she had been taking before pregnancy.
   A. Allison states, "I cannot give myself a shot! Why can't I just take the medication orally?" *DISCUSS* how you would respond as to the purpose of heparin and why it must be used instead of the Coumadin she is used to taking.

   B. *INDICATE* the information that the nurse should give Allison to ensure safe use of the heparin.

3. Jean is a primigravida at 4 weeks' gestation. She has been an epileptic for several years and her seizures have been controlled with Dilantin. Jean expresses concern regarding how her medication use will affect her pregnancy and her baby. She wants to stop taking the Dilantin. *DESCRIBE* the approach you would take in addressing Jean's concern and the course of action she is contemplating.

ONLINE LEARNING ACTIVITIES

Imagine that you have a cardiac disorder (choose one that is described in the text and choose a cardiac classification) and are considering getting pregnant (or if a male student imagine that you and your partner, who has a cardiac disorder, are planning to get pregnant). Search the Internet to help you make an informed decision about pregnancy. Prepare a report that describes your decision-making process in terms of the following:

- Information gathered regarding your (or your partner's) cardiac disorder and cardiac classification
- Risks you (or your partner) and your baby could encounter if you decide to become pregnant
- Care management regimen you would have to follow if pregnancy is your decision; consider each period of pregnancy
- Based on your experience researching a medical disorder to make an informed decision, how would you counsel your clients if they wish to use the Internet for this purpose?

Obstetric Critical Care

CHAPTER REVIEW ACTIVITIES

FILL IN THE BLANKS: Insert the term that corresponds to each of the following descriptions.

1. _____ is the gradient controlling whether fluid remains inside the _____ or moves into the _____. The force to keep fluid inside the vessel is the pulling pressure of the _____, or _____ present in the plasma. Pregnancy produces a decrease in the _____ values owing to the _____ state that reduces the concentration of plasma _____. The force exerted to push fluids through the membrane is the _____ pressure and is measured as the _____.

2. Normal arterial blood gas values for pregnancy reflect a chronic state of compensated _____.

3. In terms of clot formation, pregnancy is a _____ state. The risk for thrombus formation increases whenever _____ develops as can occur with _____ or _____.

4. _____ is a measure of the tension required for the _____ of blood into the circulation. _____ of arterial vessels and development of _____ results in a decrease in _____ and _____ during pregnancy. As a result, both systolic and diastolic blood pressure _____ during pregnancy.

5. _____ is the volume of blood ejected from the left ventricle in one minute. It is the product of _____, the volume of blood ejected from the left ventricle during one cardiac cycle and the _____, both of which _____ during pregnancy.

6. The four major determinants of cardiac output are _____, _____, _____, and _____.

TRUE OR FALSE: Circle "T" if true or "F" if false for each of the following statements. Correct the false statements.

T   F   7. Maternal adaptations to pregnancy alter a woman's physiologic status and make her hemodynamically different from the nonpregnant woman.

T   F   8. The medical records of critically ill pregnant women are more likely to be subjected to legal review than are the medical records of other clients.

T   F   9. The number of women requiring obstetric critical care has been steadily decreasing in recent years.

T   F   10. When a pregnant woman is standing, her cardiac output is higher than when she is in the supine position or sitting.

T   F   11. Cardiac output begins to decrease rapidly to prepregnancy levels immediately after the woman gives birth.

T   F   12. During pregnancy, the maternal heart rate increases approximately 20% or 10 to 15 beats per minute.

T   F   13. The maternal cardiac output increases as much as 50% during pregnancy.

T   F   14. Pregnancy is a cardiovascular state of low flow and high resistance.

T   F   15. A pregnant woman will exhibit signs of hypovolemic shock more quickly than a nonpregnant woman.

T   F   16. When caring for a woman with a pulmonary artery catheter, all connection sites should be inspected once a shift.

T   F   17. Women who have survived childhood illnesses and become pregnant represent a major group of women requiring obstetric critical care.

T   F   18. The most common diagnosis for admission to an Obstetric Intensive Care Unit is severe trauma as a result of accidents or battering.

T   F   19. Pulmonary edema is more likely to occur when there is an increase in the pulmonary capillary wedge pressure (PCWP) and a decrease in the colloid osmotic pressure (COP).

T   F   20. An arterial pressure catheter provides continuous measurements of systolic, diastolic, and mean arterial blood pressures.

T   F   21. The most common risk associated with an intraarterial line is hemorrhage and clot formation at the site.

T   F   22. A blood pressure taken with a sphygmomanometer should be assessed periodically to verify the accuracy of the arterial pressure catheter reading.

T   F   23. Oliguria is a urine output of less than 50 ml/hour for 2 consecutive hours.

T   F   24. The most common cause of traumatic injuries during pregnancy is battering or abuse.

T   F   25. Most cases of trauma during pregnancy occur during the first and the second trimesters.

T   F   26. Trauma is the leading nonobstetric cause of maternal mortality.

T   F   27. Trauma increases the risk for preterm labor.

T   F   28. When maternal survival occurs, fetal death is usually the result of abruptio placentae occurring within 12 hours of the accident.

T   F   29. All female trauma victims of childbearing age should be considered pregnant until proven otherwise.

30. *EXPLAIN* the rationale for the health care option of the obstetric critical care unit.

31. *IDENTIFY* the factors present during labor and the postpartum period that are responsible for altering the cardiac output. *INDICATE* how cardiac output is altered.
    Labor

32. Oxygen delivery to and use by peripheral tissues must be adequate; therefore its assessment is an essential aspect of the care of a critically ill pregnant woman. DESCRIBE each of the following techniques that monitor oxygenation. INDICATE expected values as part of your description.
    A. **Arterial blood gas analysis**

    B. **Pulse oximeter**

    C. **Svo$_2$**

MULTIPLE CHOICE: Circle the one correct option and state the rationale for the option chosen.

33. The nurse caring for a pregnant woman would recognize which of the following arterial blood gas values as normal for a pregnant woman?
    A. pH: 7.35
    B. Po$_2$: 105 mm Hg
    C. Pco$_2$: 50 mm Hg
    D. Bicarbonate: 16 mEq/L

34. A pulmonary catheter will be used as one of the monitoring techniques used during the care of a critically ill pregnant woman. As part of the protocol for a pulmonary artery catheter insertion and care the nurse would:
    A. Ensure that a signed informed consent is on the woman's chart
    B. Assist the woman into a supine position with the head of the bed elevated slightly to facilitate catheter insertion
    C. Keep hydralazine on hand in case an arrhythmia develops
    D. Perform catheter site care every 48 hours

35. The blood pressure of a woman with severe preeclampsia is 180/120. Her mean arterial pressure (MAP) would be:
    A. 120 mm Hg
    B. 130 mm Hg
    C. 140 mm Hg
    D. 180 mm Hg

Chapter 34: Obstetric Critical Care   313

36. A critically ill pregnant woman is to have an arterial pressure catheter inserted to monitor her systolic, diastolic, and MAP. Prior to insertion, the nurse performs an Allen test and reports the results to the physician who will be inserting the catheter. In performing this test the nurse should have:
   A. Lowered the woman's dominant hand
   B. Occluded the ulnar and radial artery simultaneously
   C. Instructed the woman to keep her fist clenched
   D. Released pressure on both arteries at the same time noting the time for capillary refill

CRITICAL THINKING EXERCISES

1. Annie is a pregnant woman in her 28th week of pregnancy. She was in an automobile accident and as a result was admitted to an obstetric critical care unit for observation and treatment of severe injuries.
   A. Annie's physician orders arterial blood gases and the insertion of an arterial pressure catheter into the radial artery to evaluate her cardiopulmonary status. *DESCRIBE* the protocol that should be followed before obtaining the arterial blood sample and inserting the arterial pressure catheter.

   B. Annie's blood gas values are: pH 7.43, Po_2 106, Pco_2 30, and Hco_3 22. *ANALYZE* these values to determine if each is within the normal range for a pregnant woman.

   C. The Glasgow Coma Scale is used to help determine Annie's neurologic integrity and the extent of any head injury Annie may have sustained during the automobile accident. *IDENTIFY* the three major assessment categories of the scale and *GIVE* one example of how you would evaluate each.

   D. Because continuous monitoring of Annie's cardiovascular status and function is required, a pulmonary artery catheter will be inserted. The pulmonary artery catheter is used to identify changes in the hemodynamic values from the _____. Annie should be placed in a _____ position with a _____ to facilitate placement of the catheter because the neck veins will become _____. Preparation of Annie for this procedure should include _____, _____, _____, and _____. The use of a pulmonary artery catheter, along with an _____ catheter, and a _____ will provide adequate data to assess _____, _____, and _____ status.

E. SPECIFY the positions you would use to enhance Annie's cardiac output. SUPPORT your answer.

F. DESCRIBE the supportive care measures required by Annie and her family.

2. Trauma continues to be a common complication during pregnancy that may require obstetric critical care.
   A. DISCUSS the significance of this complication using statistical data to describe the scope of the problem in terms of incidence, timing during pregnancy, and forms of trauma.

   B. INDICATE the effects trauma can have on pregnancy.

   C. EXPLAIN how each of the following physiologic and anatomic adaptations to pregnancy can affect the type and extent of injuries a woman could experience as a result of trauma.
   Location of bladder and uterus

   Elevation of progesterone levels

   Changes in hemodynamic (cardiopulmonary) function

D. *DESCRIBE* the potential impact of trauma on the fetus.

E. *SPECIFY* the potential effects of each of the following mechanisms of trauma.
Blunt abdominal trauma

Penetrating abdominal trauma

Thoracic trauma

F. Priorities of care for the pregnant woman following trauma must be to _____ and _____ first and then consider _____. This method of approach in care management is important because _____ survival is dependent on _____ survival.

G. *OUTLINE* the major components of the primary and secondary survey of a pregnant woman who has experienced trauma.

Primary Survey	Secondary Survey

Online Learning Activities

Access the Lowdermilk, Perry **Evolve** website at
http://evolve.elsevier.com/Lowdermilk/MatWmnHlth/ and enter the **Student** portion through the
Learning Resources section to assist you in searching the medical literature for nursing research
studies related to the needs of families when a family member is being cared for in an ICU and
nursing support measures that have been effective in meeting these needs. If possible find research
studies that address the unique needs of the families of pregnant women who are critically ill.

- Create an annotated bibliography of at least four nursing research studies
- Choose one research study and complete a bibliography card that includes the following:
  - Hypothesis; research question
  - Summary of the methodology used and key findings
  - Reliability of the study and its findings
  - Recommendations for further research
- Describe how nurses working with critically ill pregnant women can use the results of these studies
  to provide the families of these women with the type of support measures and services that they
  need

Mental Health Disorders and Substance Abuse

CHAPTER REVIEW ACTIVITIES

FILL IN THE BLANKS: Insert the term that corresponds to each of the following descriptions.

1. _____ are defined as disorders that have as their dominant feature a disturbance in the prevailing emotional state.
2. _____ are the most common mental disorder. These disorders include _____, _____, _____, and _____.
3. _____ are irrational fears that lead a person to avoid common objects, events, or situations.
4. _____ results in repeated, unprovoked episodes of intense fear, which develop without warning and are not related to any specific event.
5. _____ refers to a mental health disorder characterized by recurrent, persistent, and intrusive thoughts that cause anxiety that a person tries to control by performing repetitive behaviors.
6. _____ can occur as a result of rape. Symptoms include reexperiencing the _____ event, persistent avoidance of _____, and _____, as well as difficulty _____, _____, or _____ outbursts, difficulty _____, _____, and exaggerated _____.
7. The definition of postpartum depression without psychotic features is intense and pervasive _____ with severe and labile _____. The incidence is from _____ to _____ of new mothers. These symptoms rarely disappear without outside help. A distinguishing feature of postpartum depression is _____, which often flares up with little provocation. Many of these outbursts are directed against _____ or the _____. A prominent finding of postpartum depression is _____ of the infant often caused by abnormal _____. Women often have severe _____, _____, and spontaneous _____ long after the usual duration of baby blues.
8. Postpartum psychosis is a syndrome most often characterized by _____, _____, and thoughts by the mother of _____. Symptoms of this syndrome often begin within _____ after birth although the mean time to onset is _____ and almost always within _____ of the birth. Characteristically, the woman begins to complain of _____, _____, and _____ and may have episodes of _____ and _____. Later, _____, _____, _____, _____ statements, and _____ concerns about the baby's health and welfare may be present.

Chapter 35: Mental Health Disorders and Substance Abuse   319

Delusions, when present, often are related to the _____, and in severe cases auditory hallucinations may command the mother to _____.

9. A specific illness included in depression with psychotic features is _____, formerly called manic-depressive illness. This mood disorder is preceded or accompanied by _____ episodes and is characterized by _____, _____, or _____ moods.

10. _____ are discrete periods in which there is a sudden onset of intense apprehension, fearfulness, or terror.

TRUE OR FALSE: Circle "T" if true or "F" if false for each of the following statements. Correct the false statements.

T F 11. It is estimated that substance abuse is a problem in approximately 10% of all pregnancies.

T F 12. Every pregnant woman should be screened at least verbally for substance abuse at the first prenatal visit.

T F 13. Most states require that health care practitioners test mother and newborns for the presence of drugs.

T F 14. A woman with a history of physical or sexual abuse is at increased risk to develop a problem with abuse of alcohol or drugs.

T F 15. Major depression and anxiety disorders commonly occur with substance abuse.

T F 16. Methadone maintenance is an unsafe treatment option for pregnant women seeking treatment for heroin addiction.

T F 17. Prenatal alcohol exposure is the single greatest preventable cause of mental retardation.

T F 18. Limiting any alcohol intake to a maximum of one to two glasses of wine every couple of days is recommended as a means of preventing fetal alcohol syndrome (FAS).

T F 19. Disulfiram (Antabuse) is an effective substance to use during pregnancy for alcohol detoxification.

T F 20. Women who smoke marijuana have increased carbon monoxide levels in their blood, which reduces the oxygen supply to the fetus.

T F 21. Abruptio placentae and acute onset of preterm labor are possible outcomes of intravenous cocaine use.

T F 22. The use of acupuncture has shown promise in the treatment of heroin abuse during pregnancy.

T F 23. Sleep disorders are common manifestations of withdrawal from psychoactive substances.

T F 24. Mood disorders are characterized by a disturbance in the prevailing emotional state.

T F 25. Postpartum blues often persist for 2 to 4 months after the birth of a baby.

T F 26. Infant cognitive development is adversely affected when a postpartum mood disorder results in the disruption of mother-infant interaction.

T F 27. Rejection of the infant, often caused by abnormal jealousy, is a prominent feature of mood disorders.

T F 28. Women who have marital relationship problems are more likely to develop postpartum depression.

T F 29. Once a woman has had a postpartum episode with psychotic features, there is little risk it will occur again with a subsequent pregnancy.

T   F   30. Women with postpartum depression may experience suicidal ideation and obsessional thoughts regarding violence to their newborns.

T   F   31. Women with postpartum depression almost always require pharmacologic intervention.

T   F   32. Mothers with low self-esteem are more likely to experience postpartum depression than mothers with high self-esteem.

T   F   33. A postpartum mood disorder (depression) with psychotic features occurs in 5 to 10 women per 1000 live births.

T   F   34. Women experiencing a panic attack are in danger of harming their babies.

35. *SPECIFY* the criteria used to diagnose major depression.

36. *STATE* risk factors for postpartum depression for which the nurse must be alert when assessing women and their families after the birth of a baby.

37. *EXPLAIN* why diagnostic assessment of pregnant women for depression is difficult. *STATE* the cues for which the nurse could look in an effort to facilitate diagnosis of depression.

38. A common nursing diagnosis for a woman with postpartum depression who is hospitalized would be: Altered maternal-infant attachment related to limited ability of the mother to interact with and care for her infant, secondary to postpartum depression. *IDENTIFY* the nursing measures appropriate for this nursing diagnosis.

39. *CITE* measures and activities that nurses should teach pregnant women and their families to use in an effort to prevent postpartum depression.

40. The CAGE questionnaire is a frequently used assessment tool to screen for substance abuse.
    A. *STATE* the purpose for the CAGE questionnaire.

B. *INDICATE* the question represented by each letter:

   C

   A

   G

   E

C. *SPECIFY* how the answers should be interpreted or scored for this assessment tool.

41. *CITE* the several predisposing factors associated with cocaine use during pregnancy.

42. *EXPLAIN* the process of change including the importance of readiness to make a change.

MULTIPLE CHOICE: Circle the one correct option and state the rationale for the option chosen.

43. Nurses caring for postpartum women experiencing mood disorders need to be aware of the safety of pharmacologic agents administered to help women cope with the effects of the mood disorders. Which of the following medications would be safe for women who wish to continue breastfeeding?
    A. amitriptyline (Elavil)
    B. haloperidol (Haldol)
    C. doxepin (Sinequan)
    D. lithium carbonate (Eskalith)

44. Which of the following measures would be least effective in preventing postpartum depression?
    A. Share feelings and emotions with family members and her partner
    B. Recognize that emotional problems after having a baby are not unusual
    C. Care for the baby by herself to increase her level of self-confidence and self-esteem
    D. Ask friends or family members to take care of the baby while she sleeps or has a "date" with her partner

45. A priority question to ask a woman experiencing postpartum depression would be:
    A. Have you thought about hurting yourself?
    B. Does it seem like your mind is filled with cobwebs?
    C. Have you been feeling insecure, fragile, or vulnerable?
    D. Does the responsibility of motherhood seem overwhelming?

322   Chapter 35: Mental Health Disorders and Substance Abuse

46. The nurse should recognize that a complication of pregnancy associated with the intravenous use of cocaine would be:
   A. Prolonged, difficult labor
   B. Premature separation of the placenta
   C. Nutritional excess leading to obesity
   D. Premature rupture of the membranes

47. When conducting a health history interview during a pregnant woman's first prenatal visit, the nurse must determine if the woman is substance dependent. The nurse's first question should relate to the woman's use of:
   A. Alcohol
   B. Caffeine
   C. Cocaine
   D. Over-the-counter medications

CRITICAL THINKING EXERCISES

1. Mary, a 35-year-old primiparous woman beginning her second week postpartum, is bottle feeding her baby. She and her husband Tom moved from Buffalo, where they lived all their lives, to Los Angeles 2 months ago to take advantage of a career opportunity for Tom. They live in a community with many other young couples who are also starting families. Last month they joined the Catholic church near their home. Tom tries to help Mary with the baby but he has to spend long hours at work to establish his position. Mary's prenatal record reveals that she often exhibited anxiety about her well-being and that of her baby. During a home visit by a nurse, as part of an early discharge program, Mary tells the nurse that she always wants to sleep and just cannot seem to get enough rest. Mary is very concerned that she is not being a good mother and states "Sometimes I just do not know what to do to care for my baby the right way and I am not even breastfeeding my baby. It seems that Tom enjoys spending what little time he has at home with the baby and not with me. I even find myself yelling at him for the silliest things." The nurse recognizes that Mary is exhibiting behaviors strongly suggestive of postpartum depression.

   A. *INDICATE* the signs and symptoms that Mary exhibited to lead the nurse to suspect postpartum depression.

   B. *SPECIFY* the predisposing factors for postpartum depression that are present in Mary's situation.

C. *WRITE* several questions that the nurse could ask Mary to determine the depth of the postpartum depression that she is experiencing.

D. *WRITE* one nursing diagnosis that is reflective of Mary and Tom's current situation.

E. *DESCRIBE* the measures the nurse could use to help Mary and Tom cope with postpartum depression.

2. Substance abuse results in serious maternal and fetal damage.
   A. *CREATE* a profile of a woman who is at risk for developing a problem with substance abuse.

   B. *IDENTIFY* several barriers that limit a pregnant woman's access to treatment for a substance abuse problem.

   C. *DISCUSS* the approach the nurse should take during the first prenatal interview to screen a pregnant woman for alcohol and drug abuse.

   D. *EXPLAIN* the considerations that should guide the nurse when planning care and setting expected outcomes for the pregnant woman who abuses alcohol or illicit drugs.

E. *INDICATE* the nursing measures appropriate for the woman who is dependent on a psychoactive substance(s) during pregnancy, childbirth, and the postpartum period.

F. *COMPLETE THE FOLLOWING TABLE* by specifying the harmful effects that use of each of the following substances can have on the pregnant woman and her fetus/newborn.

Substance	Maternal Effects	Fetal/Newborn Effects
Alcohol		
Marijuana		
Cocaine		
Opiates		
Methamphetamine		

3. Imagine that you are an advanced practice nurse who specializes in the treatment of men and women who are alcohol and drug dependent. You have been hired to establish a treatment program specifically designed for pregnant women. *OUTLINE* the approach you would take to ensure that the program you establish takes into consideration the unique characteristics of women who abuse alcohol and drugs.

ONLINE LEARNING ACTIVITIES

1. Access the Lowdermilk, Perry **Evolve** website at **http://evolve.elsevier.com/Lowdermilk/MatWmnHlth/** and enter the **Student** portion through the **Learning Resources** section. Use Chapter 35 as a starting point in a search of the Internet for sites that inform and support women who are experiencing postpartum depression and their families. Prepare a report that includes the following:
   - List of the relevant sites that you found
   - Description of one site in terms of the following:
     - Sponsoring person(s), agency, organization
     - Clarity, accuracy, accessibility (ease of use), value, and depth of information provided
     - Nature of the support services offered
     - Currency—frequency of site updates
     - Variety of links to other relevant sites
     - Ability of persons using this site to obtain additional information and individualized support through such services as e-mail and chat rooms
   - Discuss how you would use these sites as one tool to extend the support a woman with postpartum depression needs into her home

2. Use the Evolve site as a starting point to search the Internet for information about alcohol and substance treatment programs in the United States that are designed to treat pregnant women with a substance abuse problem. Contact at least two of these agencies. Prepare a report of your findings that includes the following:
   - List of programs found
   - Description for each of the treatment programs you contacted in terms of the following:
     - Mission and philosophy of care
     - Treatment approaches used and services offered; support services offered to families of these women
     - Effectiveness of treatment approaches and support services
     - Qualifications of health care professionals caring for the women
     - Typical number of women cared for and the common substances abused
     - Cost of care

CHAPTER 36

Labor and Birth Complications

CHAPTER REVIEW ACTIVITIES

MATCHING: Match the description of medications used as part of the management of preterm labor in Column I with the appropriate medication listed in Column II.

COLUMN I

_____ 1. Beta-adrenergic agonist, often administered intravenously, is the only drug approved by the FDA for the purpose of suppressing uterine contractions.

_____ 2. An antenatal glucocorticoid used to accelerate fetal lung maturity when there is risk for preterm birth.

_____ 3. Beta-adrenergic agonist often administered subcutaneously using a syringe or pump.

_____ 4. A calcium channel blocker that relaxes smooth muscles including those of the contracting uterus. It is administered orally.

_____ 5. Classification of drugs used to suppress uterine activity.

_____ 6. A CNS depressant that is used during preterm labor for its ability to relax smooth muscles. It is administered intravenously.

_____ 7. A nonsteroidal antiinflammatory medication that relaxes smooth muscles as a result of prostaglandin inhibition. It is administered rectally or orally.

COLUMN II

A. Tocolytic
B. Betamethasone
C. Ritodrine (Yutopar)
D. Terbutaline (Brethine)
E. Magnesium sulfate
F. Nifedipine (Procardia)
G. Indomethacin

MATCHING: Match the description of medications used for the management of cervical ripening and uterine stimulation in Column I with the medication listed in Column II.

COLUMN I

_____ 8. Tocolytic medication administered subcutaneously to suppress hyperstimulation of the uterus.

_____ 9. Classification of hormones that can be used to ripen the cervix and/or stimulate uterine contractions.

_____ 10. Cervical ripening agent in the form of a vaginal insert that is placed in the posterior fornix of the vagina.

_____ 11. Cervical ripening agent in the form of a gel which is inserted into the cervical canal just below the internal os.

_____ 12. Pituitary hormone used to stimulate uterine contractions in the augmentation or induction of labor.

_____ 13. Natural cervical dilator made from seaweed.

_____ 14. Cervical ripening agent used in the form of a tablet that can be administered orally but more commonly intravaginally.

COLUMN II

A. Oxytocin (Pitocin)

B. Misoprostol (Cytotec)

C. Dinoprostone (Cervidil)

D. Dinoprostone (Prepidil)

E. Terbutaline (Brethine)

F. Prostaglandin

G. Laminaria tent

FILL IN THE BLANKS: Insert the term that corresponds to each of the following descriptions.

15. _____ is any birth that occurs before the completion of 37 weeks of pregnancy. _____ refers to birth that occurs before completion of 32 weeks of pregnancy.

16. _____ is defined as cervical changes and uterine contractions occurring between 20 and 37 weeks of pregnancy.

17. Preterm birth describes _____ regardless of the weight of the infant whereas low birth weight describes only _____.

18. Low birth weight can be caused by _____ or _____, a condition of fetal growth not necessarily correlated with initiation of labor; and _____ or pregnant women who are _____.

19. _____ can be used to predict who might experience preterm labor. The two most commonly used are _____ and _____.

20. _____ are glycoproteins found in plasma and produced during fetal life. Their appearance between _____ and _____ weeks of gestation could predict preterm labor. The negative predictive value is _____ whereas the positive predictive value is _____. The test is done during a _____ examination.

21. _____ is a form of estrogen produced by the fetus that is present in plasma at 9 weeks' gestation. Levels have been shown to _____ before preterm birth. The negative predictive value is _____ whereas the positive predictive value is _____.

22. _____ is another possible predictor of imminent preterm labor. It is determined by _____. A shortened _____ of less than _____ in _____ pregnancies can predict some instances of preterm labor.

23. _____ is the rupture of the amniotic sac and leakage of amniotic fluid beginning at least 1 hour before the onset of labor at any gestational age.

24. _____ is the rupture of the amniotic sac and leakage of fluid before 37 weeks' gestation. _____ often precedes this rupture but the cause remains unknown. _____ is the serious side effect of rupture of the amniotic sac at this time that makes it a major complication of pregnancy. _____ is an intraamniotic infection of the chorion and amnion that is potentially life threatening for the fetus and the woman.

25. _____ is defined as a long, difficult, or abnormal labor and is caused by various conditions associated with the _____ affecting labor.

26. _____ is described as abnormal uterine contractions that prevent the normal progress of _____, _____ (_____ powers), or _____ (_____ powers).

27. _____, or primary dysfunctional labor, often is experienced by an anxious first-time mother who is having _____ and _____ contractions that are ineffective in causing _____ or _____ to progress. These contractions usually occur in the _____ phase of the first stage of labor. _____ is usually prescribed for the management of this type of dysfunctional labor.

28. _____ or secondary uterine inertia usually occurs when a woman initially makes normal progress into the active phase of labor, then uterine contractions become _____ and _____ or _____.

29. _____ can occur whenever there are contractures of the pelvic diameters that reduce the capacity of the bony pelvis, including the inlet, midpelvis, outlet, or any combination of these planes.

30. _____ results from obstruction of the birth passage by an anatomic abnormality other than that involving the bony pelvis. The obstruction may result from _____, _____, _____, and a full _____ or _____.

31. _____ may be caused by anomalies, excessive fetal size and malpresentation, malposition, or multifetal pregnancy. _____, also called _____, is related to excessive fetal size. The most common fetal malposition is persistent _____. _____ is the most common form of malpresentation.

32. _____ is the gestation of twins, triplets, quadruplets, or more infants.

33. Six abnormal labor patterns have been identified and classified by Friedman (1989) according to the nature of _____ and _____. These patterns are _____, _____, _____, _____, _____, and _____. _____ is defined as a labor that lasts less than 3 hours from the onset of contractions to the time of birth. It may result from _____ that are _____ in intensity.

34. _____ is an attempt to turn the fetus from a breech or shoulder presentation to a vertex presentation for birth by exerting gentle, constant pressure on the abdomen.

35. A _____ is the allowance of a reasonable period of spontaneous active labor (e.g., 4–6 hours) so that the safety of a vaginal birth for the mother and fetus can be assessed.

36. _____ is the chemical or mechanical initiation of uterine contractions before their spontaneous onset for the purpose of bringing about the birth.

37. _____ is a rating system used to evaluate the inducibility of the cervix. The five characteristics assessed are _____, _____, _____, _____, and _____. If the score is low, _____ can be applied to the cervix to soften and thin or _____ the cervix.

38. _____ is the artificial rupture of the membranes. It can be used to _____ labor when the cervix is ripe or to _____ labor if the progress begins to slow.

39. _____ is the stimulation of uterine contractions after labor has started spontaneously but progress is unsatisfactory. Common methods include _____ infusion, _____, and _____ stimulation.

40. A _____ is one in which an instrument with two curved blades is used to assist the birth of the fetal head.

41. _____ or _____ is a birth method involving the attachment of a vacuum cup to the fetal head and then using negative pressure to assist in the birth of the head.

42. _____ is the birth of the fetus though a transabdominal incision of the uterus.

43. A _____ or _____ pregnancy is one that extends beyond the end of week 42 of gestation.

44. _____ is an uncommon obstetric emergency in which the head of the fetus is born but the anterior shoulder cannot pass under the pubic arch. Two major causes are _____ or maternal _____.

45. _____ occurs when the cord lies below the presenting part of the fetus. Contributing factors to its occurrence include a _____, _____, _____, or _____. When this condition is present, the woman is assisted into a position such as _____, _____, or _____. In these positions gravity keeps pressure of the _____ off of the cord.

46. An _____ occurs when amniotic fluid containing particles of debris enters the maternal circulation and obstructs pulmonary blood vessels, causing respiratory distress and circulatory collapse. Amniotic fluid is more dangerous when it contains thick _____ because it can clog the pulmonary veins more completely than other debris.

TRUE AND FALSE: Circle "T" if true or "F" if false for each of the following statements. Correct the false statements.

T F 47. Preterm labor and birth are the most serious complications of pregnancy because they lead to 50% of all neonatal deaths.

T F 48. The preterm birth rate was 15% in the year 2000.

T F 49. Preterm birth is more dangerous than low birth weight because shortened gestational time results in immature body systems.

T F 50. The rate of preterm births among Caucasian women is nearly double the rate of African-American women in the United States.

T F 51. Risk-scoring systems are excellent predictors of women who will go into labor prematurely.

T F 52. Fetal fibronectin is more likely to predict women who will not go into preterm labor than women who will go into preterm labor.

T F 53. Salivary estriol has a high positive predictive value for preterm labor.

T F 54. Endocervical length measurement has demonstrated predictive value for preterm labor in multiple gestation pregnancies.

T F 55. Early recognition of preterm labor is essential if measures to suppress labor and enhance fetal lung maturation are to be successful.

T F 56. Research evidence confirms that bed rest is highly effective in preventing preterm birth.

T F 57. It is now thought that the best reason to use tocolytics is to gain the time needed to administer antenatal glucocorticoids.

T F 58. Dysfunctional labor can occur as a result of maternal factors such as fluid and electrolyte imbalance.

T F 59. The most common type of uterine dysfunction is hypotonic uterine dysfunction.

T F 60. A breech presentation is most common in term pregnancies.

T F 61. Since 1980, the twin birth rate has increased by more than 50%.

T F 62. Dystocia is the primary cause for cesarean birth.

T F 63. A diagnosis of secondary arrest of active labor is made when there has been no change in cervical dilation for 2 hours or more for both nulliparous and multiparous women.

T F 64. Ripening of the cervix with a prostaglandin preparation usually results in a higher success rate for induction of labor.

T F 65. Prepidil gel is inserted into the posterior fornix of the vagina.

T F 66. Oxytocin is discontinued immediately and the primary health care provider notified if uterine hyperstimulation or a nonreassuring FHR occurs during labor stimulation.

T F 67. Research has consistently proven that the one-to-one support provided by a doula reduces the risk for cesarean birth for laboring women who receive this support.

T F 68. The incidence of postterm pregnancy in the United States is approximately 25%.

T F 69. Assisting the laboring woman into a hands-and-knees position can help to resolve shoulder dystocia.

T F 70. The maternal mortality rate for amniotic fluid embolism is as high as 50%.

71. *IDENTIFY* two factors for each of the following risk categories for preterm labor and birth.
Demographic risks

Biophysical risks

Behavioral-psychosocial risks

72. *EXPLAIN* why bed rest may be more harmful than helpful as a component of preterm birth care management.

73. *DESCRIBE* each of the five factors that cause labor to be long, difficult, or abnormal. Explain how they interrelate.

74. *EXPLAIN* the treatment approach of therapeutic rest.

75. Angela (1–0–0–0–0) is experiencing hypertonic uterine dysfunction, Bernice (3–1–0–1–1) is experiencing hypotonic uterine dysfunction, and Gloria (2–0–0–1–0) is having difficulty bearing down effectively. *COMPLETE THE FOLLOWING TABLE* by contrasting each woman's labor in terms of causes/precipitating factors, maternal-fetal effects, change in pattern of progress, and care management.

	Angela (Hypertonic)	Bernice (Hypotonic)	Gloria (Inadequate Expulsion)
Causes/precipitating factors			
Maternal-fetal effects			
Changes in progress of labor			
Care management			

76. Nurses caring for women during labor must always be alert for clinical manifestations of amniotic fluid embolism.
    A. *IDENTIFY* the factors that would increase a woman's risk for this life-threatening complication.

B. *LIST* the signs of amniotic fluid embolism (AFE) in each of the following categories for which the nurse must be alert when assessing pregnant women.

Respiratory distress

Circulatory collapse

Hemorrhage

C. *OUTLINE* the recommended care management of a woman experiencing an amniotic fluid embolism (AFE).

77. *IDENTIFY* four indications for oxytocin induction and four contraindications to the use of oxytocin to stimulate the onset of labor.

Indications

Contraindications

MULTIPLE CHOICE: Circle the one correct option and state the rationale for the option chosen.

78. When assessing a woman during pregnancy, the nurse needs to be alert for signs that would indicate risk for preterm labor and birth. Which of the following factors exhibited by a pregnant woman is associated with preterm labor and birth?
   A. Age: 30
   B. Obstetric history: 3–2–0–0–2
   C. Children are 2 and 4 years of age
   D. Currently being treated for her second bladder infection in 4 months

79. A woman calls the prenatal clinic to report that she has been experiencing uterine contractions for the past hour at a frequency of every 8 to 10 minutes. One of the actions the nurse would tell this woman to take would be to:
    A. Lie down on her left side
    B. Count contractions for 2 more hours
    C. Reduce fluid intake
    D. Report to the clinic for evaluation as soon as someone can bring her

80. Bed rest for prevention of preterm birth is least likely to result in:
    A. Bone demineralization
    B. Weight gain
    C. Fatigue
    D. Anxiety and depression

81. A woman's labor is being suppressed using intravenous magnesium sulfate. Which of the following measures should be implemented during the infusion?
    A. Limit fluid intake to 1000 ml or less per day
    B. Assess fetal heart rate for tachycardia
    C. Ensure that calcium gluconate is available should toxicity occur
    D. Assist woman into a comfortable semirecumbent position

82. The physician has ordered that dinoprostone (Cervidil) be administered to ripen a pregnant woman's cervix in preparation for an induction of her labor. In fulfilling this order the nurse would:
    A. Insert the Cervidil into the cervical canal just below the internal os
    B. Tell the woman to remain in bed for at least 15 minutes
    C. Call the woman's physician if she reports a history of asthma
    D. Remove the Cervidil if the woman begins to experience uterine contractions

83. A nulliparous woman experiencing a postterm pregnancy is admitted for labor induction. Assessment reveals a Bishop score of 9. The nurse would:
    A. Call the woman's primary health care provider to order a cervical ripening agent
    B. Mix 20 U of Pitocin in 500 ml of 5% glucose in water
    C. Piggyback the Pitocin solution into the port nearest the drip chamber of the primary IV tubing
    D. Begin the infusion at a rate between 0.5 to 2 mU/minute as determined by the induction protocol

84. A woman's labor is being induced. The nurse assesses the woman's status and that of her fetus and the labor process just before an infusion increment of 2 mU/minute. The nurse would discontinue the infusion and notify the woman's primary health care provider if which of the following had been noted during the assessment?
    A. Frequency of uterine contractions: every 1½ minutes
    B. Variability of FHR: present
    C. Deceleration patterns: early decelerations noted with several contractions
    D. Intensity of uterine contractions at their peaks: 80 to 85 mm Hg

85. A multiparous woman is in the first stage of the labor. In reviewing her partogram, the nurse-midwife notes that the woman's cervix has dilated from 5 cm to 6 cm over 2 hours. The nurse-midwife would recognize this woman's labor pattern as:
    A. Prolonged latent phase
    B. Protracted active phase
    C. Secondary arrest
    D. Precipitous labor

86. A laboring woman's vaginal examination reveals the following: 3 cm, 50%, LSA, 0. The nurse caring for this woman would:
    A. Place the ultrasound transducer in the left lower quadrant of the woman's abdomen
    B. Recognize that passage of meconium would be a definitive sign of fetal distress
    C. Expect the progress of fetal descent to be slower than usual
    D. Assist the woman into a knee-chest position for each contraction

CRITICAL THINKING EXERCISES

1. Imagine that you are a nurse-midwife working at an inner-city women's health clinic. You are concerned about the rate of preterm labor and birth among the pregnant women who come to your clinic for care. *OUTLINE* a Preterm Labor and Birth Prevention program that you would implement at your clinic to reduce the rate of preterm labors and birth.

2. Sara, a primiparous woman (2–0–1–0–1) at 22 weeks' gestation, comes to the clinic for her scheduled prenatal visit. She is anxious because her last labor began at 26 weeks and she is worried that this will happen again. "I had no warning the last time—is there anything I can do this time to have my baby later or at least know that labor is starting so I can let you know?"
   A. *IDENTIFY* the signs of preterm labor that the nurse-midwife should teach Sara.

   B. *EXPLAIN* how the nurse-midwife could help Sara implement a plan to reduce her risk for preterm labor.

   C. Three weeks later, Sara calls the clinic and tells her nurse-midwife that she has been having uterine contractions about every 9 minutes or so for the last hour. *DESCRIBE* what the nurse-midwife should tell Sara to do.

D. Conservative measures do not work and Sara's uterine contractions progress. She is admitted for possible tocolytic therapy. *SPECIFY* the criteria that Sara must meet before tocolysis can be safely instituted.

E. Sara is started on a tocolysis regimen that involves the intravenous administration of Ritodrine. *OUTLINE* the nursing care measures that must be implemented during the infusion to ensure the safety of Sara and her fetus.

F. The nurse is preparing to give Sara a dose of betamethasone as ordered by the physician.
   1) *STATE* the purpose of this medication.

   2) *EXPLAIN* the procedure that the nurse should follow in fulfilling this order.

3. Debra has been experiencing signs of preterm labor. After a period of hospitalization, her labor was successfully suppressed and she was discharged to be cared for at home. Debra is receiving terbutaline via a subcutaneous pump. She will record her uterine activity twice a day with an ambulatory tokodynamometer device. Debra must also remain on bed rest with only bathroom privileges.
   A. *IDENTIFY* two nursing diagnoses that would be appropriate related to Debra's home care regimen for preterm labor suppression.

   B. *OUTLINE* what the nurse should teach Debra regarding the care and maintenance of the terbutaline subcutaneous pump that is being used.

   C. *IDENTIFY* the side effects of terbutaline that the nurse should teach Debra prior to discharge.

D. *DESCRIBE* the instructions that Debra should be given regarding home uterine activity monitoring.

E. Debra has two children who are 5 years old and 8 years old. *SPECIFY* the suggestions you would give to help Debra and her children cope with the bed rest requirement ordered by Debra's primary health care provider.

4. Denise, a primigravida, has reached the second stage of her labor with her fetus at zero station and positioned LOP. She is experiencing intense low back pain. Denise did not attend any childbirth classes and is having difficulty pushing effectively. No anesthesia has been used.
   A. *IDENTIFY* the factors that can have a negative effect on the secondary powers of labor (bearing down efforts).

   B. *DESCRIBE* how you would help Denise to use her expulsive forces to facilitate the descent and birth of her baby.

   C. *SPECIFY* the positions that would be recommended based on the position of the presenting part of Denise's fetus.

5. Anne, a primigravida, attended Lamaze classes with her husband, Mark. They were looking forward to working together during the labor and birth of their baby. Because of fetal distress, an emergency low segment cesarean section with a transverse incision was performed after 18 hours of labor. Even though Anne and her son are in stable condition and she is glad that "everything turned out okay for her son," she expresses a sense of failure, stating, "I could not manage to give birth to my son in the normal way and now I never will!"
   A. *LIST* the preoperative nursing measures that should have been implemented to prepare Anne physically and emotionally for the unexpected cesarean birth.

B. *SPECIFY* the assessment measures that are critical when Anne is in the recovery room following her birth.

C. *STATE* the postoperative nursing care measures that Anne requires.

D. *IDENTIFY* the nursing diagnosis reflected in Anne's statement "I could not manage to give birth to my baby in the normal way and now I never will." *SPECIFY* the support measures the nurse could use to put her cesarean birth into perspective.

6. A vaginal examination reveals that Marie's fetus is RSA. *SPECIFY* the considerations that the nurse should keep in mind when providing care for Marie.

7. Angela (2–0–0–1–0) is at 42 weeks' gestation and has been admitted for induction of her labor.
   A. Assessment of Angela at admission included determination of her Bishop's score. *STATE* the purpose of the Bishop's score and *IDENTIFY* the factors that are evaluated.

   B. Angela's score was 5. *INTERPRET* this result in terms of the planned induction of her labor.

   C. Angela's primary health care provider ordered that Cervidil be inserted. *STATE* the purpose of the Cervidil, method of application, and potential side effects that can occur.

D. Before induction of her labor, Angela's primary health provider performs an amniotomy. *SPECIFY* the nursing responsibilities before, during, and after this procedure.

E. *INDICATE* which of the following actions reflect appropriate care (A) for Angela during the induction of her labor with intravenous oxytocin. If the action is not appropriate (NA), state what the correct action would be.

_____ 1) Assist Angela into a lateral or upright position.
_____ 2) Apply an external electronic fetal monitor and obtain a 15- to 20-minute baseline strip of FHR and pattern.
_____ 3) Explain to Angela what to expect and techniques used.
_____ 4) Prepare a primary line with an isotonic electrolyte solution.
_____ 5) Attach the secondary line of dilute oxytocin (10 U in 1000 ml) to the distal port (farthest from the venipuncture site) of the primary IV.
_____ 6) Begin infusion at 4 mU/min.
_____ 7) Increase oxytocin by 1–2 mU/min at 5- to 10-minute intervals after the initial dose until the desired pattern of contractions is achieved.
_____ 8) Stop increasing the dosage and maintain level of oxytocin when contractions occur every 2 to 3 minutes, last 40 to 90 seconds, and reach an intrauterine pressure between 40 and 90 mm Hg if internal monitoring is being used.
_____ 9) Monitor maternal blood pressure and pulse every 15 minutes and with every increment in dose.
_____10) Monitor FHR pattern and uterine activity every 15 minutes and with every increment in dose.
_____11) Limit IV intake to 1500 ml/8 hours.

F. *STATE* the major side effects of Pitocin for which the nurse must be alert when managing Angela's labor.

G. The nurse notes a hyperstimulation pattern when evaluating Angela's monitor tracing. *LIST* the actions the nurse should take in order of priority.

8. Lora is a 37-year-old nulliparous woman beginning her 42nd week of pregnancy. She and her primary health care provider have decided on a conservative, "watchful waiting" approach because neither she nor her fetus is experiencing distress.

A. To help Lora make this decision, the risks she and her fetus face as a result of a postterm pregnancy were explained. *IDENTIFY* the risks that Lora should have considered in making her decision.

B. *STATE* the clinical manifestations that Lora is likely to experience as her pregnancy continues.

C. *STATE* one nursing diagnosis appropriate for Lora's current situation.

D. *OUTLINE* the typical care management measures that should be implemented to ensure the safety of Lora and her fetus.

E. *SPECIFY* the instructions that the nurse should give to Lora regarding her self care as she awaits the onset of labor.

ONLINE LEARNING ACTIVITIES

1. Access the Lowdermilk, Perry **Evolve** website at **http://evolve.elsevier.com/Lowdermilk/MatWmnHlth/** and enter the **Student** portion through the **Learning Resources** section to assist you in searching the medical literature for research studies related to the effectiveness of tocolytics for the suppression of preterm labor and the recommendations for their safe administration.
   - Create an annotated bibliography of at least five research studies
   - Choose one research study and complete a bibliography card that includes the following:
     - Hypotheses; research question

- Summary of methodology used and key findings
- Reliability of the study and its findings
- Recommendations for further research
- Discuss how the results of these studies could be used to develop an evidence-based protocol for the use of tocolytics that is effective and safe for women in preterm labor and their fetuses

2. Access the Lowdermilk, Perry **Evolve** website at **http://evolve.elsevier.com/Lowdermilk/MatWmnHlth/** and enter the **Student** portion through the **Learning Resources** section to assist you in searching the medical literature for nursing research studies related to the impact of cesarean birth on a woman's physical and emotional recovery.
   - Create an annotated bibliography list of at least five nursing research studies
   - Choose one nursing research study and complete a bibliography card that includes the following:
     - Hypotheses; research question
     - Summary of the methodology used and key findings
     - Reliability of the study and its finding
     - Recommendations for further research
   - Develop a support plan for women following emergency and planned cesarean birth that is based on the findings of the research studies
   - Continue your search of the Internet for sites that support women following cesarean birth. Include a list of these sites in a handout entitled *Healthy Recovery following Cesarean Birth*. The handout should also include a summary of the supportive measures validated by research

CHAPTER 37

Postpartum Complications

CHAPTER REVIEW ACTIVITIES

FILL IN THE BLANKS: Insert the term that corresponds to each of the following descriptions of childbirth complications.

1. _____ is the loss of more that 500 ml following vaginal birth or 1000 ml of blood after cesarean birth. Additional criteria that may be used are a _____ change in _____ between admission for labor and postpartum or a need for _____. The leading cause is _____. _____ occurs within 24 hours after birth. _____ occurs more than 24 hours after birth but less than 6 weeks postpartum.
2. Marked hypotonia of the uterus is called _____.
3. A _____ is the accumulation of blood in the connective tissue as a result of blood vessel damage. _____ are the most common type. _____ are usually associated with a forceps-assisted birth, an episiotomy, or primigravidity. The woman often complains of persistent _____ or _____ pain or a feeling of pressure in the _____.
4. _____ refers to the turning of the uterus inside out after birth. The primary presenting signs are _____, _____, and _____. Contributing factors include _____ implantation of the placenta, _____ pressure, _____ applied to the umbilical cord, _____, _____, and an abnormally adherent _____.
5. _____ is the delayed return of the enlarged uterus to normal size and function. Recognized causes of this delay include _____ and _____.
6. _____ is an emergency situation in which profuse blood loss (hemorrhage) can result in severely compromised perfusion of body organs. Death may occur.
7. A _____ is suspected when bleeding is continuous and there is no identifiable cause. _____ is an autoimmune disorder in which antiplatelet antibodies decrease the life span of the platelets. _____ is a type of hemophilia and is probably the most common of all hereditary bleeding disorders. _____ is a pathologic form of clotting that is diffuse and consumes large amounts of clotting factors.
8. A _____ is the formation of a blood clot or clots inside a blood vessel and is caused by _____ or partial _____ of the vessel. _____ involves the superficial saphenous venous system. For _____, involvement varies but can extend from the foot to the iliofemoral region. _____ occurs when part of a blood clot dislodges and is carried to the pulmonary artery, where it occludes the vessel and obstructs blood flow to the lungs.

9. _____ refers to any clinical infection of the genital canal that occurs within 28 days after miscarriage, induced abortion, or childbirth. The first symptom is usually a _____ of 38° C or more on _____. Common infection sites are _____, _____, _____, _____, and _____.

10. _____ is the most common cause of postpartum infection. It usually begins at the _____ site.

11. _____ is an infection of the breast affecting approximately 1% of women, soon after childbirth, most of whom are _____. This infection is almost always _____ and develops well after the _____ has been established.

TRUE OR FALSE: Circle "T" if true or "F" if false for each of the following statements. Correct the false statements.

T   F   12. Early postpartum hemorrhage is often the result of cervical lacerations.

T   F   13. One of the causes of late postpartum hemorrhage is subinvolution associated with retained placental fragments.

T   F   14. When a woman hemorrhages, changes in her baseline vital sign values may not be reliable indicators of shock in the immediate postpartum period because of the physiologic adaptations that occurred during pregnancy and in the postpartum period.

T   F   15. Most cervical lacerations are shallow with minimal bleeding.

T   F   16. Pitocin can be given orally for several days after birth to enhance uterine contraction in women who experienced early postpartum hemorrhage.

T   F   17. Prostaglandin F_{2a} (Hemabate) should be used with caution or not at all if the postpartum woman has asthma.

T   F   18. Subinvolution of the uterus is the second major cause of early postpartum hemorrhage.

T   F   19. Uterine atony is associated with an "over-stretched" uterus associated with such conditions as macrosomia or multiple gestation.

T   F   20. Placenta accreta refers to a placenta that perforates the uterus.

T   F   21. Uterine inversion occurs most frequently in primiparous women with abruptio placentae.

T   F   22. The woman with a third or fourth degree laceration should not be given rectal suppositories or enemas.

T   F   23. Administration of blood and blood components can lead to febrile reactions and fluid overload.

T   F   24. Aspirin or aspirin-containing analgesics can be safely used if a woman is receiving heparin because aspirin enhances its effect.

T   F   25. Puerperal infection is the major cause of maternal morbidity and mortality in the United States.

T   F   26. Clinical manifestations of mastitis usually develop in the second to fourth week postpartum.

T   F   27. Lactation must be suppressed once mastitis is diagnosed.

MULTIPLE CHOICE: Circle the one correct option and state the rationale for the option chosen.

28. Methergine 0.2 mg is ordered to be administered intramuscularly to a woman who gave birth vaginally 1 hour ago for a profuse lochial flow with clots. Her fundus is boggy and does not respond well to massage. She is still being treated for preeclampsia with intravenous magnesium sulfate at 1 g/hour. Her blood pressure, measured 5 minutes ago, was 155/98 mm Hg. In fulfilling this order the nurse would:
    A. Measure the woman's blood pressure again 5 minutes after administering the medication
    B. Question the order based on the woman's hypertensive status
    C. Recognize that Methergine is the best choice to counteract the uterine relaxation effects of the magnesium sulfate infusion the woman is receiving.
    D. Tell the woman that the medication will lead to uterine cramping

29. A postpartum woman in the fourth stage of labor received Hemabate 0.25 mg intramuscularly. The expected outcome of care for the administration of this medication would be:
    A. Relief from the pain of uterine cramping
    B. Prevention of intrauterine infection
    C. Reduction in the blood's ability to clot
    D. Limitation of excessive blood loss that is occurring after birth

30. The nurse responsible for the care of postpartum women should recognize that the first sign of puerperal infection would most likely be:
    A. Fever greater than 38° C or higher after the first 24 hours following birth
    B. Increased white blood cell count
    C. Foul-smelling profuse lochia
    D. Bradycardia

31. A breastfeeding woman's cesarean birth occurred 2 days ago. Investigation of the pain, tenderness, and swelling in her left leg led to a medical diagnosis of deep vein thrombosis (DVT). Care management for this woman during the acute stage of the DVT would involve:
    A. Explaining that she will need to stop breastfeeding until anticoagulation therapy is completed
    B. Administering warfarin orally
    C. Placing the woman on bed rest with her left leg elevated
    D. Fitting the woman with an elastic stocking so that she can exercise her legs

32. STATE the twofold focus of medical management of hemorrhagic shock.

33. IDENTIFY four priority nursing interventions for postpartum hemorrhage.

34. *STATE* the standard of care for bleeding emergencies.

CRITICAL THINKING EXERCISES

1. Andrea is a multiparous woman (6–5–1–0–7) who gave birth to full-term twins vaginally 1 hour ago. Pitocin was used to augment her labor when hypotonic uterine contractions protracted the active stage of her labor. Special forceps were used to assist the birth of the second twin. Currently her vital signs are stable, her fundus is at the umbilicus, midline and firm, and her lochial flow is moderate to heavy without clots.

   A. Early postpartum hemorrhage is a major concern at this time. *STATE* the factors that have increased Andrea's risk for hemorrhage at this time.

   B. *IDENTIFY* the priority nursing diagnosis at this time.

   C. During the second hour after birth the nurse notes that Andrea's perineal pad became saturated in 15 minutes and a large amount of blood had accumulated on the bed under her buttocks. *DESCRIBE* the nurse's initial response to this finding. *STATE* the rationale for the action you described.

   D. The nurse prepares to administer 10 U of Pitocin intravenously as ordered by Andrea's physician. *EXPLAIN* the guidelines the nurse should follow in fulfilling this order.

   E. During the assessment of Andrea the nurse must be alert for signs of developing hypovolemic shock. *CITE* the signs the nurse would be watching for.

F. *DESCRIBE* the measures that the nurse should use to support Andrea and her family in an effort to reduce their anxiety.

2. Nurses working on a postpartum unit must be constantly alert for signs and symptoms of puerperal infection in their clients.
   A. *LIST* the factors can increase a postpartum woman's risk for puerperal infection.

   B. *IDENTIFY* the infection prevention measures that should be used when caring for postpartum women.

   C. *STATE* the typical clinical manifestations of endometritis for which the nurse should be alert when assessing postpartum women.

   D. *IDENTIFY* two nursing diagnoses that would be appropriate for a women diagnosed with endometritis.

   E. *DESCRIBE* the critical nursing measures that are essential in care management related to puerperal infection.

3. Sara, a primiparous breastfeeding mother at 2 weeks postpartum, calls her nurse-midwife to tell her that her right breast is painful and she is not "feeling well."
   A. *EXPLAIN* the assessment findings the nurse-midwife would be alert for to indicate if Sara is experiencing mastitis.

B. A medical diagnosis of mastitis of Sara's right breast is made. *STATE* two nursing diagnoses appropriate for this situation.

C. *DESCRIBE* the treatment measures and health teaching that Sara needs regarding her infection and breastfeeding because she wishes to continue to breastfeed.

D. *IDENTIFY* several behaviors that Sara should learn to prevent recurrence of mastitis.

4. Susan is a 36-year-old obese multiparous woman (4–3–0–1–3) who experienced a cesarean birth 2 days ago. A major complication of the postpartum period is the development of thromboembolic disease.
   A. *STATE* the risk factors for this complication that Susan presents.

   B. When assessing Susan on the afternoon of her second postpartum day, the nurse notes signs indicative of deep vein thrombosis (DVT). *LIST* the signs the nurse most likely observed.

   C. A medical diagnosis of DVT is confirmed. *STATE* one nursing diagnosis appropriate for this situation.

   D. *OUTLINE* the expected care management for Susan during the acute phase of the DVT.

E. Upon discharge Susan will be taking warfarin for at least 3 months. *SPECIFY* the discharge instructions that Susan and her family should receive.

ONLINE LEARNING ACTIVITIES

Access the Centers for Disease Control and Prevention (CDC) and the National Center for Health Statistics (NCHS) websites to gather statistical information regarding the postpartum complications of hemorrhage and infection. Create a chart for each complication that includes the following:
- Incidence of the complication in your state and in the nation as a whole
- Characteristics of women who develop the postpartum complication
- Impact of the complication on a woman's postpartum recovery and future childbearing
- Types of treatments commonly used to treat the complication

CHAPTER 38

Acquired Problems of the Newborn

CHAPTER REVIEW ACTIVITIES

TRUE OR FALSE: Circle "T" if true or "F" if false for each of the following statements. Correct the false statements.

T   F   1. Birth injury is increasing as a major cause of infant mortality.

T   F   2. The Apgar score can alert nurses to the possibility that a birth injury occurred.

T   F   3. Cephalhematoma may result in hyperbilirubinemia from the breakdown of accumulated red blood cells.

T   F   4. Subconjunctival hemorrhage present at birth requires immediate treatment to prevent permanent ocular damage.

T   F   5. The presentation of the fetus can affect the type and location of birth injuries.

T   F   6. Petechiae and ecchymoses will blanch when digital pressure is applied.

T   F   7. The bone most frequently fractured during the birth process is the femur.

T   F   8. Neonatal spinal cord injuries are almost always a result of a difficult birth from the breech presentation.

T   F   9. Lazy colon syndrome resulting in failure to pass meconium can occur in up to 50% of infants of diabetic mothers.

T   F   10. The fetal mortality rate from an episode of maternal ketoacidosis can be as high as 50% or more.

T   F   11. Glucose control before conception has little effect on the incidence of congenital anomalies in the infant of a woman with pregestational diabetes.

T   F   12. The woman infected with toxoplasmosis during pregnancy has a 90% chance of transmitting the infection to her fetus.

T   F   13. Newborns infected with toxoplasmosis in utero are at risk for developing congenital heart defects.

T   F   14. A major mode of transmission of gonorrhea to the fetus/newborn is via passage through an infected birth canal during birth.

T   F   15. Maternal infection with syphilis is most dangerous during the first trimester as organogenesis takes place.

T   F   16. Penicillin is the antibiotic choice for treating syphilis.

T   F   17. Even with adequate treatment, the neonate infected with syphilis may experience complications as late as 15 years of age.

T   F   18. Infants born to mothers who had chickenpox 5 days before the birth should be given varicella-zoster immune globulin (VZIG) at birth.

T   F   19. Women positive for the hepatitis B virus should not breastfeed their newborn.

T F 20. Prenatal treatment of HIV-positive women has reduced the risk for transmission of the virus to the fetus from 25% to 8%.

T F 21. Major teratogenic effects of rubella involve the cardiovascular and the sensory systems.

T F 22. The infant infected with the rubella virus may be a serious source of infection to susceptible individuals particularly women in their childbearing years.

T F 23. Newborns infected with cytomegalovirus must begin receiving penicillin therapy within 24 hours of birth.

T F 24. Snuffles is a common assessment finding exhibited by infants infected with herpes simplex virus.

T F 25. A primary maternal infection with the herpes simplex virus (HSV) after 32 weeks' gestation presents a greater risk to the fetus/newborn than a recurrent HSV infection.

T F 26. The most common cause of neonatal sepsis and meningitis in the United States is group B streptococcus.

T F 27. Hepatitis B during pregnancy is associated with an increased risk for preterm birth.

T F 28. To prevent a chlamydial infection of the eyes, silver nitrate should be instilled over the cornea of the newborn's eyes immediately after birth.

T F 29. Infants diagnosed with fetal alcohol effect (FAE) could develop learning, speech, and behavioral problems.

T F 30. Maternal heroin use, especially during the first trimester, results in a high rate of congenital anomalies.

T F 31. Marijuana use during pregnancy may result in shortened gestation and a higher incidence of intrauterine growth restriction (IUGR).

T F 32. Newborns exposed to cocaine in utero begin a process of withdrawal within 24 hours of birth.

T F 33. Cigarettes, caffeine, and marijuana may potentiate the fetal effects of maternal alcohol consumption during pregnancy.

34. Birth injuries, although decreasing in incidence, are still an important source of neonatal morbidity.
   A. *IDENTIFY* the factors that increase fetal vulnerability to injury and trauma at birth.

   B. Baby boy Timothy's right clavicle was fractured during birth as a result of shoulder dystocia. *DESCRIBE* the signs Timothy most likely exhibited to alert the nurse that his clavicle was fractured.

C. *EXPLAIN* to Timothy's parents the most likely care approach related to his fracture.

35. *FILL IN THE BLANKS:* Insert the term that corresponds to the following descriptions of diabetes mellitus during pregnancy and the effect on the newborn.

As a result of stricter control of maternal _____ and improved _____ and _____ intensive care, there has been a(n) _____ in the perinatal mortality rate in diabetic pregnancy. The incidence of congenital anomalies is still _____ higher than for infants born to mothers without diabetes. During early pregnancy, congenital anomalies are caused by fluctuations in _____ levels and episodes of _____. Later in pregnancy, maternal _____ forces high levels of _____ to cross the placenta, stimulating the fetal pancreas to release increased amounts of _____. This event results in excessive fetal _____, termed _____. In addition, if the blood of a pregnant diabetic woman becomes more _____ than fetal blood, as occurs during _____, _____ or _____, exchange will be diminished. There are indications that some neonatal conditions, namely _____, _____, _____, _____, and perhaps fetal _____ may be eliminated or the incidence decreased if maternal _____ levels are maintained within narrow limits.

36. *IDENTIFY* the most common congenital anomalies experienced by infants with diabetic mothers in terms of each of the following:
Cardiac

Central nervous system

Musculoskeletal

37. Baby boy Robert, weighing 11 pounds 4 ounces, was born 1 hour ago. His mother had gestational diabetes mellitus.

A. *DESCRIBE* the typical characteristics exhibited by a macrosomic infant such as Robert.

B. Robert, as a macrosomic infant, is most at risk for the complications of _____, _____, _____, and _____.

C. *DESCRIBE* the warning signs for each of the potential complications of which the nurse should be aware when assessing Robert during the first 24 hours after his birth.

38. *STATE* the infections(s) represented by each letter in the acronym TORCH.

T

O

R

C

H

39. Sepsis is one of the most significant causes of neonatal morbidity and mortality.

   A. *COMPLETE THE FOLLOWING TABLE* by identifying the modes of infection transmission during each of the periods below.

Period	Modes of Transmission
Prenatal	
Perinatal	
Postnatal	

   B. *IDENTIFY* the major risk factors that, if present, should alert the nurse to the increased potential for infection in the neonate.

   C. *LIST* the signs a neonate might exhibit that would indicate that sepsis is present.

   D. *DESCRIBE* two effective nursing measures for each of the following categories.

   PREVENTION   **CURE**   **REHABILITATION**

40. When assessing a newborn after birth the nurse notes the following: limited movement of left arm with crepitus at the shoulder, absence of Moro reflex on left side. The nurse would suspect:
    A. Brachial paralysis
    B. Fracture of the clavicle
    C. Phrenic nerve injury
    D. Intracranial hemorrhage on the right side of the brain

41. The nurse is caring for a newborn whose mother had gestational diabetes during pregnancy. His estimated gestational age is 41 weeks and his weight indicates that he is macrosomic. When assessing this newborn the nurse would be alert for which of the following?
    A. Fracture of the femur
    B. Hypercalcemia
    C. Blood glucose level of 38 mg/dl
    D. Signs of a congenital heart defect

42. When caring for a pregnant woman who is HIV positive the nurse would recognize that which of the following would increase the risk of virus transmission to the fetus or newborn?
    A. Rupture of the membranes 1 hour or less before birth
    B. Postterm birth
    C. Cesarean birth
    D. Low maternal CD4 T-lymphocyte count

43. The care management of a newborn whose mother is HIV positive would most likely include:
    A. Isolating the newborn in a special nursery
    B. Cleansing of skin with soap, water, and alcohol prior to invasive procedures such as vitamin K administration
    C. Wearing gloves for routine care measures such as feeding
    D. Initiating zidovudine treatment once the newborn's HIV status is determined

CRITICAL THINKING EXERCISES

1. Baby girl Susan was born 2 hours ago. Her mother tested positive for HBsAg antibodies as a result of infection with hepatitis B Virus (HBV).
   A. DESCRIBE the protocol that should be followed in providing care for Susan.

   B. Susan's mother asks the nurse if she can breastfeed her baby daughter. DISCUSS the nurse's response to this mother's question.

2. Baby boy Andrew is a full-term newborn who was just born by spontaneous vaginal delivery. Genital herpes recurred in his mother, and her membranes ruptured before the onset of labor.

   A. *IDENTIFY* the four modes of transmission for HSV to the newborn. *INDICATE* the mode most likely to have transmitted the infection to Andrew.

   B. *LIST* the clinical signs Andrew would exhibit as evidence of a disseminated and localized HSV infection.

   C. *DESCRIBE* the recommended nursing measures related to each of the following:
   Management after birth, prior to discharge

   Vidarabine eye ointment and intravenous acyclovir therapy

3. Baby girl Mary is 1 day old. Her mother is HIV positive but received no treatment during pregnancy.

   A. *DISCUSS* Mary's potential for HIV infection.

   B. *IDENTIFY* the modes of transmission of HIV to Mary.

   C. *OUTLINE* the protocol that most likely will be followed to determine if Mary is HIV positive.

D. Name the opportunistic infections, if contracted by Mary, that would strongly suggest that she is infected with HIV.

E. *DESCRIBE* the care measures recommended for Mary.

F. Mary's mother wishes to breastfeed Mary because she has read that it can prevent infection. *DISCUSS* the nurse's response to this mother's question.

4. Baby boy Thomas, at 2 days of age, has developed thrush.
   A. *DESCRIBE* the signs most likely exhibited by Thomas that led to this diagnosis.

   B. *NAME* the modes of transmission for this infection.

   C. *DISCUSS* the care management required by Thomas as a result of his yeastlike fungal infection.

5. Jane, a newborn, has been diagnosed with fetal alcohol syndrome (FAS) as a result of moderate to sometimes heavy binge drinking by her mother throughout pregnancy.
   A. *DESCRIBE* the characteristics Jane most likely exhibited to establish the diagnosis of FAS.

   B. *STATE* three long-term effects Jane could experience as she gets older.

C. *DESCRIBE* two nursing measures that could be effective in promoting Jane's growth and development.

6. Maternal substance abuse can be harmful to fetal and newborn health status, as well as growth and development.
   A. *DESCRIBE* the assessment findings associated with newborn withdrawal from each of the following substances.
   HEROIN

   METHADONE

   B. Susan has just been born. Her mother used cocaine during pregnancy. *IDENTIFY* the effects Susan may exhibit as a result of exposure to cocaine while in utero.

7. Tony is a 2-hour-old newborn. It is suspected that his mother abused drugs during pregnancy.
   A. *LIST* the signs associated with neonatal abstinence syndrome that the nurse should observe for when assessing Tony.

   B. Tony begins to exhibit signs that confirm that his mother used heroin during pregnancy. *CITE* two nursing diagnoses that would be appropriate for Tony.

   C. *OUTLINE* the care management that Tony and his mother will require as Tony progresses through withdrawal.

ONLINE LEARNING ACTIVITIES

Access the Lowdermilk, Perry **Evolve** website at
http://evolve.elsevier.com/Lowdermilk/MatWmnHlth/ and enter the **Student** portion through the
Learning Resources section to assist you in a search of the Internet for current requirements for
mandatory testing of maternal and newborn HIV status. Contact several state governments including
your own to determine these requirements. Prepare a paper that includes the following:

- Summary of the requirements of the state governments you contacted
- Discussion of the following points related to mandatory testing:
  - Rationale for mandatory testing
  - Legal and ethical implications of such testing
- Role of the nurses involved in women's health in implementing testing requirements including
  appropriate counseling and support measures

CHAPTER 39

Hemolytic Disorders and Congenital Anomalies

CHAPTER REVIEW ACTIVITIES

FILL IN THE BLANKS: Insert the congenital disorder represented by each of the following descriptions.

1. _____ A group of disorders that results from the absence of or change in a protein, usually an enzyme and mediated by the action of a certain gene (autosomal recessive inheritance). Examples include phenylketonuria and galactosemia.

2. _____ A small brain is present in a normally formed head.

3. _____ Urinary meatus opens below the glans penis or anywhere along the ventral surface of the penis, scrotum, or peritoneum; _____: urethral meatus opens on the dorsal surface of the penis; _____: abnormal development of the bladder, abdominal wall, and pubic symphysis that causes the bladder, urethra, and ureteral orifices to be exposed.

4. _____ Enlargement of the ventricles of the brain as a result of an imbalance between production and absorption of cerebrospinal fluid (CSF). It is characterized by a bulging anterior fontanel, an abnormal increase in the circumference of the head, and an increasing CSF pressure.

5. _____ Ventricular septal defects and tetralogy of Fallot are two common forms of this type of congenital disorder.

6. _____ The most common form of clubfoot. The foot points downward and inward, the ankle is inverted, and the Achilles tendon is shortened, all making the foot appear C shaped.

7. _____ The most common congenital anomaly of the nose requiring emergency surgery after birth. It consists of a bony or membranous septum between the nose and the pharynx.

8. _____ A form of spina bifida cystica (a neural tube defect) in which an external sac containing the meninges and cerebrospinal fluid protrudes through a defect in the vertebral column.

9. _____ A covered (with a peritoneal sac) defect of the umbilical ring into which varying amounts of the abdominal organs may herniate; _____ is the herniation of the bowel through a defect in the abdominal wall to the right of the umbilical cord. No protective sac covers the intestines.

10. _____ The passageway from the mouth to the stomach ends in a blind pouch or narrows into a thin cord; thus a continuous passageway to the stomach is not present.

Chapter 39: Hemolytic Disorders and Cogenital Anomalies   361

11. _____ A type of neural tube defect characterized by the absence of both cerebral hemispheres and the overlying skull. It is incompatible with life.
12. _____ Disorder characterized by displacement of the abdominal organs into the thoracic cavity.
13. _____ A form of spina bifida cystica (a neural tube defect) in which an external sac containing the meninges, cerebrospinal fluid, and nerves protrudes through a defect in the vertebral column.

TRUE OR FALSE: Circle "T" if true or "F" if false for each of the following statements. Correct the false statements.

T   F   14. When physiologic jaundice is experienced by Caucasian and African-American infants, the level of unconjugated bilirubin in the serum peaks at a higher level than in Asian or Native American infants.

T   F   15. Preterm newborns are at increased risk for developing pathologic jaundice.

T   F   16. For the full-term infant a serum bilirubin of 15 mg/dl is considered the upper limit beyond which the risk for kernicterus increases.

T   F   17. Kernicterus usually appears within 24 to 48 hours following birth.

T   F   18. The most common cause of pathologic hyperbilirubinemia is hemolytic disorders in the newborn.

T   F   19. ABO incompatibility is more common than Rh incompatibility but causes less severe problems in the affected infant.

T   F   20. At birth an indirect Coombs' test is performed on the newborn's cord blood to determine if the fetus has produced antibodies to its mother's blood.

T   F   21. Major congenital disorders are the leading cause of death among infants in the United States.

T   F   22. Certain congenital heart defects may not become apparent until the infant or child exhibits symptoms when exposed to stressors such as growth demands or infection.

T   F   23. The cause for congenital heart defects is readily identified in the majority of diagnosed infants.

T   F   24. Closure of spina bifida cystica is usually delayed until the infant is approximately 6 months of age.

T   F   25. An infant with a left-sided diaphragmatic hernia should be positioned on its left side and with its head and chest elevated.

T   F   26. Clubfoot occurs more frequently in females than in males.

T   F   27. Surgical repair of a cleft palate usually takes place when the affected infant is 6 to 12 weeks old.

28. *DESCRIBE* the physiologic basis for ABO incompatibility.

29. Congenital anomalies affect the health and well-being of infants.
   A. *FILL IN THE BLANKS:* Insert the term that corresponds to the following descriptions related to congenital anomalies.

   A disease or disorder that is transmitted from generation to generation is termed _____ or _____. A _____ disorder is one that is present at birth and can be caused by _____ or _____ factors, or both. Many defects appear to be of _____ inheritance, which is the interaction of multiple _____, with _____ factors that affect development. Examples of this form of inheritance are _____, _____, _____, _____, and _____ or _____.

   B. *SPECIFY* the assessment techniques and considerations that guide prenatal diagnosis of congenital anomalies.

   C. *EXPLAIN* why observation of the amount of amniotic fluid can be helpful in the perinatal diagnosis of certain congenital anomalies.

   D. *INDICATE* how each of the following types of postnatal tests can be used to diagnose an infant with a congenital anomaly.
   Biochemical tests

   Cytologic studies

   Dermatoglyphics

30. Congenital heart defects are a major cause of death in the first year of life.
   A. *LIST* several maternal factors that are associated with a higher incidence of congenital heart defects.

B. *IDENTIFY* the four physiologic classifications of congenital heart defects and *GIVE* one example for each classification.

C. *DESCRIBE* the signs that may be exhibited at birth by an infant with a congenital heart defect.

MULTIPLE CHOICE: Circle the one correct option and state the rationale for the option chosen.

31. The nurse is caring for a full-term newborn who is Rh positive. His mother (3–2–0–1–2), who is Rh negative, was never treated to prevent sensitization with her previous pregnancies. When assessing the newborn the nurse must be alert for signs indicative of pathologic hyperbilirubinemia. Which of the following signs would alert the nurse to this pathologic disorder?
    A. Jaundice in face including sclera beginning at 36 hours after birth
    B. Serum bilirubin level on the second day of life of 16 mg/dl
    C. Serum bilirubin concentration of 2 mg/dl in cord blood
    D. Total serum bilirubin level increase of 3 mg/dl in 24 hours

32. An Rh-negative woman (2–2–0–0–2) just gave birth to an Rh-positive baby boy. The direct and indirect Coombs test results are both negative. The nurse would:
    A. Prepare to administer RhoGAM to the newborn within 24 hours of his birth
    B. Observe the newborn closely for signs of pathologic jaundice
    C. Recognize that RhoGAM is not needed because both Coombs test results are negative
    D. Administer 300 mg of Rh_O (D) immune globulin intramuscularly to the woman within 72 hours of her baby's birth

33. The nurse will be assisting the physician with an exchange transfusion to be performed for a newborn male with pathologic jaundice that has been unresponsive to phototherapy. As part of the protocol for this procedure the nurse would:
    A. Keep the newborn NPO for 6 to 8 hours prior to the procedure
    B. Expect that 95% to 100% of the newborn will be exchanged with donor blood
    C. Implement measures to maintain the newborn's body temperature to prevent hypothermia
    D. Observe the newborn closely for signs of hypercalcemia

34. A newborn female has been diagnosed with myelomeningocele. Which of the following would be an important nursing measure to protect the newborn from injury and further complications during the preoperative period?
    A. Maintain the newborn in a lateral or prone position
    B. Tell the parents that they cannot hold their newborn
    C. Cover the sac with Vaseline gauze to keep it moist and intact
    D. Place a collection bag over the genitalia to collect urine

CRITICAL THINKING EXERCISES

1. Pathologic jaundice or hyperbilirubinemia is a serious health problem with the potential for severe complications that can permanently affect the life and health of the infant.

   A. *COMPLETE THE FOLLOWING TABLE* by contrasting physiologic and pathologic jaundice in terms of time of onset, time of resolution, and expected serum levels of unconjugated bilirubin.

Jaundice	Onset	Resolution	Serum Bilirubin Levels
Physiologic			
Pathologic			

   B. The yellowish discoloration of the skin, mucous membranes, sclera, and other organs is called _____. The deposit of bilirubin in the brain results in bilirubin encephalopathy, which is also called _____.

   C. *EXPLAIN* the underlying physiologic process that leads to hyperbilirubinemia in the newborn.

   D. *LIST* the potential causes for pathologic jaundice or hyperbilirubinemia.

   E. *IDENTIFY* the measures found to be effective in preventing hyperbilirubinemia.

Chapter 39: Hemolytic Disorders and Cogenital Anomalies   365

F. Baby boy James has developed pathologic hyperbilirubinemia as a result of red blood cell destruction by maternal Rh-positive antibodies. He is being prepared for an exchange transfusion.

1) *EXPLAIN* the rationale for this procedure.

2) *STATE* two nursing diagnoses related to James and his parents at this time.

3) *OUTLINE* the nursing care measures required as James undergoes an exchange transfusion.

G. Clinical manifestations of bilirubin encephalopathy or _____ typically appear between _____ and _____ days after birth. During the first phase of the disorder, the newborn is _____ and _____, with a poor _____ and depressed or absent _____. These signs are followed by a _____, _____, _____, and _____. Often _____ and _____ occur. These signs occur over a period of _____ hours. About _____ of the affected infants survive but many suffer from permanent neurologic sequelae.

2. Angela, who is Rh negative, had a spontaneous abortion at 13 weeks' gestation, which resulted in what she said was just a heavier than usual menstrual period. Six months later she becomes pregnant again.

A. *DESCRIBE* the physiologic basis for Rh incompatibility and the occurrence of sensitization.

B. An indirect Coombs' test is positive. *STATE* the meaning of this finding.

C. *INDICATE* if Angela is or is not a candidate for RhoGAM. *SUPPORT* your answer.

D. *DESCRIBE* RhoGAM (Rh immunoglobulin) and its use.

E. Angela's fetus is at risk for erythroblastosis fetalis and hydrops fetalis. *EXPLAIN* each of these conditions.

Erythroblastosis fetalis

Hydrops fetalis

F. *DESCRIBE* the treatment approaches that can be used to prevent intrauterine fetal death and early neonatal death for Angela's baby.

3. Baby girl Jennifer was born with spina bifida cystica, myelomeningocele. *DESCRIBE* the measures the nurse should use to manage Jennifer's care and help her parents cope with this congenital anomaly.

4. Baby boy Thomas was just born. He is exhibiting signs that the nurse-midwife and the neonatologist believe are consistent with a diaphragmatic hernia.
   A. *IDENTIFY* the clinical manifestations that Thomas most likely exhibited to cause his health care providers to suspect diaphragmatic hernia.

B. *STATE* the priority nursing diagnosis for Thomas.

C. *OUTLINE* the essential care measures during the immediate postbirth period.

5. Baby girl Denise was born with a cleft lip and palate.
   A. *STATE* three nursing diagnoses faced by Denise and her parents. *DISCUSS* the rationale for each nursing diagnosis stated.

   B. *OUTLINE* several nursing measures that will need to be implemented to ensure Denise's well-being until surgical repair can be accomplished.

ONLINE LEARNING ACTIVITIES

Access the Lowdermilk, Perry **Evolve** website at **http://evolve.elsevier.com/Lowdermilk/MatWmnHlth/** and enter the **Student** portion through the **Learning Resources** section to assist you in contacting the March of Dimes website. Prepare a report that includes the following:

- Summary of the types of information and services provided in terms of prevention, detection, and treatment of congenital disorders
- Services directed to health care professionals
- Services directed to persons affected by congenital disorders and their parents and family
- How the professional nurse can use the March of Dimes website to improve the quality of health care they provide to persons affected by congenital disorders and their parents and family

CHAPTER 40

Nursing Care of the High Risk Newborn

CHAPTER REVIEW ACTIVITIES

MATCHING: "Complications Associated with Oxygen Therapy" Match the description in Column I with the appropriate term in Column II.

COLUMN I

_____ 1. Disorder of developing blood vessels in the eye often associated with oxygen tensions that are too high for the level of retinal maturity initially resulting in vasoconstriction and continuing problems after the oxygen is discontinued.

_____ 2. Acute inflammatory disease of the gastrointestinal mucosa commonly complicated by perforation.

_____ 3. Occurs when fetal shunt between the pulmonary artery and the aorta fails to constrict after birth or reopens after constriction has occurred.

_____ 4. Chronic pulmonary iatrogenic condition caused by barotrauma from pressure ventilation and oxygen toxicity.

_____ 5. One of the most common types of brain injury encountered in the neonatal period and among the most severe in both short-term and long-term outcomes.

COLUMN II

A. Bronchopulmonary dysplasia (BPD)

B. Retinopathy of prematurity (ROP)

C. Patent ductus arteriosus (PDA)

D. Periventricular-intraventricular hemorrhage (PV-IVH)

E. Necrotizing enterocolitis (NEC)

TRUE OR FALSE: Circle "T" if true or "F" if false for each of the following statements. Correct the false statements.

T F   6. An extremely low birth weight infant is one whose weight at birth is 2000 g or less.

T F   7. Eight months after birth, an infant born at 30 weeks' gestation would be considered to be the corrected age of 5.5 months.

T F   8. The incidence of physical and emotional abuse is slightly higher toward the infant who, because of preterm birth or illness, was separated from the mother for a period of time after birth.

T F   9. Preterm infants are at risk for polycythemia.

T F 10. Sudden infant death syndrome (SIDS) is much more likely to develop in preterm infants than in term infants.

T F 11. For preterm infants a PaO_2 of less than 60 mm Hg or an oxygen saturation of less than 92% indicates the need for oxygen therapy.

T F 12. Surfactant is administered intravenously to a preterm infant.

T F 13. Infants born before 36 weeks' gestation require exogenous surfactant administration to survive extrauterine life.

T F 14. Infants who need oxygen should have their respiratory status assessed accurately every 1 to 2 hours.

T F 15. Acrocyanosis is an assessment finding indicative of an underlying respiratory disorder.

T F 16. A decrease in rectal temperature is often an early sign of cold stress in the newborn.

T F 17. High risk infants usually have lower caloric, nutrient, and fluid requirements than those of the term, normal newborn.

T F 18. The flow rate for a gavage tube feeding should approximate that of an oral feeding (1 ml/minute).

T F 19. Sucking on a pacifier during gavage or between oral feedings can improve the preterm newborn's oxygenation.

T F 20. Not all postmature infants exhibit signs of dysmaturity.

T F 21. When meconium is present in the amniotic fluid at birth, the infant's mouth and nose should be suctioned while still on the perineum before the infant's first breath.

T F 22. Hypoglycemia is defined as a blood glucose level of less than 40 mg/dl in preterm infants during the first 3 days of life.

23. *EXPLAIN* the purpose of exogenous surfactant administration to the preterm newborn.

24. *DESCRIBE* kangaroo care.

25. The preterm infant is vulnerable to a number of complications related to immaturity of body systems. COMPLETE THE FOLLOWING TABLE by identifying the potential problems and their physiologic basis for each of the physiologic functions listed.

Physiologic Function	Potential Problems	Physiologic Basis
Respiratory function		
Cardiovascular function		
Maintaining body temperature		
Central nervous system function		
Maintaining adequate nutrition		
Maintaining renal function		
Maintaining hematologic status		
Resisting infection		

26. When providing care, nurses need to consider the pain experienced by newborns especially those who are at high risk and require numerous invasive procedures.
    A. *EXPLAIN* the CRIES pain assessment tool.

    B. *DESCRIBE* infant behaviors that could indicate that the infant has a memory of painful experiences.

    C. *STATE* the consequences of mismanaged infant pain.

    D. *DISCUSS* how each of the following strategies can be used to manage the pain experienced by newborns:
    Nonpharmacologic management

    Pharmacologic management

27. Respiratory distress syndrome (RDS) is a lung disorder usually associated with preterm birth.
    A. Respiratory distress syndrome (RDS) is caused by a lack of _____, which leads to progressive _____, loss of _____, and a _____ imbalance, with uneven distribution of _____.
    B. Clinical signs of RDS include _____, _____, _____, _____, _____, increased work of _____, _____, _____ or _____ acidosis, and _____ and _____. These symptoms usually appear immediately after _____ or within _____. Physical examination reveals poor _____, _____, _____, use of _____, and occasionally _____.
    C. RDS is usually self-limiting with respiratory symptoms abating after _____ hours. The disappearance of symptoms coincides with _____ production.
    D. Treatment of RDS involves establishment and maintenance of adequate _____ and _____, administration of _____, and maintenance of a _____ environment.

MULTIPLE CHOICE: Circle the one correct option and state the rationale for the option chosen.

28. Preterm infants are at increased risk for developing respiratory distress. The nurse should assess for signs that would indicate that the newborn is having difficulty breathing. A sign of respiratory distress would be:
    A. Use of abdominal muscles to breathe
    B. Respiratory rate of 40 breaths per minute or greater
    C. Periodic breathing with a 5- to 10-second respiratory pause followed by 10 to 15 seconds of rapid breathing
    D. Seesaw breathing pattern

29. When caring for a preterm infant at 30 weeks' gestation, the nurse should recognize the newborn's primary nursing diagnosis would be:
    A. Risk for infection related to decreased immune response
    B. Impaired gas exchange related to deficiency of surfactant
    C. Ineffective thermoregulation related to immature thermoregulation center
    D. Imbalanced nutrition: less than body requirements related to ineffective suck and swallow

30. Preterm newborns are vulnerable to cold stress. An early sign of cold stress would be:
    A. Decrease in rectal temperature
    B. Apneic spells
    C. Mottling with acrocyanosis
    D. Bradycardia

31. A nurse is preparing to insert a gavage tube and feed a preterm newborn. As part of the protocol for this procedure the nurse would:
    A. Determine the length of tubing to be inserted by measuring from tip of nose to lobe of ear to midpoint between xiphoid process and umbilicus
    B. Coat the tube with water-soluble lubricant to ease passage
    C. Insert tube through the nose as the preferred route for most infants
    D. Check placement of tube by injecting 2 to 3 ml of sterile water into the tube and listening for gurgling with a stethoscope

CRITICAL THINKING EXERCISES

1. Oxygen therapy is a vital component in the care of the newborn experiencing respiratory distress.
    A. IDENTIFY the criteria that should be used to determine if there is a need for supplemental oxygen.

B. *CREATE* a set of general guidelines that reflects the recommended principles for safe and effective administration of oxygen to a compromised newborn.

C. *COMPLETE THE FOLLOWING TABLE* by specifying the indications for each of the following methods of oxygen therapy and describing the care measures required to ensure their safe and effective administration.

Method	Indications	Nursing Measures
Hood		
Nasal cannula		
Continuous positive airway pressure		
Mechanical ventilation		

2. Baby girl Jane has been receiving oxygen therapy. Her health care providers are preparing to begin the process of weaning her from the oxygen.
   A. *DESCRIBE* signs that would indicate that Jane is ready to be weaned from oxygen therapy.

   B. *OUTLINE* the guidelines that should be followed when weaning Jane from oxygen therapy.

3. Anne, a 3-pound 12-ounce (1705-gm) preterm newborn at 32 weeks' gestation, is admitted to the neonatal intensive care unit (NICU) after her birth for observation and supportive care. Anne's nutritional needs are a critical concern in her care. Oral formula feedings are attempted first.

A. *STATE* the assessment data that the nurse should document after each of Anne's feedings to indicate feeding method effectiveness.

B. The acceptable weight loss limit during Anne's first week of life is up to _____ of her birth weight. After the first week, Anne's loss or gain during each 24-hour period should not exceed _____ of the previous day's weight. Possible causes for weight loss include increased _____ or _____, increased _____ losses, inadequate _____ or incorrect _____ administration, and problems with _____.

C. The nurse determines that Anne's suck is weak and she becomes too fatigued during oral feedings to obtain sufficient nutrients and fluid. The nurse confers with the neonatologist and a decision is made to provide intermittent gavage feedings with occasional oral feedings. *DESCRIBE* the guidelines the nurse should follow when inserting the gavage tube.

D. *STATE* the priority nursing diagnosis for Anne.

E. *DISCUSS* the principles the nurse should follow before, during, and after a gavage feeding to ensure safety and maximum effectiveness.

F. *OUTLINE* the protocol that should be followed when advancing Anne back to full oral feeding.

4. The neonatal intensive care unit (NICU) is a stressful environment for preterm infants and their families.
   A. *IDENTIFY* the common sources of stress facing infants and their families in an intensive care environment.
      Infant stressors

      Family stressors

   B. Nurses working in the ICN must be aware of infant cues and adjust stimuli accordingly. *LIST* infant cues that indicate overstimulation and infant cues that indicate a relaxed state.
      Overstimulation

      Relaxed state

   C. *IDENTIFY* specific measures that can be used to protect infants from overstimulation and yet provide appropriate stimulation to meet the developmental and emotional needs of infants.

   D. *SPECIFY* the guidelines that should be followed regarding infant positioning.

   E. *DESCRIBE* the measures a nurse can use to help parents and family cope with their infant's death.

5. Mary and Jim are parents of a preterm baby boy.
   A. *STATE* the parental tasks that need to be accomplished by Mary and Jim, as parents of a preterm infant.

   B. *IDENTIFY* two nursing diagnoses related to Mary and Jim as parents of a preterm infant.

   C. *DESCRIBE* the nursing measures that should be used to support Mary and Jim and facilitate their progress through the stages and tasks of parenting a preterm infant.

6. Marion is beginning her 43rd week of pregnancy.
   A. *SUPPORT THIS STATEMENT:* Perinatal mortality is significantly higher in the postmature fetus and neonate.

   B. *STATE* the assessment findings that are typical of a postmature infant.

   C. *DESCRIBE* the two major complications that can be experienced by a postmature infant.

7. Janet, a pregnant woman at term, is in labor. On the basis of serial ultrasound findings, her fetus is estimated to be smaller than it should be as a consequence of Janet's heavy smoking during pregnancy and her high-risk status related to preeclampsia.
   A. *LIST* the assessment findings that are characteristic of a small for gestational age (SGA) infant.

B. *IDENTIFY* four major complications facing Janet's baby during labor, birth, and the postpartum period.

C. *DESCRIBE* the physiologic basis for each potential complication and the signs and symptoms indicative of its presence.

8. Marion is at 24 weeks' gestation and is in preterm labor. Her primary health care provider determines that preterm birth is inevitable and has elected to transport Marion to a tertiary center before she gives birth to maximize the survival potential of her unborn infant.
   A. *EXPLAIN* the advantages of transport before birth.

   B. Marion gives birth before she can be transported. Her baby will now be transported to the tertiary center once stable. *INDICATE* the needs of this preterm baby that must be stabilized prior to transport.

   C. *IDENTIFY* the measures that the nurse should use to support Marion and her family as her newborn is transported to the tertiary center.

ONLINE LEARNING ACTIVITIES

Access the Centers for Disease Control and Prevention (CDC) and the National Center for Health Statistics (NCHS) websites to gather statistical information related to preterm, postterm, small for gestational age, and large for gestational age infants. Create a chart for each category of infant that includes the following:
- Incidence in your state and in the nation as a whole
- Characteristic of women who would give birth to this category of infant
- Impact of this infant's gestational age or birth weight on its health and well-being—consider morbidity and mortality statistics for this category of infant

Based on an analysis for the data collected, suggest strategies that could increase the rate of term births of infants that are appropriate for gestational age.

CHAPTER 41

Grieving the Loss of a Newborn

CHAPTER REVIEW ACTIVITIES

1. Mary, a pregnant woman at 24 weeks' gestation, has been admitted to the labor unit following a prenatal visit at her health care provider's office. Fetal death is suspected and eventually confirmed. *IDENTIFY* the phase of grief response represented by each of the comments made by Mary as she reacts to her loss. *DESCRIBE* each phase in terms of expected duration, behaviors typically exhibited, and emotions experienced.

   A. "The doctor says he cannot find my baby's heart beat or feel my baby move. He thinks my baby has died. I know you will hear my baby's heart beat since you have a monitor here. My baby is okay—I just know it!!"

   B. "I know this never would have happened if I had quit my job as a legal secretary. My mom told me that pregnant women should take it easy. If I had listened I would have my baby in my arms right now!"

   C. "Since my baby died I just cannot seem to concentrate on even the simplest things at home and at work. I always seem to feel tired and out of sorts."

   D. "It is going to be hard. I will always remember my little baby boy and the day he was supposed to be born. But I know that my husband and I have to go on with our lives."

2. *DISCUSS* the meaning for each of the following:
   Bereavement (grief)

   Anticipatory grief

   Bittersweet grief

   Complicated bereavement

3. Worden (1991) identified four tasks of mourners. *IDENTIFY* the four tasks and state nursing actions that could help a grieving family accomplish each task.

4. *EXPLAIN* how a father's grief response may differ from that of his partner, the mother.

5. *IDENTIFY* each of the five components of the caring framework as developed by the research of Swanson and Kauffman. *EXPLAIN* how you would use these components to support grieving parents.

6. *DESCRIBE* how you, as a nurse, would help parents and other family members actualize the loss of their newborn.

7. Nurses working with families experiencing loss must be able to distinguish normal grieving behaviors from those that indicate complicated bereavement.
A. *IDENTIFY* those behaviors that characterize complicated bereavement.

B. *DESCRIBE* the approach a nurse should take if signs of complicated bereavement are noted.

MULTIPLE CHOICE: Circle the one correct option and state the rationale for the option chosen.

8. A woman gave birth to twin girls, one of whom was stillborn. Which of the following nursing actions would be least helpful in supporting the woman as she copes with her loss?
   A. Remind her that she should be happy that one daughter survived and is healthy
   B. Assist the woman to take pictures of both babies
   C. Encourage the woman to hold the deceased twin in her arms to say good-bye
   D. Offer her the opportunity for counseling to help her with her grief and that of her surviving twin as she gets older

9. During the acute distress phase of the grief response parents are most likely to experience:
   A. Fear and anxiety about future pregnancies
   B. Difficulty with cognitive processing
   C. Search for meaning
   D. Sadness and depression

10. A 17-year-old woman experiences a miscarriage at 12 weeks' gestation. When she is informed about the miscarriage she begins to cry stating that she was upset about her pregnancy at first and now she is being punished for not wanting her baby. The nurse's best response would be:
   A. "You are still so young, you probably were not ready for a baby right now."
   B. "This must be so hard for you—I am here if you want to talk."
   C. "At least this happened early in your pregnancy before you felt your baby move."
   D. "God must have a good reason for letting this happen."

CRITICAL THINKING EXERCISES

1. Jane (2–1–0–0–1) is a 21-year-old woman admitted with vaginal bleeding at 13 weeks' gestation. She experiences a miscarriage. Jane is accompanied by her husband Tom. Her 5-year-old daughter is at home with Jane's mother.
   A. *DESCRIBE* the approach you would take to develop a plan of individualized support measures for Jane as she and her family cope with their loss.

B. *CITE* questions and observations you would use to gather the information required to create an individualized plan of care.

C. *FORMULATE* three nursing diagnoses appropriate for Jane and her family.

D. *IDENTIFY* the therapeutic communication techniques you should use to help Jane and Tom acknowledge and express their feelings and emotions about their loss.

E. At discharge, Jane is crying. She tells you, "I know it must have been something I did wrong this time since my first pregnancy was okay. We wanted to give our daughter a baby brother or sister." *INDICATE* whether the following responses would be therapeutic (T) or nontherapeutic (N). *SPECIFY* how you would change the responses determined to be nontherapeutic.

_____ 1) "You are still young. As soon as your body heals, you will be able to try to have another baby."

_____ 2) "What can I do that would help you and Tom cope with what happened?"

_____ 3) "Do not worry. I am sure you did everything you could to have a healthy pregnancy."

_____ 4) "It was probably for the best. Fetal loss at this time is usually the result of defective development."

_____ 5) "You sound like you are blaming yourself for what happened. Let's talk about it."

_____ 6) "This must be difficult for you and your family."

_____ 7) "If it had to happen it is best that it happened this early in the pregnancy before you and your family became attached to the fetus."

_____ 8) "You really should concentrate on your little daughter rather than thinking so much about the baby you lost."

_____ 9) "I feel sad about the loss that you and Tom are experiencing."

_____ 10) "Would you and Tom like to speak to our hospital's chaplain before you are discharged?"

2. Angela gave birth vaginally to a stillborn fetus at 38 weeks' gestation. In addition to emotional support, her physical needs must be recognized and met. *IDENTIFY* these physical needs and how you would meet them.

3. Anita gave birth to a baby boy who died shortly thereafter as a result of multiple congenital anomalies, including anencephaly. She and her husband Bill are provided with the opportunity to see their baby.

    A. *DISCUSS* how the nurse can help Anita and Bill make a decision that is right for them about seeing their baby.

    B. Anita and Bill decide to see their baby. *SPECIFY* the measures the nurse can use to make the time Anita and Bill spend with their baby as easy as possible and to provide them with an experience that will facilitate the grieving process.

4. Tara is at 16 weeks' gestation. A sonogram reveals that her fetus has anencephaly. Her primary health care provider recommends a therapeutic abortion. *DISCUSS* the role of the nurse in supporting Tara as she makes her decision about the abortion and copes with her grief.

ONLINE LEARNING ACTIVITIES

Contact two of the web sources listed at the end of the chapter for when a baby dies. Describe each site in terms of the following:

- Clarity, accuracy, accessibility (ease of use), value, and depth of information provided
- Currency—frequency of site updates
- Nature of support services offered
- Variety of links to other relevant sites
- Ability of persons visiting the site to obtain additional information and individualized support through such services as e-mail and chat rooms

Discuss how nurses working with grieving parents could use these sites to extend support into the homes of parents.

Answer Key

CHAPTER 1: CONTEMPORARY MATERNITY NURSING AND WOMEN'S HEALTH CARE

Chapter Review Activities

1. C, 2. D, 3. F, 4. A, 5. G, 6. B, 7. E

8. Maternity nursing
9. Women's health nursing
10. Evidence-based practice

11. Outcomes-oriented care, cost, length of stay, client satisfaction

12. *Healthy People 2010*, quality and years of healthy life; health disparities

13. Standards of practice
14. Telemedicine
15. Best practice
16. Clinical benchmarking
17. Risk management
18. Integrative health care

19. *Factors contributing to infant mortality:* limited maternal education, young maternal age, unmarried, poverty, lack of prenatal care, poor nutrition, smoking, alcohol and drug use, poor maternal health habits

20. F, 21. T, 22. T, 23. F, 24. T, 25. F, 26. T, 27. F, 28. F, 29. T, 30. T, 31. F, 32. T, 33. T, 34. F, 35. F, 36. T

37. *Three major changes in childbirth practices; how changes improved care:* see Childbirth Practices section; discuss three of the following: increase in nurse-midwives as primary obstetric care providers, use of regional anesthesia/analgesia, family-centered birthing, childbirth education classes, early discharge, doulas, settings for birth, early discharge programs, neonatal security measures, more natural management of second stage of labor

38. *Factors/social conditions affecting health of women:* see Health of Women section; discuss race, violence, incidence of HIV/AIDS, poverty

Critical Thinking Exercises

1. *Nursing director of inner city prenatal clinic:* see Trends in Fertility and Birth Rate sections; answer should include:
   - Biostatistics and contributing factors
   - Factors associated with high risk pregnancy
   - Benefits of prenatal care; impact of inadequate prenatal care
   - Importance of self-care and consumer involvement; devise ways to encourage participation in prenatal care

2. *High technology will not reduce rate of preterm birth and LBW infants:* discuss the following topics when formulating answer:
   - Factors associated with LBW and IMR
   - Factors that escalate rate of high risk pregnancy

- high-tech care: what it can and cannot do

High-tech care is no longer the solution; answer should reflect factors associated with IMR, the high cost of care management for high risk pregnancies and compromised infants as compared to the cost and effectiveness of early, ongoing, comprehensive prenatal care

3. *Three proposed changes with rationale:* changes proposed should reflect efforts toward improving access to care, using research-based approaches and standards to guide care, and creating health-care services that address the factors associated with poor pregnancy outcomes

4. *Self-care approaches:* see Involving Consumers and Promoting Self-care section; care measures proposed should include health teaching regarding nutrition and stress management; anticipatory guidance for pregnancy, parenting, and menopause; self-assessment measures such as BSE; guiding decision making by providing information regarding the pros and cons of care choices available; communication and counseling techniques should be used; substance abuse counseling; referral to support groups

5. *Barriers to prenatal care:* see Limited Access to Care section; address solutions to the following barriers: inability to pay, lack of transportation, dependent child care, minority status, cultural beliefs, young maternal age, homeless, unmarried

CHAPTER 2: COMMUNITY CARE: THE FAMILY AND CULTURE

Chapter Review Activities

1. B, 2. E, 3. D, 4. C, 5. F, 6. A, 7. B, 8. E, 9. C, 10. D, 11. A

12. Culture
13. Subculture
14. Cultural relativism
15. Acculturation
16. Assimilation
17. Ethnocentrism
18. Cultural competence
19. Present-orientation
20. Future-orientation
21. Past-orientation
22. Personal space
23. Family
24. Nuclear
25. Extended
26. Binuclear
27. Single parent, economically, socially
28. Reconstituted (blended)
29. Homosexual
30. Family Systems theory
31. Family Lifecycle theory
32. Family Stress theory, internal, external
33. Community
34. Aggregate

35. Primary prevention, immunizations, infant care seat education, education to prevent tobacco use

36. Secondary prevention, health screening
37. Tertiary prevention
38. Primordial prevention
39. Clinical integration
40. Third-party payer

41. T, 42. F, 43. F, 44. F, 45. T, 46. T, 47. T, 48. T, 49. T, 50. F, 51. T, 52. T, 53. F, 54. F, 55. T, 56. T, 57. F, 58. F, 59. T

60. *Theoretical approaches to care of families:* see Theoretical Approaches to Understanding Families section and Table 2-1 for a description of each approach and examples regarding nurses use of these approaches.

61. *Discuss purpose of incorporating cultural aspects when providing culturally competent care:* see Childbearing Beliefs and Practices section;

A. Communication: consider language; need for a translator; dialect, interpersonal style, volume of speech, meaning of touch and gestures

B. Space: include feelings of territoriality; recognize that comfort zone must be established in terms of touch, proximity to others, and handling of possession; ensure that client is in control of personal space to ensure a sense of autonomy and security

C. Time: consider past, present, and future orientations and how this could affect meeting appointment times and health care practices, beliefs, and goals

D. Family roles: parent role; roles for grandparents and siblings; father's participation in pregnancy, childbirth, and child care

62. *Process for providing culturally competent care:* see Developing Cultural Competence section and Cultural Considerations box; incorporate the components of culturally competent care and pathway for cultural competence in answer; use questions in Cultural Considerations box to assess a client's cultural beliefs.

63. *Identify six population groups of women vulnerable to reproductive health risks:* pregnant adolescents, substance abusers, violence-prone families, mentally ill, persons with STIs or other communicable diseases, and those with malnutrition.

64. *State three characteristics of refugees that increase their vulnerability:* see Refugees and Immigrants section; include in answer such characteristics as grief of leaving homeland and loss of family members; effects of surviving trauma of war and refugee camps; experiencing multiple health problems such as infection, malnutrition, stress disorders; cultural differences including inexperience with Western medicine.

65. *Nurses' use of the telephone to provider health services:* see Telephonic Nursing Care section; include warm lines, advice lines, telephonic nursing assessment, consultation, and education, and communication via the Internet.

66. B is correct; negative images of homosexuals in our society rather than the findings of research influence how people view what will happen to children raised by gay or lesbian parents; this is not a rare family form.

67. A is correct; B, C, and D reflect the characteristics of families with closed boundaries; they are more prone to crises because they have a narrow network to help them in times of stress.

68. B is correct; providing explanations, especially when performing tasks that require close contact, can help to avoid misunderstandings; touching the client, making eye contact, and taking away the right to make decisions can be interpreted by clients in some cultures as invading their personal space.

69. D is correct; A, B, and C are incorrect interpretations based on the woman's culture and customs; Native-Americans often use cradle boards and avoid handling their newborn often; they should not be fed colostrum.

Critical Thinking Exercises

1. *Imagine that you are a nurse working in a multicultural prenatal clinic:* use Table 2-2 and Box 2-2 to formulate your answer; consider components of communication, space, time, roles; identify the degree to which each woman/family adheres to their culture's beliefs and practices; do not stereotype.

2. Pamela, a Native American pregnant woman:
   A. *Questions to ask:* see questions listed in the Cultural Considerations box.
   B. *Communication approach to use:* see Childbearing Beliefs and Practices section; include concepts of communication patterns, space, time, and family roles when formulating your answer.
   C. *Identify Native American beliefs and practices:* see Table 2-2 to formulate your answer; remember to determine her individual beliefs and practices to avoid stereotyping.

3. *Describe cultural beliefs and practices of Hispanic family—recent birth of twin girls:* Table 2-2 outlines parenting guidelines for several ethnic groups including those Hispanic families are likely to follow.

4. *Refugee couple from Bosnia seeking prenatal care:* (see Refugees and Immigrants; Cultural Factors related to Family Health; and Childbearing Beliefs and Practices sections).
   • Consider the process of working with a translator; be sure to show respect for this couple by addressing questions and comments to them and not to the translator.
   • Box 2-1 outlines steps to follow when using a translator including preparation measures, meeting the translator, interaction during the interview, and consultation with translator after the interview.
   • Consider the stressors faced by refugees and the health care needs they present.
   • Research Bosnia: cultural beliefs and practices and the current political turmoil that led this couple to come to the United States at this time.

5. Home care nurse must become familiar with neighborhoods and their resources:

   A. *Walking survey:* walking survey involving use of observation skills during a trip through a community (see Box 2-4).
   B. *Use of findings:* discuss how each of the survey's components reflect a community's strengths and problems; strengths could be used to provide clients with needed support; nurse could mobilize community leaders to solve identified problems; try using the survey to assess your community and the community in which your college is located.

6. Marie, a single parent of two children, is homeless (see Homeless Women section).
   A. *Discuss types of health problems to which they are most vulnerable:* infections, injury, chronic illnesses such as asthma and circulatory problems, anemia and other nutritionally related disorders such as obesity, dental caries, and diabetes.
   B. *Marie's vulnerability for pregnancy:* victimization, economic survival, lack of access to health care and birth control measures, need for closeness and intimacy, doubt fertility.
   C. *Principles to guide nurse when providing care:* treat with respect and dignity, case management to coordinate care to meet multiple needs, flexible appointment times providing service when they come in, make each interaction count, be purposeful, keep her empowered, help her to reconnect with her support system if possible and appropriate.

7. Consuelo, pregnant wife of a migrant worker and mother of two (see Migrant Women section)
   • Begin by confirming that she is pregnant.
   • Consider risks she faces including an increased risk for miscarriage, inadequate prenatal care, and infant mortality.
   • Exposure to teratogens.

- Inadequate availability and use of contraceptives, increased rate of STIs including HIV, and poor nutrition are major concerns that need to be addressed.

8. *List questions for a postpartum follow-up telephone call:* see Telephonic Nursing Care section; include questions guided by expected postpartum physical and emotional changes; ask her how she is feeling and managing, condition of her newborn (eating, sleeping, eliminating), response of other family members to newborn, sources of happiness and stress, adequacy of help and support being received and need for additional support or referrals.

9. *Home visit to a postpartum woman at 36 hours after birth:* see Boxes 2-5 and 2-6, and Care Management—the first home care visit section to answer each component of this exercise, including the approach you would take to prepare, your actions during the visit, safety precautions and infection control measures you would follow, how you would end the visit, and the interventions you would follow after the visit including documentation of assessments, actions, and responses.

10. Angela, a pregnant woman with hyperemesis gravidarum (see Home Care along the Perinatal Continuum of Care section for A and B and Care Management and Intervention subsection for C).
    A. *Criteria for discharge readiness:* include criteria related to Angela's health status and that of her fetus, availability of qualified home care professionals, family resources, and cost-effectiveness of discharging her to home care.
    B. *Information needed to institute high-tech care in the home:* medical diagnosis and prognosis, prescribed therapies, medication history, drug dosing

information, potential ancillary supplies, type of infusion access device that will be used, and available systems of social support.
    C. *Home environment criteria:* do a walk-through inspection to determine physical features of the home; access to the home; sanitary conditions; adequacy of area to store, prepare, and administer prescribed treatment; presence of utilities; safety features; and access to transportation and emergency support.

11. *Cost-effectiveness of a home health care service for postpartum women and their families:* see Perinatal Services section; include in your answer
    - Ability to observe first hand the home environment and family dynamics in a familiar or natural setting; natural; adequacy of resources; safety.
    - Teaching can be tailored to the woman, her family, and to her home.
    - Less expensive than a day in the hospital; travel time and other expenses must be considered.
    - Prevention, early detection, and treatment measures can be offered.
    - Long-term positive effects on parenting and child health.
    - Use research findings and recommendations of professional organizations to validate proposal.

CHAPTER 3: GENETICS

Chapter Review Activities

1. Q, 2. H, 3. C, 4. F, 5. S, 6. G, 7. D, 8. M, 9. R, 10. L, 11. A, 12. P, 13. J, 14. B, 15. O, 16. I, 17. K, 18. N, 19. E

20. Congenital disorders
21. Genetic testing
22. Direct (molecular) testing
23. Linkage analysis
24. Biochemical testing
25. Cytogenic testing

26. Carrier screening tests

27. Predictive testing; presymptomatic; predispositional

28. Gene-expression profiling
29. Pharmacogenomics
30. Gene therapy (Gene transfer)

31. F, 32. T, 33. F, 34. T, 35. F, 36. F, 37. T, 38. F, 39. F, 40. T, 41. T, 42. F, 43. F, 44. F, 45. F, 46. T, 47. F

48. *Identify five main genetics-related nursing activities:* see Genetics-Related Nursing Activities section.

49. *Advances in genetics as a result of the Human Genome Project* (see Human Genome Project section); explore the public data base created by the project and disseminated on the Internet site of the NCBI.

50. *ELSI risks* (see ELSI section): consider type of information gained, anxiety and altered relationships engendered by the information, confidentiality and discrimination/stigmatization issues.

51. *Factors influencing decision regarding genetic testing* (see Factors Influencing the Decision to Undergo Genetic Testing section): factors can include family pressures, responsibility to others, access to testing, cultural/ethnic beliefs.

52. *Explain each type of inheritance and give an example:*
    - Unifactorial inheritance: inheritable characteristic is controlled by a single gene that can be dominant or recessive; Marfan syndrome, Huntington's chorea, cystic fibrosis
    - Multifactorial inheritance: congenital disorder resulting from a combination of genetic and environmental factors; cleft lip and palate, congenital heart defects.
    - X-linked inheritance: transmission of abnormal genes on the X-chromosome; can be recessive or dominant; both males and females can be affected but females are usually carriers and if expressed in the female it tends to be less severe because females also have a normal gene on their second chromosome.

53. D is correct; genotype is the entire genetic makeup whereas phenotype is the manner in which the genotype is expressed in the person's physical appearance.

54. A is correct; autosomal dominant inheritance is unrelated to exposure to teratogens; each pregnancy has the same potential for expression of the disorder; there is no reduction if one child is already affected; if the gene is inherited, the disorder is always expressed.

55. D is correct; there is a 25% chance females will be carriers; if males inherit the X-chromosome with the defective gene, the disorder will be expressed and they can transmit the gene to female offspring; females are affected if they receive the defective gene from both parents.

56. D is correct; cystic fibrosis, as an inborn error of metabolism, follows an autosomal recessive pattern of inheritance; two defective genes (one from each parent) are required for the disorder to be expressed; she does not have the disorder and the father does not have the defective gene— therefore none of their children will have the disorder but there will be a 50% chance they will be carriers of the defective gene.

Critical Thinking Exercises

1. *Support of statement that nurses should have basic understanding of genetics* (see Nursing and Genetics section): answer should reflect the rapid advance in genetic based treatment and the ability to diagnose

genetic disorders; emphasize the nurse's role as teacher and advocate.

2. *Questions to determine if risk factors for inheritable disorders are present:* ask questions that would elicit information regarding health status of family members, abnormal reproductive outcomes, history of maternal disorders, drug exposures, and illnesses, advanced maternal and paternal age, and ethnic origin

3. Couple facing a genetic disorder:
   A. *Nurse's role in determining genetic risk:* Tay-Sachs is an autosomal-recessive disorder that follows a unifactorial pattern of inheritance; Mr. G. needs to be tested because he must also be a carrier to produce a child with the disorder; emphasize the nurse's role in terms of emotional support, facilitation of the decision-making process, and interpretation of diagnostic test results and how they can influence future childbearing decisions. Consider factors that can influence the decision to participate or not participate in testing.
   B. *Inheritance possibility when both parents carry the defective recessive gene:* there is a 25% chance child will be normal, a 25% chance that child will express the disorder, and a 50% chance that child will be a carrier; this pattern is the same for every pregnancy; there is no reduction in risk from one pregnancy to another.
   C. *Education and emotional support:* discuss the nature of this disorder, extent of risk, and consequences if the child inherits the disorder; options available including amniocentesis, continuing or not continuing the pregnancy if the child is affected; use of reproductive technology or adoption; be sensitive to cultural and religious beliefs; encourage expression of feelings; refer for further counseling or support groups as appropriate.

CHAPTER 4: ALTERNATIVE AND COMPLEMENTARY THERAPIES

Chapter Review Activities

1. E, 2. H, 3. B, 4. F, 5. D, 6. J, 7. C, 8. A, 9. G, 10. I

11. Holistic healing, body, mind, spirit

12. Alternative and complementary therapies, client, internal environment, body, mind, spirit, natural healing

13. Energy healing
14. Holism
15. Holistic nursing, biopsychosocial, spiritual
16. Spirituality
17. Standard (Western, allopathic) medicine
18. Traditional Chinese medicine

19. T, 20. T, 21. F, 22. T, 23. T, 24. F, 25. T, 26. F, 27. T

28. *Barriers preventing full integration of traditional and alternative health care approaches:* see Integrative Health Care section; lack of research to validate effectiveness; opposing/competing philosophies and paradigms; health care cost concerns; inconsistent state licensing laws; biases, attitudes, and prejudices.

29. *Explain touch as a powerful healing tool; cite examples:* see Touch and Energetic Healing and Applications in Women's Health Care sections;
    - Natural (intuitive) to touch what is hurt and needs comfort; laying on of hands to heal.
    - Touch is vital to human development, has a positive impact on immune function, reduces heart rate, BP, anxiety.
    - Examples: massage, acupressure, therapeutic touch, healing touch.
    - Nausea and vomiting (acupressure).

- Labor progress, satisfaction, and anxiety (massage, acupressure, therapeutic touch).

30. *Mind as a healing tool:* see Mind-Body Healing section; include in your answer how the mind is used in each modality and identify how the modality can be used to enhance health care.

31. *Use of herbs:* see Alternative Pharmacologic Modalities section;
    - Recognize that herbs vary in potency and concentration; dosage is important; read labels carefully and use only as directed and for the purpose recommended.
    - Inform health care providers and pharmacist when herbs are going to be used or are being used; interaction with health problem or medications taken can occur.

Critical Thinking Exercises

1. Health care consumers are turning to alternative and complementary therapies
   A. *Factors responsible for this trend:* see Introduction.
      - Depersonalization and increasing reliance on technology and specialization; harried health care providers, increased costs, and disease focus.
      - Growing appreciation of health and how mind, body, and spirit are connected.
   B. *Alternative approaches:* offer human-centered care focusing on the mind, body, and spirit; value human input and autonomy; honor and respect individual's beliefs, values, and desires.
   C. *Nursing's response:* see Nurse's Role section and Boxes 4-2 and 4-3; discuss holistic nursing and how nurses are supported and educated for this role; explain specific modalities nurses use including therapeutic touch.

   D. *Concepts shared by most therapies:* see Overview of Alternative and Complementary Modalities section; include a description of the commonalities namely:
      - Emphasis on client as a whole being
      - Importance of nutrition, rest, relaxation, exercise, and emotional health
      - Belief that signs and symptoms of disease reflect deeper processes on an emotional and spiritual level

2. *Woman experiencing perimenopausal symptoms:* see Applications in Women's Health Care—Gynecology section;
   - Review Marie's history including health problems, medications used, and allergies.
   - Ask Marie if she has some ideas in mind: what she has heard about and is interested in using.
   - Outline options available and how they could help her problems including: homeopathy, plant-based estrogens, herbs, vitamin E, Chinese herbs; refer to an herbalist if Marie wishes to have a specific preparation developed for her individual concerns.
   - Discuss the potential benefits of participating in a yoga program (see Box 4-5).
   - Refer Marie to Internet sites and support groups that emphasize the safe and effective use of alterative approaches for relief of perimenopausal symptoms.

3. *Alternative therapies/approaches for pregnancy and childbirth:* see Applications in Women's Health Care—Pregnancy and Obstetric Care section; examples:
   - Nausea and vomiting (acupressure, acupuncture, herbal and homeopathic remedies)
   - Labor (prepared childbirth approaches, therapeutic touch and healing, massage, biofeedback, guided imagery)

CHAPTER 5: ASSESSMENT AND HEALTH PROMOTION

Chapter Review Activities

1. Mons pubis
2. Labia majora
3. Labia minora
4. Prepuce
5. Frenulum
6. Fourchette
7. Clitoris
8. Vestibule
9. Perineum
10. Vagina, rugae, Skene, Bartholin
11. Fornices
12. Uterus, cul de sac of Douglas
13. Corpus
14. Isthmus
15. Fundus
16. Endometrium
17. Myometrium
18. Cervix
19. Endocervical, internal os, external os
20. Squamocolumnar junction; Papanicolaou
21. Uterine (fallopian) tubes

22. Ovaries, ovulation, estrogen, progesterone, androgen

23. Breasts
24. Tail of Spence
25. Nipple
26. Areola
27. Montgomery glands (tubercles)
28. Acini
29. Lactiferous sinuses (ampullae)

30. T, 31. F, 32. F, 33. T, 34. T, 35. F, 36. F, 37. T, 38. F, 39. T, 40. T, 41. F, 42. F, 43. T, 44. F, 45. T, 46. F, 47. F, 48. F, 49. T, 50. F, 51. T, 52. T, 53. F, 54. F, 55. T, 56. F, 57. T, 58. T, 59. F, 60. F, 61. F, 62. F, 63. T, 64. T, 65. T, 66. T, 67. T

68. **External Female Genitalia:** A. mons pubis; B. prepuce of clitoris; C. frenulum of clitoris; D. labia minora; E. vestibule; F. fourchette; G. perineum; H. anus; I. vaginal orifice; J. labia majora; K. vestibule; L. urethra; M. glans of clitoris
    Perineal Body: A. posterior fornix; B. buttocks; C. rectum; D. anus; E. perineal body; F. vagina; G. urethra; H. symphysis pubis; I. Bladder; J. anterior fornix; K. uterus; L. cul de sac of Douglas
    Cross Section of Uterus: A. fundus; B. body (corpus of the uterus); C. endometrium; D. myometrium; E. internal os of cervix; F. external os of cervix; G. vagina; H. endocervical canal; I. lateral fornix of vagina; J. cardinal ligament; K. uterine blood vessels; L. broad ligament; M. ovary; N. fimbriae; O. infundibulum of uterine tube; P. ampulla of uterine tube; Q. ovarian ligament; R. isthmus of uterine tube; S. interstitial portion of uterine tube
    Breast (sagittal section): A. clavicle; B. intercostal muscle; C. pectoralis major; D. alveolus; E. ductule; F. duct; G. lactiferous duct; H. lactiferous sinus; I. nipple pore; J. suspensory ligament of Cooper; K. 6th rib; L. 2nd rib
    Breast (anterior dissection): A. acini cluster; B. lactiferous (milk) duct; C. lactiferous sinus (ampulla); D. nipple pore; E. areola; F. Montgomery gland (tubercle)
    Female Pelvis: A. 7th lumbar vertebrae; B. iliac crest; C. sacral promontory; D. sacrum; E. acetabulum; F. obturator foramen; G. subpubic arch under symphysis pubis; H. ischium; I. pubis; J. ilium; K. sacroiliac joint

69. Menstrual cycle
    Diagram of Menstrual Cycle: A. gonadotropin releasing hormone (Gn-RH); B. follicle stimulating hormone (FSH); C. luteinizing hormone (LH); D. follicular phase; E. luteal phase; F. Graafian follicle; G. ovulation; H. corpus luteum; I. estrogen; J. progesterone; K. menses; L. proliferative phase; M. secretory phase; N. ischemic phase; O. hypothalamic-pituitary cycle; P. ovarian cycle; Q. endometrial cycle

Answer Key 393

70. *Guidelines for performing a Pap smear:* guidelines for each component of the procedure are outlined in the Procedure Box—Papanicolaou Smear

71. *Characteristics of a palpated lump:* location, size, mobility, consistency, tenderness, type of borders

72. *Breast self-examination technique:* see Teaching for Self-Care Box: BSE; A. –; B. –; C. +; D. +; E. +; F. –; G. +; H. +; I. +

73. D is correct; clean gloves are required only if open lesions are present and when compressing the nipple if discharge is anticipated; fingers should not be lifted; two hands are used for women with large, pendulous breasts.

74. C is correct; self-examination should not be used for self-diagnosis but rather to detect early changes and seek guidance of a health care provider if changes are noted.

75. B is correct; do not ask questions during the examination because it may distract the client, interfering with relaxation measures she may be using; offer explanations only as needed during the examination.

76. A is correct; all women should be screened because abuse can happen to any woman; abuse often escalates during pregnancy; the most commonly injured sites are head, neck, chest, abdomen, breasts, and upper extremities. If abuse is suspected the nurse needs to assess further to encourage disclosure and then assist the woman to take action and formulate a plan. Nurses should follow the laws of their state with regard to reporting instances of abuse.

77. B is correct; bone mineral density testing should be initiated at 65 years of age or older unless risk factors are present; endometrial biopsies are not recommended on a routine basis for most women but women at risk for endometrial cancer should have one done at menopause; mammograms should be done annually for women 50 years of age and older.

78. A is correct; all women not just specific groups should participate in preconception care 1 year before planning to get pregnant.

Critical Thinking Exercises

1. *Importance of preconception care:* see Preconception Counseling and Care section; this nurse should
   - Define preconception counseling and what it entails; stress the importance of both partners participating
   - Identify impact of a woman's health status and lifestyle habits have on the developing fetus during the first trimester
   - Describe how preconception counseling can assist a couple to choose the best time to begin a pregnancy

2. Establishing a woman's health clinic:
   A. *Services to be offered* (see Reasons for Entering the Health Care System section): pregnancy services including preconception counseling and care; health promotion early detection; fertility control; infertility; sexuality services including safer sex and early detection and treatment of STIs; menstrual problems; puberty- and menopause-related services.
   B. *Barriers* (see Barriers to Seeking Health Care section): discuss financial, cultural, and gender issues as barriers; use barriers to create strategies including advocating for universal health insurance, providing culturally sensitive services, improving access including transportation and child care provisions and longer hours open, innovative incentives.
   C. *Services to meet goal of health promotion and prevention:* use Fig. 5-17 to guide your answer and identify services to emphasize:

- Consider common risk factors for health problems and behaviors that increase risk for health problems.
- Create programs that address age-specific issues for example puberty, teen pregnancies, menopause.

3. *Woman requesting advice regarding diet and exercise to lose weight* (see Nutrition and Exercise sections):
   - BMI falls in the high end of the overweight range (see Box 5-4).
   - Review risks for health disorders that are associated with being overweight.
   - Start with 24-hour to 3-day nutritional recall; based on analysis of woman's current nutritional habits suggest use of food guide pyramid, emphasize complex carbohydrates and foods high in iron and calcium, reduce fat intake, insure adequate fluid intake avoiding those high in sugar, alcohol, or caffeine; use weight changes and activity patterns to determine adequacy of caloric intake.
   - Aerobic exercise: discuss weight-bearing vs. non-weight-bearing exercises as well as frequency and duration of exercise sessions for maximum benefit.

4. Woman experiencing stress
   A. *Physical and emotional signs of stress:* see Stress section and Box 5-5 for a listing of typical physical, behavioral, and psychologic signs of stress.
   B. *Stress management* (see Stress Management section):
      - Help Alice to formulate her goals in life and to set priorities; work on time management to allow for relaxing times.
      - Discuss her interests, hobbies to be incorporated into a stress management program designed for her; develop alternatives to alcohol and smoking for relaxation such as biofeedback, guided imagery, yoga.
      - Refer to support group for stress management.

- Suggest literature and Internet sites that may be beneficial.
   C. *Smoking cessation:* (see Substance Use Cessation section and Box 5-7)
      - Use the four A's formula of ask, assess, advise, assist.
      - Have Alice describe her smoking: how much, how long, triggers to smoking.
      - Discuss how she stopped before.
      - Suggest a variety of strategies available to stop smoking, helping her to make a decision on a method that is right for her.

5. *Woman's concern regarding violence against women* (see Violence against Women and Health Protection sections):
   - Discuss woman's current circumstances and what she does now to protect herself.
   - How she changed her behavior based on the experiences of her friends; how she helped or did not help them; her evaluation of how the legal and health care system met the needs of her friends; discuss what could have and should have been done to help her friends.
   - Discuss protective and legal services including hot lines, emergency centers; facilitate access to services to promote assertiveness, self-defense techniques, self-help groups.

6. *State how culture, age, physical and emotional disorders, and abuse can influence health assessment of women:* see specific subsection for each factor in Health Assessment section.

7. Nurse responses to concerns and questions of women
   A. *How to get ready for first GYN examination:* explain what will occur and each guideline to follow for preparation and why each is important for the accuracy of the test; tell her to avoid douching, vaginal medications, and intercourse for 24–48 hours before the examination; she should not be menstruating.

B. *Signs indicating ovulation*: mid-cycle spotting and pain (mittelschmerz), breast swelling and tenderness, elevated basal body temperature, cervical mucus changes (spinnbarkeit), and other changes in behavior and emotions individual to each woman (premenstrual signs)

C. *Breast characteristics across the life span*: see Table 5-1, which outlines characteristics of breasts of adolescent, adult, and postmenopausal women.

D. *Douching*: vaginal secretions are usually acidic and protect the reproductive tract from infection; a douche may alter this acidity and injure the mucosa, thereby increasing the risk for infection; gentle and regular front to back washing with mild soap and water is all that is necessary to be clean.

8. *Woman anxious about first GYN examination*:
   - Explain each component of the examination, how it is done, why it is performed, and how it will feel.
   - Show her the instruments that will be used.
   - Encourage her to verbalize what she is feeling, her concerns and questioning.
   - Teach her simple relaxation measures such as deep breathing.
   - Ensure her privacy and modesty and tell her how it will be maintained throughout the examination.

9. Health history of a new client at a Women's Health Clinic
   A. *Components*: see History section for a list and description of components.
   B. *Writing questions*: use components of health history as a guide; write questions that are open ended, clear, concise, address only one issue, and progress from general to specific.
   C. *Therapeutic communication techniques with examples* (see Interview, Cultural Considerations, Communication Variables, and Women with Special Needs sections):
      - Use facilitation, reflection, clarification, empathetic responses, confrontation, interpretation.
      - Be sensitive and nonjudgmental in your approach; use a relaxed, confident, professional manner.
      - Consider the culture of the client and any special needs including those related to sensory deficit.
      - Use full name of client; introduce yourself.
      - Consider comfort and privacy of the environment in which the interview will take place.

10. *Teaching self-examination techniques*: each technique involves cognitive, psychomotor, and affective learning; use a variety of methodologies including discussion (when, how often, why, expected and reportable findings, who to call, what will be done if abnormal findings are experienced); explore feelings regarding self-examination; provide literature with illustrations; demonstrate and have client redemonstrate using practice models and then client themselves as appropriate.
    Breast self-examination: see Teaching for Self-Care Box—BSE
    Vulvar (genital) self-examination: see Vulvar Self-Examination section

11. *Culturally sensitive approach to women's health care*:
    - Approach woman in a respectful and calm manner.
    - Consider modifications in the examination to maintain her modesty.
    - Incorporate communication variations such as conversational style, pacing, spacing, eye contact, touch, time orientation.
    - Take time to learn about the woman's cultural beliefs and practices regarding well woman assessment and care.

12. *Screening for abuse when providing well woman care*:

A. *Adjusting the environment:* provide for comfort and privacy; assess the woman alone without her partner or adult children present.

B. *Abuse indicators:* see Abused Women section for identification of several indicators of possible abuse and areas of the body most commonly injured including during pregnancy, specific somatic complaints, and behaviors including a pattern of canceling health care appointments.

C. *Questions to ask:* see Fig. 5-10, which lists the four questions that all women should be asked in a very direct manner.

D. *Approach if abuse is confirmed:*
   - Acknowledge the abuse and affirm that it is unacceptable and common; tell her that you are concerned and that she does not deserve it.
   - Communicate that it can recur; cite the cycle of violence (see Chapter 6); tell her that help is available; empower her to use this help.
   - Help her to formulate an escape plan.

13. *Describe events in each cycle composing the menstrual cycle:* see Hypothalamic-pituitary cycle, Ovarian cycle, and Endometrial cycle subsections of the Menstrual cycle for a full description of the events and changes characteristic of each cycle.

14. *Assisting with a pelvic examination:* see Procedure Boxes—Assisting with Pelvic Examination and Papanicolaou Smear and Pelvic Examination section to formulate your answer.
   A. *Client preparation and support:* teach about what is to occur as part of the examination, assist to change clothes, tell her to empty her bladder, and assist her to get into the position required for the examination; tell her how to relax and provide privacy; inform and support her throughout the examination; assist her with cleansing, getting into an upright position, and dressing as needed

after the examination; discuss any questions or concerns the woman may have related to the examination.
   B. *Assist the health care provider:* assist with preparing and supporting the client, preparing equipment, and taking care of specimens including correct labeling and sending to the lab.

Chapter 6: Violence Against Women

Chapter Review Activities

1. Intimate partner violence (IPV), rape, physical assault, stalking

2. Wife battering, spouse abuse, domestic, family violence, economic, sexual, intimidation, isolation, stalking, terrorizing

3. Repeated, increasing tension, battery, calm, remorse, "honeymoon"

4. Machismo, toughness, hardness

5. 18, 3-year, disrobing, nudity, masturbation, fondling, digital penetration, anal, oral, vaginal

6. Incest, 18, sexual assault
7. Sexual assault, rape, touches, kisses, hugs, petting, intercourse

8. Rape, intercourse, penile penetration, sex organ, labia, statutory, date/acquaintance, marital, gang, stranger, psychic

9. Molestation
10. Sexual harassment

11. Rape-trauma, anxiety, stress, emotional, psychologic, somatic, acute phase (disorganization), outward adjustment phase, long-term process (reorganization phase)

12. *Identify factors associated with abuse against women:* see Conceptual Perspectives on

Violence section; each category of factors is described.

13. *Cultural influence on violence against women*: see Cultural Considerations section; answer should reflect
    - Factors true for all cultures such as role and expected behavior of men and women, importance of family and roles within the family, to whom you go when experiencing problems, approach to health care, definition of what violence and abuse means, impact of environmental stressors and availability of resources.
    - Examples from a variety of cultures can then be given for each factor.

14. Characteristics of women who are abused and men who are abusers
    A. *Characteristics of women in abusive relationships contrasted with those who are not*: see Battered Women section; battered women tend to exhibit strong, traditional feminine characteristics whereas women in nonviolent relationships tend to be more independent, assertive, and willing to take a stand.
    B. *Characteristics of women who seek help*: see Care Management section; beaten severely and frequently, never experienced or witnessed abuse in their own families, have alternative in terms of jobs or careers
    C. *Barriers to seeking help*: see Care Management section; avoid stigma and involvement of police, fear they will not be believed or of reprisal from abuser.
    D. *Characteristics of men are likely to abuse*: see Box 6-1 for a list of many characteristics and Table 6-1 for causes of aggression.
    E. *Forms of abuse*: forms of abuse are illustrated in Fig. 6-1 and include using children, economics, male privilege, coercion and threats, intimidation, emotional abuse, exploitation, isolation, blaming; abuse can be physical, emotional, sexual.

15. *The use of the ABCDEs tool when caring of an abused woman*: see Plan of Care and Intervention section for a full description of this tool and how it is used.

16. *Strategies to prevent cycle of violence*: see Prevention subsection of Plan of Care and Interventions; answer should include educating and empowering women; referring women to support and self-help groups; educating children about gender roles and relationships, healthy ways to deal with conflict and anger, and problem-solving skills; advocating for community services, availability of counseling, and legislation for stricter laws to protect women.

17. *Factors that deter women from reporting rape*: see Sexual Assault section; stigma, embarrassment, guilt (provoked assault), fear of retribution and reaction of family members including sexual partner, dread of humiliation at a trial, discouragement of others, low conviction rate.

18. F, 19. T, 20. F, 21. T, 22. F, 23. T, 24. T, 25. T, 26. F, 27. F, 28. T, 29. F, 30. T, 31. F, 32. T

33. A is correct; characteristics of a potential batterer include defects in assertiveness, inadequate verbal skills especially with regard to expressing feelings, and an unusual amount of jealousy often expecting his partner to spend all of her time with him.

34. D is correct; battered women are often isolated as a result of fear, the stigma society places on them that they must enjoy being abused, and restrictions on their activities by their partner; typical feminine characteristics are more apparent in women in abusive relationships whereas assertiveness, independence, and willingness to take a stand are more characteristic of women who are in nonviolent relationships.

35. B is correct; anxiety and depression can lead to use of alcohol, tobacco, and drugs as a means of coping; inadequate diet results in low maternal weight gain increasing the risk for anemia and giving birth to a low birth weight newborn; the rate of spontaneous abortion, preterm birth, and stillbirth is increased; abused women are more likely to experience infections, headaches, pain, and depression.

36. A is correct; women who experience repeated and severe abuse, have never witnessed or experienced abuse in their own families, and who have alternatives such as a job or career are more likely to seek assistance.

37. C is correct; rapid mood swings are characteristic of the acute phase whereas desire to talk about the rape, nightmares, and eating disorders tend to occur during the reorganization phase; returning to her job, maintaining her household, and disinterest in discussing the rape along with denying and suppressing thoughts and feelings are other behaviors associated with the outward adjustment phase.

Critical Thinking Exercises

1. *Disproving myths regarding violence against women:* use the Introduction section for statistical information regarding the incidence and demographics of violence against women, Table 6-3, Perspectives on Violence, and Battered Women sections to disprove myths A, B, C, and D; use Battering during Pregnancy section to disprove myth E.

2. Cycles of Violence
   A. *Identify characteristics behaviors of each phase of the Cycle of Violence:* see Cycle of Violence section and Fig. 6-2 for a full description of the behaviors characteristic of each phase.

   B. *Providing anticipatory guidance:* discuss the behaviors for each phase with the woman so that she can be forewarned and understand what the behaviors mean, and that they will all occur again unless intervention occurs; help her to develop a plan to implement when Phase I is beginning to avoid Phase II outcomes.

3. Cues indicative of physical abuse
   A. *Identify cues:* see Assessment and Nursing Diagnoses section
      • injuries (minor bruising to serious injuries) to face, breasts, abdomen, buttocks; fractures requiring significant force, multiple injuries at various stages of healing, patterns left by objects used in the abuse
      • anxiety, insomnia, self-directed abuse, depression, drug or alcohol abuse
      • delay in seeking care, missed appointments, vague explanations of injuries, isolation lack of eye contact, partner does not want to leave a woman alone
   B. *Suspicion that pregnant woman is being abused:* see Assessment and Nursing Diagnoses section
      • Use appropriate communication techniques including direct questions.
      • Perform interview and examination in a private setting; female health care provider might be helpful.
      • If injuries are noted tell her that these are common in women who are abused; tell her she is not responsible for another person's abusive behavior.
      • Consider legal implications.
   C. *Abuse is confirmed:* see Plan of Care and Interventions section; use the ABCDEs of caring as a framework for helping Carol.
   D. *Why pregnancy leads to violence:*
      • Stress of pregnancy may strain relationship decrease ability to cope; increasing frustration leads to violence.

- Jealous of fetus; seen as an intruder in their relationship.
- Angry with woman, fetus.
- Attempt to end pregnancy.

E. *Approach to avoid:* avoid being judgmental, evaluating Carol's actions and responses to violence in terms of how the nurse would act in the same situation or to rush her; Carol needs to be helped at her own pace but formulating an escape plan is critical.

F. *Adverse effects of violence on pregnancy:*
- Inadequate diet and rest with low maternal weight gain, anemia; increased risk for infections, headache, pain, depression
- Use of alcohol, drugs, tobacco to cope with stress
- Increased risk for low birth weight, miscarriage, preterm birth, stillbirth
- Interference with attachment process with newborn

G. *Indicators for readiness to leave abusive relationship:*
- Exhibits capability to plan for and invest in herself
- Recognizes that abuse is part of a continuing pattern
- Expresses desire to leave; needs to leave when no abuse is occurring with reassurance of available economic and social support to make it on her own

H. *Legal responsibilities of the nurse:*
- Full documentation of the abuse should be done (see Box 6-3 for guidelines to follow).
- Know your state's requirement regarding the reporting of abuse/battering.

4. Adult woman survivor of sexual abuse as a teenager
A. *Signs of abuse:* see Sexual Abuse Care Management section and Table 6-2 for signs of the physical and psychosocial effects of sexual abuse and the onset of

posttraumatic stress syndrome/disorder; sexual abuse can have a profound effect on a woman's seeking health care when pregnant and not pregnant, sexual relationships, and response to pregnancy and childbirth.

B. *Suggested healing activities:* see Sexual Abuse Nursing Care section
- Express feelings, develop coping mechanisms.
- Seek counseling.
- Support groups for adult survivors to decrease depression, anger, guilt, and isolation.
- Improve self esteem.

5. Woman who has been raped
A. *Nurse's responsibility to assess and to collect and preserve evidence of the rape:* see Box 6-4 and Box 6-5 for Adult Sexual Assault Protocol to follow.
- Gather history allowing her to tell her story at her own pace; restate to clarify and show empathy; obtain information regarding her gynecologic and obstetric history.
- Inform her of all the steps involved in the examination and why they are needed.
- Physical examination: inspect for injuries and collect specimens; use photos and drawings as needed; document findings.
- Perform an emotional status assessment.
- Ensure that all legal steps and requirements are fulfilled including obtaining a consent.

B. *Nurse's actions to meet emotional needs:*
- Treat with dignity, courtesy, and respect.
- Maintain privacy and modesty.
- Reassure of her safety; it was not her fault and she is not alone in her experience.
- Evaluate emotional status; provide time for her to talk with someone.

- Help her to shower, put on clean clothes, rest after the examination.
C. *Phases of rape-trauma syndrome represented by behaviors listed:* C, A, A, C, B, C, A, A, B, C, B, C, A
D. *Discharge interventions:* see Discharge section
  - Provide medications (sedative, emergency contraceptive, analgesic etc.) with printed instructions as appropriate.
  - List names and numbers of resource people for assistance as needed during recovery.
  - Assist her to return home.
  - Schedule follow-up examination to assess progress of healing of injuries, repeat cultures and other tests, check for pregnancy.

CHAPTER 7: REPRODUCTIVE SYSTEM CONCERNS

Chapter Review Activities

1. Amenorrhea, pregnancy, anorexia nervosa, amenorrhea, stress, weight loss, eating, exercise, mental illness

2. Dysmenorrhea, menstruation, primary dysmenorrhea, 6 to 12 months, ovulation, estrogen, progesterone, secondary dysmenorrhea, a few days before menses

3. Premenstrual syndrome (PMS), symptoms occur in the luteal phase and resolve in a few days of menses onset, symptom-free follicular phase, symptoms are recurrent, premenstrual dysphoric disorder (PDD)

4. Endometriosis, proliferative, secretory, menstruation, inflammatory, fibrosis, adherence, dysmenorrhea, dyspareunia, diarrhea, pain with defecation, constipation, fertility

5. Oligomenorrhea, hypomenorrhea, oral contraceptive pill (OCP)

6. Metrorrhagia, intermenstrual bleeding, mittlestaining

7. Breakthrough bleeding

8. Menorrhagia, hypermenorrhea, hormonal, systemic, neoplasms, infection, contraception (IUDs), hematocrit, hemoglobin

9. Abnormal uterine bleeding (AUB)

10. Dysfunctional uterine bleeding (DUB), anovulation, luteinizing hormone (LH), progesterone, corpus luteum, menarche, menopause

11. T, 12. F, 13. T, 14. F, 15. F, 16. F, 17. F, 18. F, 19. T, 20. T, 21. F, 22. F, 23. F, 24. T, 25. T, 26. F, 27. T, 28. F, 29. T, 30. F, 31. F, 32. T, 33. F, 34. T, 35. F

36. 5, 39, 51, ovulatory cycles, menses, irregular menstrual cycles, menopause, 1, climacteric
Complete table related to changes associated with perimenopause: perimenopausal changes are fully described in separate subsections of the Menopause section.

37. Lipid metabolism, HDL, LDL; *Factors increasing a woman's risk for developing cardiovascular disease:* see Coronary Heart Disease subsection of Menopause section; factors include obesity, smoking, elevated cholesterol and BP, diabetes mellitus, family history of CAD, alcohol abuse, effects of aging on cardiovascular system.

38. Menopause Hormone Therapy (see specific subsections of Menopausal Hormone Therapy section for A, B, C, D; see Alternative Therapies section and Box 7-2 and Table 7-5 and Teaching for Self-Care box for E).
A. *Therapeutic uses:* short-term (e.g., 1 to 3 years) relief of menopausal discomforts

(e.g., hot flashes) in women who are not at risk for cardiovascular disease

B. *Side effects/adverse reactions*: headaches, nausea and vomiting, bloating, ankle and feet swelling, weight gain, breast soreness, brown spots on skin, eye irritation, and depression

C. *Risks of hormone therapy*: increased risk for breast cancer, increased risk for endometrial cancer with unopposed use of estrogen, blood clots, heart attack, stroke, gallbladder disease

D. *Nonhormonal/alternative therapies*: homeopathy, acupuncture, herbs, phytoestrogens, vitamins, other pharmacologic agents, and daily lifestyle changes can be used to relieve hot flashes, irritability, headaches, insomnia, urogenital symptoms

39. B is correct; the 13-year-old reflects several of the risk factors associated with this menstrual disorder, namely: presently in a growth period, participating in a sport that is stressful, subjectively scored, requires contour revealing clothing, and success is favored by a prepubertal body shape.

40. C is correct; A, B, and D all interfere with prostaglandin synthesis whereas acetaminophen has no antiprostaglandin properties; prostaglandins are a recognized factor in the etiology of dysmenorrhea.

41. A is correct; decreasing the ingestion of red meats as well as switching from a high-fat to a low-fat diet has been associated with symptom relief; asparagus and cranberry juice have a natural diuretic effect that can reduce edema and related discomforts; simple refined sugars not complex carbohydrates should be avoided along with salt for 7 to 10 days before menstruation to reduce fluid retention; complex carbohydrates can provide the fiber required to prevent constipation.

42. D is correct; alcohol, tobacco, and caffeine can worsen symptoms experienced whereas

exercise can provide relief as can peaches and watermelon, both of which have a natural diuretic effect; sodium intake should be less than 3 g daily.

43. C is correct; women taking danazol often experience masculinizing changes; it is taken orally for a 3- to 6-month period; ovulation may not be fully suppressed, therefore birth control is essential because this medication is teratogenic.

44. A is correct; oligomenorrhea—infrequent menses; menorrhagia—excessive bleeding during menses; hypomenorrhea—scanty bleeding at normal intervals

45. C is correct; DUB is most commonly associated with anovulatory cycles in women at the extremes of their reproductive years (puberty, perimenopause); it can also occur when women secrete low levels of progesterone; it is associated with obesity.

46. A is correct; dysmenorrhea is painful menstruation; dysuria is painful urination; dyspnea is difficulty breathing.

Critical Thinking Exercises

1. Woman with hypogonadotropic amenorrhea (see Hypogonadotropic amenorrhea section)

   A. *Risk factors exhibited*: athletic competition subjectively scored, endurance sport favoring low body weight, inappropriate body composition, nutritional deficits related to need to maintain body size, stress and vigorous exercise, need to wear body revealing clothing, prepubertal body shape or weight categories favors success or ability to participate

   B. *Nursing diagnosis*: risk for disturbed body image or anxiety related to delayed onset of menstruation and development of secondary sexual characteristics

C. *Expected outcomes:* Marie will
- verbalize understanding regarding basis for delayed onset of pubertal changes
- participate in a therapeutic regimen that will favor age-appropriate physical development

D. *Care management:*
- Stress reduction measures
- Reduce exercise or gain weight through good nutrition to alter fat-to-lean body ratio
- Involve family and coach in treatment plan
- Discuss risk for osteoporosis
- Begin hormonal treatment or calcium supplementation if needed

2. Woman with primary dysmenorrhea (see Dysmenorrhea section)

A. *Compare and contrast primary and secondary dysmenorrhea:* see Dysmenorrhea section for full description of each disorder

B. *Nursing diagnoses:* consider the areas of acute pain and ineffective role performance as the focus for nursing management of this woman's primary dysmenorrhea; use assessment data to determine which nursing diagnosis will take precedence

C. *Relief measures:* discuss basis of the problem and that it usually diminishes with age; suggest nonpharmacologic measures such as exercise, massage and effleurage, relaxation techniques and guided imagery, yoga, meditation, good nutrition including natural diuretics and decreased fat, heating pad; pharmacologic measures such as NSAIDs and oral contraceptives may be prescribed; herbal preparations may also be helpful (see Table 7-2)

3. Woman experiencing PMS (see PMS section)

A. *Typical signs and symptoms:* clinical manifestations usually related to effects of fluid retention, behavioral and emotional changes, cravings, headache, fatigue/energy level, and backache

B. *Nursing diagnosis:* nursing diagnoses could include acute pain, activity intolerance, disturbed sleep pattern, constipation or diarrhea, ineffective role performance; use assessment findings to determine those which would apply to a particular client including those that are priority

C. *Nursing approach:*
- Obtain a detailed history and encourage woman to keep a diary of physical and emotional manifestations (what occurs, when, contributing circumstances) from one cycle to another
- Individualize plan based on this woman's experiences
- Discuss nutrition, exercise, and lifestyle/career measures
- Refer to appropriate support group or for counseling if needed
- Discuss pharmacologic and herbal preparations that are available

4. Woman with endometriosis (see Endometriosis section)

A. *Clinical manifestations:* dysmenorrhea (secondary), pelvic pain and heaviness, thigh pain, elimination difficulties, dyspareunia, metrorrhagia and menorrhagia

B. *Pathophysiology of the disorder:* growth of endometrial tissue outside uterus mainly in the pelvis; implants respond to cyclical changes in hormones; bleeding of implants leads to inflammatory response, formation of scar tissue, fibrosis, anemia; impaired fertility can occur

C. *Pharmacologic management:* each medication used is discussed in Management subsection; oral contraceptives are used to create a pseudopregnancy; Gn-RH agonists and androgenic derivatives are used to create a pseudomenopause; goal is to suppress endogenous estrogen production and to cause implants to shrink and atrophy

    D. *Support measures:* educate regarding disease process; discuss treatment options; refer to support groups and counseling as appropriate, work with couple together and separately to allow for expression of feelings and concerns; review options for pregnancy since infertility can be an outcome

5. Woman at risk for osteoporosis (see Osteoporosis subsection of Menopause section)

    A. *Risk factors exhibited:* Caucasian, slender/thin, family history of osteoporosis, smokes, sedentary lifestyle, dietary risks related to inadequate calcium coupled with excess fast food, caffeine, and soft drinks

    B. *Prevention measures* (see Box 7-3): specifically address risk factors presented by the woman:
- Nutrition: increase calcium (diet, supplement), decrease caffeine, phosphorous, and fat intake
- Exercise and activity: emphasize weight bearing
- Bone density testing

    C. *Signs of osteoporosis:* decrease in height, back pain especially lower back, dowager's hump, fractures

6. Woman experiencing perimenopausal changes (see Menopause section)

    A. *Relief measures* (see specific subsection for each change, Teaching for Self-Care box—Comfort Measures, Box 7-2, Table 7-5, and Alternative Therapies, Sexual Counseling, and Support Groups sections): discuss each change, why it occurs, and several relief options; encourage the woman and her partner to be involved in the process of coping with the changes of the perimenopause period and the decisions that have to be made

    B. *Decision making regarding MHT* (see Menopausal Hormone Therapy section, Box 7-2, and Tables 7-4 and 7-5): answer should include benefits, risks, side effects, preparations and administration, and alternatives

    C. *Instructions for use of transdermal patch:* apply to trunk and upper arms, not on breasts; check site for irritation, alternate sites, apply once or twice a week to hairless, clean, dry, intact site; emphasize importance of regular and ongoing health care to monitor effects of hormone use

    D. *Use of Internet:* provide Heidi with a list of appropriate sites with which to start; give her guidelines regarding how to find sites and how to evaluate sites she finds including sponsor, currency, accuracy; caution her to seek advice of health care provider before beginning a recommended treatment or seek information if she has questions

CHAPTER 8: SEXUALLY TRANSMITTED AND OTHER INFECTIONS

Chapter Review Activities

1. Sexually transmitted diseases (STDs) or sexually transmitted infections (STIs), chlamydia, human papillomavirus (HPV), gonorrhea, herpes simplex virus II (HSV II), syphilis, human immunodeficiency virus (HIV)

2. Safer sex practices, know partner, reduce number of partners, lower risk sex, avoiding exchange of body fluids

3. Male condom, female condom
4. Chlamydia

5. Gonorrhea

6. Syphilis, primary syphilis, chancre, 5 to 90, secondary syphilis, 6 weeks to 6 months, symmetric maculopapular rash, palms, soles, lymphadenopathy, fever, chills, headache, malaise, condylomata lata, latent phase, tertiary syphilis

7. Pelvic inflammatory disease (PID), menstrual period, abortion, pelvic surgery, childbirth

8. Human papillomavirus (HPV), condylomata acuminata

9. Herpes simplex virus II (HSV II), painful lesions, fever, chills, malaise, dysuria

10. Hepatitis A virus (HAV), milk, shellfish, polluted water, person to person

11. Hepatitis B virus (HBV)
12. Hepatitis C virus (HCV)

13. Human immunodeficiency virus (HIV), cellular immune

14. Group B streptococcus (GBS)
15. Bacterial vaginosis, fishy

16. Candidiasis, pruritus, dryness, dysuria, thick, white, lumpy, cottage-cheese like, vaginal walls, cervix, labia

17. Trichomoniasis
18. TORCH
19. Toxoplasmosis
20. Rubella
21. Cytomegalovirus (CMV)

22. T, 23. F, 24. F, 25. T, 26. F, 27. F, 28. T, 29. F, 30. T, 31. T, 32. F, 33. F, 34. F, 35. T, 36. F, 37. T, 38. F, 39. F, 40. T, 41. F, 42. T, 43. T, 44. F, 45. T, 46. F, 47. T, 48. T, 49. T, 50. F, 51. F, 52. T, 53. T, 54. F

55. A is correct; because these infections are often asymptomatic they can go undetected and untreated causing more severe damage including ascent of the pathogen into uterus and pelvis resulting in PID and infertility; many effective treatment measures are available including for chlamydia.

56. B is correct; A is indicative of candidiasis; C is indicative of HSV II; D is indicative of trichomoniasis.

57. B is correct; metronidazole is used to treat bacterial vaginosis and trichomoniasis; erythromycin is effective in the treatment of chlamydia; acyclovir is used to treat herpes.

58. B is correct; A, C, and D are not used to treat GBS infection; acyclovir is used orally to treat herpes; there are no lesions with GBS.

59. D is correct; recurrent infections commonly involve only local symptoms that are less severe; stress reduction, healthy lifestyle practices, and acyclovir can reduce recurrence rate; viral shedding can occur before lesions appear.

60. *Sexual behavior categories according to degree of risk for STI transmission:* see Table 8-1 for identification of safer sex guidelines according to each category listed

61. *Common risk factors for STIs:* Box 8-2 cites many common risk behaviors according to sexual, drug use-related, and blood-related risks

62. *Infection control principles and practices:* see Box 8-4 for a full explanation of standard precautions and precautions for invasive procedures

63. *STI table:* see specific infection subsection for information related to typical clinical manifestations and management guidelines for each of the infections listed

64. *Heterosexual transmission of HIV to women* (see HIV section)

A. *Mode of transmission:* exchange of body fluids (semen, blood, vaginal)

B. *Clinical manifestations during seroconversion:* viremic, influenza-type responses such as fever, headache, night sweats, malaise, lymphadenopathy, myalgia, nausea, diarrhea, weight loss, sore throat, rash

C. *Management:* education related to disease process, measures to prevent transmission of infection and to maintain resistance to infection, healthy lifestyle practices, contraception, and signs of opportunistic infections; expert multidisciplinary care with a holistic focus; use of prophylactic medication; referrals (psychologic, legal, financial) as needed

65. *Meaning of TORCH:* see TORCH Infections section and Table 8-7 for the infections represented by each letter

Critical Thinking Exercises

1. Woman attending first visit at a women's health clinic
   A. *Write one question for each STI/HIV risk factor category* (see Box 8-2): questions should reflect risks identified, and be open-ended, clear, concise, and nonjudgmental
   B. *Major points to emphasize for STI prevention:* see Safer Sex Practices section and Table 8-1;
      - Knowing partner: questions to ask, how to assess genitalia.
      - Avoid relations with many partners or partners who have had many previous sexual partners.
      - Insist on barrier method; be prepared.
      - Do not make decisions based on appearances and unfounded assumptions.
      - Carefully examine partner.
      - Know low risk sexual practices and those that are unsafe.

C. *Measures to help client develop assertiveness and communication skills related to safer sexual practices:*
   - Emphasize importance of discussing prevention measures including condom use with partner at a time removed from sexual activity.
   - Role play using possible partner responses for woman to react to; rehearse how she will handle various situations so she can sort out her feelings and fears ahead of time.
   - Reassure that her reluctance is not unusual.

2. *Pregnant woman diagnosed as HIV positive at 4 weeks' gestation:* see HIV—counseling for HIV testing section;
   - Oral zidovudine (AZT) at 14 to 34 weeks' gestation, IV during labor, and syrup to newborn after birth
   - Breastfeeding is contraindicated

3. Woman with severe PID (see Pelvic Inflammatory Disease section)
   A. *Risk factors:*
      - Menstrual history; pathogen ascent into uterus usually occurs at end of or just after menses
      - Young age
      - IUD use coupled with unsafe sexual practices
      - Recent abortion, pelvic surgery, childbirth, dilation and curettage
      - Sexual history, risky behaviors; history of sexual partner(s) if possible; history of STIs
   B. *Diagnostic criteria:* oral temperature greater than 38.3° C, abnormal discharge cervical or vaginal discharge, elevated erythrocyte sedimentation rate, lab documentation of cervical infection, lower abdominal tenderness, bilateral adnexal tenderness, cervical motion tenderness
   C. *Nursing diagnoses during acute phase:* nursing diagnoses will most likely

include acute pain, anxiety (effect on sexuality and future fertility), impaired physical mobility, constipation/diarrhea, and impaired urinary elimination

D. *Management guidelines:*
  - Position and activity: bedrest in the semi-Fowler position to keep pelvis in the dependent position; elevate legs slightly to prevent pulling on pelvis, which would increase discomfort
  - Comfort measures: analgesics, back rub, hygiene, relaxation techniques, diversional activities, proper positioning
  - Support measures: provide time for woman to express feelings; include partner in care as appropriate; help woman to deal with effects of the PID and the potential long-term effects; use a nonjudgmental, empathetic approach
  - Health education: how to comply with treatment regimen, including taking medications effectively, refraining from intercourse until fully healed, use of contraceptives and safer sex practices

E. *Self-care during recovery phase:* see Teaching for Self-Care Box—Sexually Transmitted Infections for self-care suggestions; emphasize activity restrictions, importance of rest, good nutrition, taking medications completely, and follow-up

F. *Reproductive risks:* tubal obstructions and adhesions leading to ectopic pregnancy or infertility, chronic pelvic pain, dyspareunia

4. Woman diagnosed with gonorrhea
  A. *Essential assessment areas during health history:* Box 8-3 outlines points to emphasize during assessment
  B. *Nursing diagnosis:* anxiety related to potential effect of STI on future sexual function OR risk for ineffective sexuality pattern related to recent diagnosis of STI

C. *Management:*
  - Educate Laura about STIs including gonorrhea; discuss cure, control, and recurrence factors.
  - Discuss self-care measures: see Teaching for Self-Care Boxes—Sexually Transmitted Infections and Prevention of Genital Tract Infections.
  - Discuss safer sex practices (Table 8-1) and practice assertiveness with partners.
  - Review Genital Self Examination (see technique Chapter 5).

5. *Reducing pain of condylomata associated with HPV infection:* see HPV—management section
  - Bath with oatmeal solution
  - Keeping area clean and dry; use of a cool dryer
  - Wearing cotton underwear, loose-fitting clothing
  - Healthy lifestyle to enhance immune system and healing process

6. Woman diagnosed with herpes simplex virus II (see HSV—management section)
  A. *Measures to relieve pain and prevent secondary infection:*
    - Correct use of antiviral medications (Table 8-2) including avoidance of pregnancy if medication is teratogenic (e.g., acyclovir).
    - Cleanse lesions BID with saline; use a warm sitz bath with baking soda.
    - Keep dry with cool hair dryer or pat dry; use hydrogen peroxide, Burows solution or oatmeal baths.
    - Use alternative treatments such as cool, wet black tea bags or compresses with an infusion of clove or peppermint oil.
    - Cotton underwear, loose clothing.
    - Oral analgesics; limited use of topicals to decrease discomfort (e.g., thin layer of lidocaine ointment or anesthetic spray).
    - Diet and lifestyle to enhance healing.

B. *Preventing/reducing recurrence:*
- Educate regarding etiology, signs of recurrence, transmission, treatment, precipitating factors for reactivation of virus.
- Keep diary to identify stressors, recurrences, helpful measures.
- Stress reduction measures, avoid heat, sun, or hot baths, use a lubricant during intercourse to reduce friction.

7. *Measures to prevent transmission of hepatitis B virus:* immunoprophylaxis for household members and sexual contacts; maintain high levels of personal hygiene; careful disposal of items contaminated with blood or body fluids including saliva; safer sex measures

8. Woman concerned about exposure to HIV (see HIV section)
    A. *Risky behaviors* (see Box 8-2): exposure to contaminated body fluids including semen and blood; discuss sexual practices and partners as well as possible IV drug use
    B. *Testing procedure:* see Screening and Diagnosis and Counseling for HIV testing sections for full description of types of tests and testing protocol, counseling required, and legal implications; nurse should witness an informed consent, tell woman how long it will take for results to be available, consider ethical issues of confidentiality and privacy, and use a nonjudgmental, empathetic approach
    C. *Counseling protocol:* counseling should occur before and after testing, by the same person, in a private area with no interruptions; all assessments, actions, and responses should be documented:
        - Pretest: personalized risk assessment; explain meaning of test results, informed consent, plan for reducing risk and preventing infection
        - Posttest: inform regarding results, review meaning of result obtained, reinforce self-care/prevention measures; refer for treatment if positive result is obtained
    D. *Instructions following a negative test result:* use Sonya's risky behaviors as a basis for discussing prevention measures including safer sex practices; discuss impact HIV could have on her health and that of her fetus when pregnant

CHAPTER 9: CONTRACEPTION AND ABORTION

Chapter Review Activities

1. Coitus interruptus
2. Natural family planning
3. Fertility awareness methods
4. Calendar method
5. Basal body temperature (BBT)
6. Spinnbarkeit
7. Symptothermal
8. Spermicide
9. Condom
10. Diaphragm
11. Cervical cap
12. Contraceptive sponge
13. Monophasic pill
14. Multiphasic pill
15. Norplant system
16. Mifepristone (RU 486)
17. Intrauterine device (IUD)

18. Sterilization, oviducts, ligation, electrocoagulation, bands, clips, sperm ducts (vas deferens), vasectomy

19. Induced abortion, elective abortion, therapeutic abortion

20. F, 21. T, 22. T, 23. T, 24. T, 25. F, 26. F, 27. F, 28. F, 29. F, 30. T, 31. T, 32. T, 33. F, 34. F, 35. T, 36. T, 37. T, 38. F, 39. T, 40. F, 41. F, 42. F, 43. F, 44. F, 45. T, 46. T, 47. T, 48. F, 49. T, 50. T, 51. F, 52. F

53. A is correct; oral contraception provides no protection from STIs, therefore a condom and spermicide are still recommended to prevent transmission; B, C, and D reflect appropriate actions and recognition of side effects.

54. B is correct; cervical mucus is thickened thereby inhibiting sperm penetration; ovulation and the development of the endometrium are also inhibited; there is no protection from STIs; the overall effectiveness rate is nearly 100% if used correctly.

55. A is correct; although B, C, and D are all temporary side effects, the most common is the irregular pattern of bleeding that occurs especially during the first year of use; women report that this bleeding is also the most distressing side effect.

56. C is correct; the string should be checked after menses, before intercourse, at the time of ovulation, and if expulsion is suspected; a missing string or one that becomes longer or shorter should be checked by a health care professional.

57. D is correct; maximum spermicide effectiveness lasts no longer than 1 hour; foams and jellies/creams have a nearly instant effect whereas tablets and suppositories require 10 to 30 minutes to dissolve and film about 5 minutes; douching or rinsing should not occur for at least 6 hours after the last act of coitus.

58. B is correct; spermicide should not be applied around the rim because a seal will not form to keep the cap in place; use during menses increases the risk for toxic shock syndrome; checking the cap's position is all that is required before each subsequent act of coitus.

59. Couple making decision about contraceptive method to use:

A. *Factors influencing effectiveness:* see full list in Box 9-1

B. *Meaning of braided:* see Legal Tip— Informed Decision in Assessment and Nursing Diagnosis section; benefits, risks, alternatives, inquiries, decisions, explanations, documentation

60. *Purpose for self-assessment of cervical mucus:*
   - Alert couple about reestablishment of ovulation after breastfeeding or discontinuing oral contraceptives.
   - Determine if cycles are ovulatory at any time including menopause, when planning pregnancy, or for timing infertility treatments and diagnostic procedures.

61. *Periodic abstinence or natural family planning as a method of birth control*
   A. ovulation, abstaining from unprotected intercourse, irregular menstrual periods (cycles)
   B. 5, 22
   C. Drop, 0.05°, progesterone, rise, 0.2° to 0.4°, 2 to 4 days, thermal shift
   D. Cervical mucus ovulation detection, cervical mucus, amount, consistency
   E. Basal body temperature (BBT), cervical mucus, libido, spotting, mittelschmerz, fullness, tenderness, fullness, cervix, dilation, softening, rising
   F. Luteinizing hormone (LH), 12 to 24

62. *Use of nonprescription barrier methods:*
   A. C
   B. C
   C. C
   D. I
   E. C
   F. I
   G. I

63. *Use of diaphragm:*
   A. C
   B. I

C. C
D. C
E. C
F. I
G. I
H. I

64. *Cite four factors for seeking an abortion* (see Abortion section): preserve life and health of the mother, genetic disorders of the fetus, rape/incest, pregnant woman's request

Critical Thinking Exercises

1. Toxic shock syndrome (see Toxic Shock Syndrome section)
   A. *Prevention measures when using diaphragm:* prompt removal 6 to 8 hours after intercourse; avoid use during menses; awareness of danger signs of TSS
   B. *Clinical manifestations:* see Nurse Alert; fever of sudden onset greater than 38.4° C, hypotension, rash

2. Woman seeking assistance with making choice regarding birth control method
   A. *Nursing Diagnosis:* deficient knowledge related to methods of contraception OR anxiety related to lack of knowledge regarding contraception
   B. *Approach for nurse to use to assist with decision making:*
      - Assess her level of knowledge regarding how her body works; sexual practices including beliefs, practices, number of partners, frequency of coitus.
      - Fully describe different methods; determine preferences for or objections to methods described.
      - Level of contraceptive involvement desired: comfort with touching genitalia, myths and misconceptions, religious and cultural factors.
      - Health status as determined with heath history, physical examination, and laboratory testing as appropriate.

3. Woman choosing to use combination estrogen-progestin oral contraceptive (see Hormonal Methods section).
   A. *Mode of action* (see Oral Contraceptive section): suppression of hypothalamus and anterior pituitary, which diminishes secretion of FSH and LH and as a result follicles do not mature and ovulation is inhibited; altered maturation of endometrium; thickening of cervical mucus
   B. *Advantages:* see Advantages subsection; easy to use, not connected with intercourse, improves sexual response, regular predictable menses with decreased blood loss, decrease in dysmenorrhea and PMS, some protection from GYN problems such as endometrial and ovarian cancer, functional ovarian cysts, benign breast disease, ectopic pregnancy; may improve acne
   C. *Absolute/relative contraindications:* see Disadvantages and Side Effects section: the WHO recommends not using OCPs for the following conditions: history of thromboembolic disorders, cerebral vascular or coronary artery disease, breast cancer, estrogen depended tumors, pregnancy, impaired liver function/tumor, smokers older than 35 years of age, lactation less than 6 weeks postpartum; headaches with focal neurologic symptoms, hypertension (greater than 160/100 mm Hg), surgery with prolonged immobility or on legs, diabetes with vascular changes
   D. *Cite side effects in terms of estrogen excess/deficit and progestin excess/deficit:* side effects in these categories are fully discussed in the Disadvantages and Side Effects section
   E. *Signs and symptoms requiring woman to stop taking the OCP and notifying her health care provider:* see Signs of Potential Complications Box—Oral Contraceptives for full explanation of ACHES

F. *Instructions for the client:*
- Follow specific directions on package insert in terms of taking the pill and what to do if one or more are missed; take at same time of day.
- Use own pills not someone else's because OCPs vary.
- Discuss side effects and complications.
- Check effect of other medications being taken on the effectiveness of the OCP.
- Importance of using STI protection and of using backup method for first cycle on OCP, when certain other medications are being taken, or if pill(s) have been missed.

4. Woman using a cervical cap (see Cervical Cap section and Teaching for Self-Care Box—Use of Cervical Cap):
   A. *Factors making client a poor candidate for using cap:* abnormal Pap test results, history of TSS, vaginal or cervical infection, cannot be fitted properly, insertion/removal too difficult for the woman, allergy to latex or spermicide
   B. *Client instructions for safe and effective use:*
   - When and how to insert and remove, checking placement before each act of coitus, use of spermicide.
   - Avoid using during menses or for at least 6 weeks postpartum.
   - Check fit annually and after GYN surgery, birth, major weight loss or gain.
   - Arrange for Pap smear after 3 months of use to check for cervical dysplasia.

5. *Instructions following IUD insertion:*
   - See Signs of Complications Box—IUDs, which uses the acronym of PAINS to identify signs of problems.
   - Teach how and when to check string.
   - Stress importance of appropriate genital hygiene and sexual practices.
   - Inform when IUD needs to be replaced.

6. Couple contemplating sterilization (see Sterilization section)
   A. *Decision-making approach:* nurse acts as facilitator to help couple explore the pros and cons of sterilization itself and the options available for male and female
   B. *Preoperative and postoperative care measures and instructions for vasectomy:*
   - Preoperative: health assessment in terms of history, physical examination, and laboratory tests; preparatory instructions; witness an informed consent
   - Postoperative: prevention and early detection of bleeding and infection; self-care measures in terms of hygiene, comfort, prevention and reduction of swelling with ice packs and scrotal support; activity restrictions for a couple of days—moderate activity level
   - Caution that sterility is not immediate: an alternative method should be used until sperm count is zero for two consecutive semen analyses
   - STI protection must be considered as appropriate

7. Couple using Symptothermal Method (see Symptothermal Method section and Fig. 9-3)
   A. *Components:* BBT, cervical mucus, secondary cycle phase-related symptoms
   B. *Assessing BBT and cervical mucus:*
   - BBT: see Basal Body Temperature Method section and Fig. 9-2
   - Cervical mucus: see Teaching for Self-Care Box—Cervical Mucus Characteristics
   C. *Effectiveness:* typical effectiveness rate for all fertility awareness methods is 25% during the first year of use

8. Woman contemplating elective abortion (see Abortion section)

A. *Nursing diagnosis:* decisional conflict related to unplanned pregnancy and need to complete education
B. *Describe approach:* use therapeutic communication techniques to establish trusting relationship; discuss alternatives available to her and the consequences of each; nurse facilitates decision-making process and the client makes the decision; make appropriate referrals to help her with the decision
C. *Purpose of laminaria and procedure for vacuum aspiration:*
   - Laminaria is used to dilate cervix after 8 weeks' gestation; inserted 4 to 24 hours before the procedure.
   - Aspiration: vaginal area cleansed; procedure takes 5 minutes; prepare her for menstrual-like cramping and sound of machine.
D. *Nursing diagnoses:* consider fear/anxiety, anticipatory grieving, risk for infection, acute pain
E. *Nursing measures for care and support:* assess physical condition checking for bleeding and ability to void, keep her informed, provide support and comfort measures, rest for 1 to 3 hours prior to discharge; provide time for her to talk about her feelings about the experience and make referrals as needed
F. *Discharge instructions:* hygiene measures to prevent infection; signs of complications (bleeding, infection); activity restrictions; resumption of sexual relations and use of birth control and safer sex measures; arrange for follow-up appointment and stress importance

9. Woman seeking assistance following unprotected intercourse (see Emergency Contraception section)
   - Explore possibility of pregnancy and options related to continuing pregnancy if it occurs, keeping baby, adoption.
   - Explore options for emergency contraception to prevent pregnancy: methods available, how each works, timing, side effects, how administered.
   - Emphasize importance of follow-up to check for effectiveness of method used and occurrence of infection.
   - Discuss methods of contraception and safer sex measures to prevent recurrence of this situation.

Chapter 10: Infertility

Chapter Review Activities

1. E, 2. F, 3. C, 4. B, 5. D, 6. A

7. In vitro fertilization and embryo transfer (IVF & ET)

8. Intracytoplasmic sperm injection
9. Gamete intrafallopian transfer (GIFT)
10. Zygote intrafallopian transfer (ZIFT)
11. Therapeutic donor insemination
12. Gestational carrier
13. Surrogate motherhood
14. Assisted hatching

15. F, 16. F, 17. T, 18. T, 19. T, 20. F, 21. T, 22. F, 23. T, 24. T, 25. T, 26. T, 27. F, 28. T, 29. T, 30. F, 31. F, 32. F

33. B is correct; spinnbarkeit refers to stretchiness of cervical mucus at ovulation to facilitate passage of sperm; there is an LH surge prior to ovulation; BBT rises in response to increased progesterone after ovulation; cervical mucus becomes thinner and more abundant with ovulation.

34. B is correct; the couple should abstain from intercourse for 2 to 4 days before expected ovulation; the test is scheduled for the expected time of ovulation; report for examination within several hours after ejaculation of semen into vagina.

35. C is correct; lubricants other than water soluble can contain spermicides or have spermicidal properties; elevation of hips and wearing boxer shorts have not been proven to affect fertility; daily hot tubs or saunas may increase scrotal temperature enough to interfere with spermatogenesis.

36. C is correct; this medication is a powerful ovulatory stimulant that can result in multiple pregnancy therefore regular ovarian ultrasound and monitoring of estradiol levels are required to prevent hyperstimulation; it is administered intramuscularly and is used when clomiphene fails to induce ovulation.

37. B is correct; danazol is used to create a pseudomenopause when a woman has endometriosis in order to cause the implants to atrophy and shrink thereby increasing the chance that a woman will be fertile after treatment.

38. Couple receiving care for infertility (see Infertility section)
    A. *Identify/describe components for normal fertility*: normal male and female reproductive tract, hormonal support for gametogenesis, timing for intercourse, adequate sperm and ova, patent tubal system for passage of sperm and ova
    B. *Support statement that assessment for infertility must involve both partners*: see Box 10-6, which outlines findings favorable for fertility indicating male and female factors; cite statistics revealing that a female factor causes 50%, a male factor causes 35%, unexplained factors and unusual causes 15%

39. *Impact of male smoking on fertility*: depending on number of cigarettes smoked each day, smoking can result in abnormal sperm, decrease number of sperm, and chromosomal damage

40. *Medications used in the treatment of infertility*: use Table 10-3 and Medical section of Plan of Care and Interventions to describe the mode of action and purpose for each medication listed

41. *Cite surgical procedures to treat infertility*: see Surgical section of Plan of Care and Interventions; remove tumors and release scar tissue adhesions; hysterosalpingogram to release blockage; laparoscopy to release adhesions, destroy endometrial implants, repair tubes; reconstructive surgery of uterus; repair of varicocele and microsurgery to restore sperm ducts; cryosurgery, cautery to destroy abnormal cervical tissue

42. Subfertility, conceive, sterility, pregnant, impregnated a woman, pregnant
    A. *Probable causes of male and female infertility*: see Female Infertility and Male Infertility sections and Boxes 10-1 and 10-2 for a discussion of several factors implicated in each type of infertility
    B. *Religious and cultural beliefs*: see Box 10-3 and Cultural Considerations Box for several examples

Critical Thinking Exercises

1. Couple undergoing testing for infertility
   A. *Nursing support measures*: see Psychosocial section of Plan of Care and Interventions; help couple to
      - Express feeling and openly discuss sexuality issues
      - Make decisions regarding diagnostic tests and treatment options
      - Grieve the loss of fertility and inability to have biologic children if that is the outcome
      - Refer to support groups and adoption agencies as appropriate
   B. *Female and male assessment*: see text sections and Boxes 10-5 and 10-7 for a full explanation of the components for each assessment

C. *Procedure for semen analysis:* see Semen Analysis section of Assessment of Male Infertility; emphasize need to abstain from ejaculation for 2 to 5 days before test, not to use spermicide or use a plastic sheath that does not contain spermicide, to collect specimen in a clean container, to protect it from extremes of heat and cold, and to transport to lab within 2 hours of ejaculation

D. *Semen characteristics evaluated:* see Box 10-8 for a full list of characteristics in terms of liquification, volume, pH, density, and morphology

E. *Postcoital test instructions:* see Assessment of Couple section; instructions should include purpose of test, when to have intercourse (at ovulation), what to do afterwards, when to come for examination; caution that vagina must be free of infection and couple should abstain for 2 to 4 days before the test

2. *Concerns engendered by assisted reproductive technologies:* see Reproductive Alternatives section, Box 10-9, and Table 10-4
  • Who should pay; insurance coverage; access for wealthy vs. poor couples
  • Children: who are their biologic parents, medical history
  • Availability to married couples only
  • Ownership of ovum, sperm, embryos
  • Attempt to create the "perfect" child
  • Risk for multiple gestation with potential for reduction elective abortion

3. Woman scheduled for a diagnostic laparoscopy (see Laparoscopy section of Diagnostic Tests)
  A. *Timing:* early in menstrual cycle to avoid disturbing a possible fertilized ovum
  B. *Preprocedure care measures:* NPO for 8 hours, void before procedure, bowel preparation may be required

C. *Purpose and process of the procedure:*
  • Diagnostic: visualize and assess structures to determine if abnormalities are present
  • Therapeutic: relieve blockage, release adhesions, remove or destroy implants
  • Process: small incisions in abdomen to allow passage of laparoscope; instillation of carbon dioxide to enhance visualization of structures

D. *Postprocedure care measures:*
  • Assessment of status: vital signs, LOC, incision sites, signs of bleeding, infection, pain, elimination (especially voiding)
  • Prevention of aspiration, administer IV fluids, comfort measures, assist with elimination
  • Usually discharged in 4 to 6 hours if stable
  • Discharge instructions: expectations regarding referred shoulder pain or subcostal discomfort from use of carbon dioxide, pain medication use, type of activity to avoid, signs of complications (infection, bleeding) and who to call

4. Couple experiencing problems with fertility:
  A. *Typical responses and nursing actions:* see Table 10-2 for description of reactions and several recommended nursing actions
  B. *Guiding the decision-making process:*
    • Discuss meaning of fertility and having biologic children for this couple and for their family; consider cultural and religious beliefs and values.
    • Fully inform couple of diagnostic tests and treatment options so informed decision can be made.
    • Review financial considerations including what insurance will cover.

- Encourage couple to define what they are willing to endure physically, and emotionally, and financially to have a biologic child; discuss alternatives to biologic children.
- Refer to support groups.

CHAPTER 11: PROBLEMS OF THE BREAST

Chapter Review Activities

1. B, 2. E, 3. G, 4. A, 5. F, 6. H, 7. D, 8. C, 9. T, 10. F, 11. T, 12. F, 13. F, 14. T, 15. F, 16. T, 17. F, 18. T, 19. F, 20. F, 21. T, 22. F, 23. T, 24. F, 25. T, 26. T, 27. T, 28. T, 29. F

30. Educating women about breast cancer (see Malignant Conditions of the Breast section)
    A. *Information regarding risk factors:* see Etiology section and Boxes 11-2 and 11-3 to determine risk factors to teach women; identify factors, degree of risk they represent alone and in combination; include research findings; discuss how risk factors can influence health care including suggestions for assessment methods and frequency, lifestyle changes, and prevention methods for very high risk women
    B. *Breast screening recommendations* (see Table 11-3):
       - Jane: BSE monthly
       - Marion: BSE monthly, clinical breast examination every 3 years
       - Denise: BSE monthly, clinical breast examination and mammography annually
    C. *Factors inhibiting women from participating in breast screening and strategies to encourage compliance* (see Clinical Manifestations and Diagnosis section and Cultural Considerations Box):

- Inhibiting factors: culture, lack of knowledge and time, fear, finances and insurance coverage
- Strategies: reminder postcards, buddy system, insurance coverage, teaching days and programs for women and health care providers, advertisements in the media, mobile clinics to bring health screening to neighborhoods, flexible clinic hours, free screening and walk-in self referrals

    D. *Manifestations suggestive of breast cancer:* often unilateral; lump or thickening of the breast, hard and fixed or soft and spongy, well-defined or irregular borders, dimpling (fixed to integument), nipple discharge (unilateral, spontaneous, intermittent, and persistent; clear, serous, bloody, colored, purulent)
    E. *Screening and diagnostic tests:* mammography, ultrasound, MRI, biopsy of tumor tissue or fluid; blood tests (CBC, liver enzymes, Ca level, alkaline phosphatase)

31. *Definitions of treatment approaches:* see appropriate subsections of Therapeutic Management section for a full description of each treatment approach

32. *Woman's concern regarding the genetic risk for breast cancer* (see Malignant Conditions of the Breast—Etiology section):
    - Tell her most cancers are not related to genetic factors.
    - Obtain a full family history regarding breast and other cancers.
    - Discuss BRCA testing and its meaning.
    - Help her to explore what she would do if results were positive.
    - Encourage BSE and clinical breast examination.

33. D is correct; breast cancer is more common among Caucasian women; it is most prevalent among women 40 years of age

and older as menopause is approached; the majority of women do not exhibit the identified risk factors; two risk factors are obesity and high-fat diets.

34. D is correct; tamoxifen reduces growth and inhibits recurrence of estrogen-sensitive breast cancer; usual dose is 20 to 40 mg, po, once or twice a day depending on dosage for a period of 5 years; because it is an antiestrogen medication it can cause signs of estrogen deficit such as hot flashes and menstrual changes.

35. B is correct; the right arm should be used as much as possible to maintain mobility and prevent lymphedema; loose nonrestrictive clothing should be worn; tingling and numbness are expected findings for as long as a few months after surgery.

36. A is correct; acute pain is a common finding; it usually begins a week before the onset of menses; leakage from nipples is not associated with this disorder; surgery is unlikely and is only attempted in a few selected cases; cancer risk increases when the lesions are proliferative with atypia and hyperplasia.

37. D is correct; fibroadenomas are generally small, unilateral, firm, nontender, movable lumps located in the upper outer quadrant; borders are discrete and well defined; discharge is not associated with this disorder.

Critical Thinking Exercises

1. Woman with fibrocystic breast change (see Fibrocystic Changes section of Benign Conditions of the Breast)
   A. *Assessment process to diagnose fibrocystic change:*
      - History and physical assessment including clinical breast examination
      - Note association of clinical manifestations with menstrual cycle and lifestyle

- Ultrasonography to determine if lumps are solid or fluid filled
- Fluid filled—fluid aspirated if necessary
- Solid—mammography if older than 50 and fine-needle aspiration
   B. *Clinical manifestations:*
      - Lumpiness and enlargement of both breasts premenstrually (1 week before)
      - Symptoms subside 1 week postmenstrually
      - Women experience dull heavy pain, fullness, tenderness
      - Cysts: soft, differentiated, mobile; manifest as painful, enlarging lumps
   C. *Nursing diagnosis:* based on assessment findings and time in menstrual cycle; can include acute pain, anxiety
   D. *Relief measures:* try several approaches and see which combination works the best—keep a diary
      - Discomfort: analgesics, support bra, heat
      - Diet: eliminate dimethylxanthine (e.g., caffeine); limit sodium
      - Avoiding alcohol and smoking can help
      - Vitamin E; mild diuretics premenstrually
   E. *Risk for cancer:* depends on type of cellular change; risk is primarily related to lesions that are proliferative with atypia and hyperplasia

2. Woman with lump in left breast
   A. *Diagnostic protocol:*
      - History and physical examination including clinical breast examination; document characteristics of the lump and other associated findings such as dimpling, increased venous pattern, enlarged lymph nodes
      - Mammography, ultrasound, MRI; compare with previous test results if available
      - Biopsy of lump tissue to confirm diagnosis

- Laboratory testing including CBC, liver enzymes, serum Ca levels, alkaline phosphatase
B. *Emotional impact of cancer diagnosis:* (see Emotional Support after Diagnosis section and Evidence-Based Practice Box)
  - Shock limits information processing
  - Impact disruption caused by diagnosis: role changes, financial, body image, sexual function, disability, pain, despair, fear, shame
  - Refer to reliable Internet resources
  - Review decision-making questions she and her family should ask (see Box 11-4)
C. *Nursing diagnoses and care management:*
  - Preoperative period:
    - Nursing diagnoses could include fear/anxiety, anticipatory grieving, risk for ineffective family and individual coping are likely to be priority diagnoses
    - Preoperative teaching and typical surgical care measures; Reach for Recovery volunteer may be asked to come and speak to woman and family
  - Immediate postoperative period:
    - Nursing diagnoses would include acute pain, risk for infection, impaired skin integrity, risk for deficient fluid volume
    - Typical postoperative care along with elevation of arm; avoid using arm for BP, IV, blood draws, and medications; follow protocol for movement and use of affected arm; check for bleeding in drainage bag, on dressing, and under arm; assist with position changes, leg exercises, and coughing and deep breathing
    - Emotional support is important for both periods
D. *Preparing Molly for self-care at home:* see Box 11-6 and Teaching for Self-Care Box—After a Mastectomy; instructions should address pain control; signs of expected changes and complications; infection prevention; wound, dressing, and drainage care; BSE; arm exercises and use of arm for activities of daily living; time for follow-up appointment
E. *Support measures:*
  - Help woman and partner deal with change in appearance; encourage open communication; meet with woman and her partner together and separately
  - Refer to community resources and support groups
  - Discuss follow-up treatments including adjuvant therapy, radiation therapy, reconstructive surgery, and complementary/alternative therapies
  - Use of prostheses
  - Ensure that health care provider is with woman and her partner when she views wound for the first time

3. *Tamoxifen therapy* (see Tamoxifen section of Adjuvant Therapy and the Medication Guide for Tamoxifen):
  - Oral antiestrogen medication; be prepared for menopause-like symptoms such as hot flashes
  - Plan should include action/purpose, dosage and how to take effectively, adverse reactions to watch for and what to do if they occur

4. Woman with breast cancer beginning chemotherapy (see Adjuvant Chemotherapy and Teaching Needs for the Client and Family Undergoing Adjuvant Therapy sections):
  A. *Teaching plan:*
    - Name of medication, route of administration, treatment schedule, timing, length of time for administration
    - Payment—insurance coverage
    - Side effects and how to manage them including use of alternative therapies
    - Importance of birth control to prevent pregnancy

- Required follow-up care
- Expected effect of treatment on her daily life; adjustments that will need to be made

B. *Nursing diagnoses:* use assessment findings to determine which diagnoses would apply and their priority for this client
- Imbalanced nutrition: less than body requirements
- Risk for infection
- Disturbed body image
- Interrupted family processes
- Ineffective role performance
- Fear/anxiety

CHAPTER 12: STRUCTURAL DISORDERS AND NEOPLASMS OF THE REPRODUCTIVE SYSTEM

Chapter Review Activities

1. C, 2. F, 3. J, 4. G, 5. H, 6. A, 7. B, 8. I, 9. D, 10. E

11. Pessary
12. Anterior repair (colporrhaphy)
13. Posterior repair (colporrhaphy)
14. Myomectomy
15. Uterine artery embolization
16. Hysterectomy
17. Bilateral salpingo-oophorectomy (BSO)
18. Colposcopy
19. Conization
20. Cryosurgery
21. Loop electrosurgical excision procedure (LEEP)
22. Radical hysterectomy
23. Total pelvic exenteration
24. Simple vulvectomy
25. Skimming vulvectomy
26. Radical vulvectomy

27. *Risk factors for reproductive tract cancers:* see Incidence and Etiology subsection for each of the cancers listed for identification of risk factors

28. *Ovarian cancer, a "silent" cancer:* symptoms are often vague with early warning signs and symptoms absent; definitive screening tests do not exist; recognizable signs that there is a problem often are not noted until disease is advanced

29. F, 30. T, 31. F, 32. T, 33. F, 34. T, 35. T, 36. F, 37. F, 38. T, 39. T, 40. F, 41. T, 42. T, 43. F, 44. F, 45. T, 46. F, 47. F, 48. T, 49. T, 50. T, 51. F, 52. F, 53. T, 54. T, 55. F

56. B is correct; a knee-chest position would be helpful for a mildly retroverted uterus; estrogen is the hormone responsible for maintaining and improving tissue tone; if surgery is needed, a vaginal hysterectomy or abdominal hysterectomy would be recommended; an anterior repair is used to correct a cystocele; Kegel exercises could be suggested to increase pelvic floor muscle tone.

57. D is correct; fibroids are dependent on estrogen for growth; therefore they will increase in size during pregnancy and shrink with menopause; menorrhagia is the most common clinical manifestation and can lead to anemia if severe; constipation, low dull abdominal pain and pressure, and backache are other common signs and symptoms as the tumors enlarge.

58. B is correct; reducing fluid intake can be dangerous because fluids are required to prevent urinary tract infection; A, C, and D are all effective in reducing urinary incontinence.

59. B is correct; only the uterus was removed therefore HRT will not be needed; douches, tub baths, and intercourse should be avoided until after the follow-up examination to determine the progress of

healing; turning, coughing, and deep breathing should be performed every 2 hours and leg exercises every 2 to 4 hours until ambulation.

60. C is correct; CIS is noninvasive and therefore cervical conization with follow-up is the appropriate treatment choice; the LEEP procedure can be used for the conization.

Critical Thinking Exercises

1. Woman diagnosed with moderate uterine prolapse along with cystocele and rectocele (see Uterine Prolapse, Cystocele and Rectocele and Care Management sections)
   A. *Clinical manifestations:* see Clinical Manifestations subsection; manifestations include bearing down/pelvic pressure, urinary and bowel elimination problems; bulging into vagina would be noted during vaginal examination; fatigue, low back pain, and dyspareunia are common
   B. *Two priority nursing diagnoses with expected outcomes:*
      • Constipation or diarrhea related to altered position of uterus, rectum, and bladder; woman will experience regular, soft-formed bowel elimination
      • Ineffective sexuality patterns related to vaginal change associated with uterine prolapse, cystocele, and rectocele; woman will openly discuss measures to enhance sexual function
   C. *Management of uterine prolapse, cystocele and rectocele:* see Plan of Care and Interventions section; answer should include use of Kegel exercises, diet (fiber and fluids), stool softeners, mild laxative, genital hygiene including sitz baths and proper use of commercial products including a pessary
   D. *Using a pessary:*
      1. *Nursing diagnosis:* risk for infection

2. *Instructions for use:* tailor instructions for the type that is used; include how to insert and remove, how to care for and cleanse, genital hygiene measures, signs indicative of infection
   E. *Postoperative care following vaginal hysterectomy and colporrhaphy* (see Postoperative Care section and Box 12-3):
      • Ensure cleanliness
      • Keep bowel and bladder empty
      • Check for pain, bleeding, infection

2. Woman with fibroids (see Benign Neoplasms—Leiomyomas section)
   A. *Clinical manifestations:* abnormal bleeding, anemia, backache and low abdominal pressure, elimination problems, dysmenorrhea; clinical manifestations become more apparent as tumors get larger
   B. Symptoms, age, childbearing potential, Gn-RH agonists such as Lupron, uterine artery embolization, myomectomy, laser surgery, electrocautery, hysterectomy

3. Woman with endometrial cancer
   A. *Nursing diagnosis for preoperative and postoperative periods* (see Endometrial Cancer Section)
      • Preoperative: fear related to diagnosis of uterine cancer and anticipated surgery; woman will openly discuss fears and concerns with health care provider and family
      • Postoperative: acute pain, risk for deficient fluid volume, risk for infection; eventually disturbed body image, ineffective sexuality patterns; an expected outcome for pain would be woman will experience reduction in pain when relief measures are implemented
   B. *Nursing care and support:*
      • Preoperative (see Preoperative Care section and Box 12-2): preoperative

Answer Key   419

teaching, typical physical measures for major abdominal surgery

- Postoperative: (see Postoperative Care section and Box 12-3; measures included in plan should be assessment of physical and emotional status, fluid intake (IV to oral), turn, coughing, deep breathing, and leg exercises, wound care, perineal care, pain relief and comfort measures, avoid positions that increase pelvic congestion

C. *Discharge instructions:* see Discharge Planning and Teaching section and Teaching for Self-Care Box—Woman who has had a Myomectomy or Hysterectomy for a full explanation of teaching topics

D. *Cultural issues* (see Cultural Considerations Box—Meaning of Cancer): body image, meaning of uterus and fertility in her culture; meaning of death; responses to pain

E. *Nursing diagnosis related to diagnosis and treatment:* Anxiety OR disturbed body image related to effects of surgery and possibility of ongoing treatment for cancer

F. *Support measures during recovery:*
- Provide time to discuss fears, ask questions, feelings regarding self as woman and sexuality.
- Involve significant others.
- Teach about effects of surgery and other treatment measures that may be used; discuss use of alternative therapies.
- Refer to support groups.

4. Woman with invasive cancer of the cervix
   A. *Nursing diagnoses with expected outcomes:*
   - Fear related to concerns about cancer and effects of radiation treatments; woman will openly express fears regarding diagnosis and treatment with health care provider and family

- Impaired skin integrity related to effects of radiation on tissue; will use appropriate measures to reduce skin breakdown and enhance healing

B. *Table regarding internal and external radiation care management:* see External Radiation Therapy and Internal Radiation Therapy sections of Nursing Management and Teaching for Self-Care Boxes: After Internal Radiation Therapy and After External Radiation Therapy to identify points to highlight when completing this table

C. *Nursing precautions for self protection:* see Radiation Therapy section and Nurse Alert for precautions to follow; emphasize wearing of film badge, use of careful isolation techniques, and planning nursing care to reduce exposure; distance, time, and shielding are three ways to control exposure

5. Woman recovering from a radical vulvectomy
   A/B. *Nursing measures to prevent infection and maintain sexual functioning:* see Nursing Care section of Cancer of the Vulva for a full list of nursing care measures for each expected outcome of care

   C. *Discharge instructions:* see Teaching for Self-Care Box—After Radical Vulvectomy to determine the critical discharge instructions that should be given to this woman

6. *Cancer during pregnancy:* see Cancer Therapy and Pregnancy section; answer should include
   - Issues and emotions regarding the mother, fetus, and impact of treatment
   - Potential for pregnancy termination
   - Review of options for treatment with their potential impact on the maternal-fetal unit

- ethical considerations for treatment and its impact on fetal well-being is a critical component of decision making

7. Woman receiving chemotherapy for treatment of advanced ovarian cancer (see Cancer of Ovary—Therapeutic Management and Nursing Implications)
   A. *Measures to relieve selected chemotherapy-related problems* (see Table 12-2): be sure to include an explanation of why the problems occur and why suggested relief measures will help
   B. *Support measures*: consider discussion of such issues as stages of grief , advanced directives, services of hospice, Internet resources, and alternative/complementary therapies

CHAPTER 13: CONCEPTION AND FETAL DEVELOPMENT

Chapter Review Activities

1. Conception
2. Gametes, sperm, ovum
3. Mitosis, diploid, 46, 23
4. Meiosis, haploid, 23
5. Gametogenesis, spermatogenesis, oogenesis
6. Fertilization, ampulla, zona reaction, diploid (46)
7. Zygote, morula, blastocyst, trophoblast

8. Implantation, endometrium, chorionic villi, trophoblast, decidua, decidua basalis, decidua capsularis

9. Embryo
10. Fetus, cephalocaudal
11. Amniotic membranes, chorion, amnion
12. Amniotic fluid, oligohydramnios, hydramnios
13. Umbilical cord, arteries, vein, Wharton's jelly, nuchal cord
14. Placenta, cotyledons, hormones, oxygen, nutrients, wastes, carbon dioxide

15. Viability
16. Ductus arteriosus
17. Ductus venosus
18. Foramen ovale
19. Hematopoiesis
20. Surfactants, lecithin-sphingomyelin
21. Quickening, 16, 20
22. Meconium
23. Dizygotic, fraternal
24. Monozygotic, identical
25. Teratogen

26. *Functions of yolk sac, amniotic fluid and membranes, umbilical cord, placenta:* see individual sections for each of these structures in the Development of the Embryo

27. F, 28. F, 29. T, 30. T, 31. F, 32. T, 33. T, 34. F, 35. T, 36. T, 37. F

38. *Complete table related to primary germ layers:* see Primary Germ Layers section of the Embryo and Fetus for identification of tissues and organs that develop from each layer

39. D is correct; feeling of movement is called quickening; the sex of a baby is determined at conception; the heart begins to pump blood by the 3rd week and a beat can be heard with ultrasound by the 8th week of gestation.

40. B is correct; the L/S ratio is a test to determine the presence of the surfactants lecithin and sphingomyelin; it becomes 2:1 indicating lung maturity at approximately 35 to 36 weeks' gestation; an elevated alpha-fetoprotein level is an indicator for an open neural tube defect; renal disorders usually are indicated by a decreased amount of amniotic fluid.

41. C is correct; the healthy newborn of a well-nourished mother will not need iron sources until about 5 months of age; iron-

fortified cereal is usually introduced at this time.

42. A is correct; if a woman's diabetes is uncontrolled, maternal hyperglycemia will produce fetal hyperglycemia and stimulate hyperinsulinemia, resulting in increased fetal growth (macrosomia or large for gestational age); lung maturation is inhibited and neonatal hypoglycemia can occur; strict control of maternal glucose levels before and during pregnancy will reduce the risk

Critical Thinking Exercises

1. A. *Progress of development at 2 months, 5 months, and 7 months*: see Table 13-1 to formulate your answer; use of illustrations and life-size models would facilitate learning
   B. *Survival after 35 weeks' gestation*: discuss how the respiratory system develops including the critical factor surfactant production; describe how surfactant helps the newborn to breathe
   C. *Quickening*: explain that this is the woman's perception of fetal movement that occurs at about 16 to 20 weeks' gestation; use Box 13-3 to describe how the fetus moves; it will not hurt but can be uncomfortable and interfere with sleep toward the end of pregnancy; fetus will develop its own sleep-wake cycle
   D. *Fetal-sensory perception*: discuss sensory capability of the fetus using Sensory Awareness section of Fetal Maturation; fetus can hear sounds such as parents' voices and respond to light touch; encourage Susan to interact with her fetus
   E. *Sex determination*: discuss function of X and Y chromosomes; sex of her fetus will become recognizable around 12 weeks' gestation
   F. *Multiple gestation—twins*: discuss monozygotic (identical) and dizygotic (fraternal) twinning and how each

occurs; emphasize that fraternal twinning tends to occur in families
   G. *Influence of activity and position on fetal growth and development* (see Placental section): discuss differences in circulation through placenta in various positions including supine, lateral, sitting, and standing; discuss the impact of excessive exercise on placental circulation; emphasize that efficient circulation through the placenta is important to ensure adequate supply of oxygen and nutrients

CHAPTER 14: ANATOMY AND PHYSIOLOGY OF PREGNANCY

Chapter Review Activities

1. C, 2. P, 3. K, 4. T, 5. S, 6. U, 7. J, 8. N, 9. V, 10. B, 11. G, 12. A, 13. O, 14. I, 15. Q, 16. E, 17. M, 18. W, 19. F, 20. H, 21. D, 22. R, 23. L

24. Gravidity
25. Parity
26. Gravida
27. Nulligravida
28. Nullipara
29. Primigravida
30. Primipara
31. Multigravida
32. Multipara
33. Viability
34. Preterm
35. Term
36. Postdate, postterm
37. Human chorionic gonadotropin (hCG)

38. *Complete table regarding signs and symptoms of pregnancy*: see Table 14-2 and Signs of Pregnancy Section to insert information into this table regarding Presumptive, Probable, and Positive signs and symptoms of pregnancy

39. *Obstetric History:* Nancy (1–1–0–1 or 3–1–1–0–1); Marsha (2–0–1–2 or 4–2–0–1–2); Linda (1–1–1–3 or 4–1–1–1–3)

40. F, 41. T, 42. F, 43. T, 44. F, 45. F, 46. T, 47. F, 48. F, 49. T, 50. T, 51. F, 52. T, 53. F, 54. T, 55. T, 56. F, 57. T, 58. T

59. Changes in vital signs as pregnancy progresses:
    - *Blood pressure and heart rate patterns:* see Box 14-3; blood pressure decreases in the second trimester by 5 to 10 mm Hg and returns to baseline during the 3rd trimester; pulse increases by 10 to 15 beats per minute; murmurs and palpitations can occur; *Respiratory patterns:* see Box 14-4; breathing becomes more thoracic in nature and volume is deeper with a slight increase in rate; some shortness of breath may be experienced in the 2nd trimester as the diaphragm is pushed up by the enlarging uterus; continues until lightening occurs; *Temperature:* baseline temperature increases by about 1°F as a result of the increase in BMR and the progesterone effect; women may complain of heat intolerance

60. *Mean arterial pressure (MAP) calculation* (see Box 14-2): use the following formula:

$$\frac{\text{systolic} + 2(\text{diastolic})}{3}$$

Answers are: 91, 81, 90, 110

61. Specify value changes for selected laboratory tests during pregnancy:
    - CBC: see Table 14-3 and Box 14-3
    - Clotting activity: see Circulation and Coagulation times section of Cardiopulmonary System and Table 14-3
    - Acid-base balance: see Acid-Base section and Table 14-3
    - Urinalysis: see Fluid and Electrolyte section and Table 14-3

62. Expected adaptations in elimination during pregnancy:
    - Renal: see Renal System section; slowed passage of urine and dilatation of the ureters as a result of progesterone increases the risk for UTIs; bladder irritability, nocturia, urinary frequency and urgency (1st and 3rd trimester after lightening)
    - Bowel: see Esophagus, Stomach, and Intestines sections; constipation and hemorrhoids; effect of increased progesterone, which decreases peristalsis, and intestinal displacement by enlarging uterus

63. *Changes in endocrine function and secretions of hormones:* see Endocrine System section for a description of each hormone and how it changes with pregnancy

64. A is correct; hCG indicates a positive pregnancy test and is a probable sign; breast tenderness and morning sickness are presumptive signs; fetal heart sounds are a positive sign of pregnancy.

65. D is correct; gravida (total number of pregnancies including the present one is 5); para (term birth of daughter at 39 weeks = 1; stillbirth at 32 weeks and triplets at 30 weeks = 2; spontaneous abortion at 8 weeks = 1; total number of living children = 4).

66. C is correct; while little change occurs in respiratory rate, breathing becomes more thoracic in nature with the upward displacement of the diaphragm; women normally experience a greater awareness to breathe and may even complain of dyspnea at rest as pregnancy progresses; supine hypotension syndrome with a decrease in systolic pressure as much as 30 mm Hg occurs as a result of vena cava and aorta compression by the uterus when the woman is in a supine position; baseline pulse rate increases by 10 to 15 beats per minute; systolic and diastolic pressure decreases by

approximately 5 to 10 mm Hg beginning in the 2nd trimester returning to 1st trimester levels in the 3rd trimester.

67. D is correct; recording cycle information assists with accuracy of diagnosis; C reflects the most common error of performing this test too soon, she will need to repeat the test in 1 week if the result is negative; first morning voided specimens should be used because they are the most concentrated and apt to have the largest amount of hCG; anticonvulsants, tranquilizers, diuretics, and promethazine can result in inaccurate results.

68. B is correct; friability refers to cervical fragility resulting in slight bleeding when scraped or touched; Chadwick sign refers to a deep bluish color of cervix and vagina as a result of increased circulation; Hegar sign refers to softening and compressibility of the lower uterine segment.

Critical Thinking Exercises

1. Responses to client concerns and questions:
   A. *Spotting after intercourse:* discuss cervical and vaginal friability and increased vascularity; makes the vagina and cervix softer and more delicate so spotting after intercourse is expected; caution that any bleeding should be reported so it can be evaluated
   B. *Use of home pregnancy test:* see Teaching for Self-Care Box—Home Pregnancy Testing; emphasize the importance of following directions because each brand of test is slightly different; use first-voided morning specimen for the most concentrated urine and notify health care provider regardless of the test result
   C. *Bladder and vaginal infections:* discuss impact of increased vaginal secretions and impact of stasis of urine that contains nutrients and has a higher pH; review prevention measures at this time
   D. *Breast changes with pregnancy:* discuss changes in beasts such as enlargement of Montgomery's glands and development of lactation structures resulting in larger breasts that are tender during the 1st trimester; changes in consistency and presence of lumpiness during BSE; changes are bilateral
   E. *Effects of pregnant woman's position:* discuss supine hypotensive syndrome and importance of the lateral position when at rest
   F. *Nosebleeds:* discuss impact of estrogen-stimulated increase in upper airway vascularity, which increases edema, congestion, and hyperemia of the tissue making nose bleeds more common
   G. *Ankle edema:* explain that the swelling of her ankles is a result of the pressure of the enlarging uterus and the dependent position of her legs; elevating her legs and exercising them helps to decrease edema; caution her to never take someone else's medications or to self-medicate herself
   H. *Posture and low back pain:* lordosis occurs as a result of the enlargement of the uterus, which decreases abdominal muscle tone and increased mobility of the pelvic joints, tilting the pelvis forward and resulting in lower back pain, a change in posture, and a shifting forward of the change of gravity
   I. *Braxton Hicks:* the woman is describing false labor contractions because they diminish with activity; these contractions facilitate blood flow and promote oxygen delivery to the fetus; compare these contractions with true labor contractions
   J. *Shortness of breath:* explain that what she is experiencing is a result of increased sensitivity of her respiratory center to carbon dioxide, compensation for a mild respiratory alkalosis, and the elevation of her diaphragm by the

enlarging uterus; assess the woman for signs of pulmonary edema to be sure the shortness of breath is physiologic rather than pathologic

2. *Blood pressure protocol:* consider the effects of maternal age, activity and stress level, health status, arm, and position; protocol should emphasize consistency in arm and position used, size of cuff, time provided for relaxation prior to measurement; repeat if finding is inconsistent with woman's baseline or is abnormal

CHAPTER 15: MATERNAL AND FETAL NUTRITION

Chapter Review Activities

1. Healthy diet before conception, folic acid (folate), neural tube defects, 400 mcg (0.4 mg)

2. Intrauterine growth restriction, low birth weight, preterm, small for gestational age (SGA), SGA, preterm birth

3. Macrosomia, fetopelvic disproportion, operative, cesarean birth, hemorrhage, infection, trauma, fetal death

4. Stage of gestation, fetuses, age, activity level, weight, energy, 300 kcal, weight gain

5. Pregnant adolescents, poor women, women adhering to unusual diets

6. Iron deficiency anemia, adolescents, African-American, lower socioeconomic status

7. Lactose intolerance

8. Pica, clay, dirt, laundry starch, ice, freezer frost, baking powder, soda, cornstarch, hemoglobin, anemia, food cravings, nutrients

9. Obstetric/gynecologic effects on nutrition, medical history, usual maternal diet, anthropometric (body) height, weight, body mass index (BMI)

10. Vegetables, fruits, legumes, nuts, seeds, grains, semi-vegetarian, lacto-ovo-vegetarians, strict vegetarians, vegans

11. *Complete table related to nutrient requirement during pregnancy:* see Table 15-1 and corresponding sections in the text to complete this activity

12. *Indicators of nutritional risk:* see Box 15-2 to identify the five risk indicators

13. *Guidelines for strict vegetarians during pregnancy:* see Cultural Influences and Vegetarian Diets section of Plan of Care and Interventions
    • These diets tend to be low in vitamins B_{12} and B_6, iron, calcium, zinc, and perhaps calories; supplements may be needed.
    • Food needs to be combined to ensure that all essential amino acids are provided.

14. *Signs of good and inadequate nutrition:* see Table 15-5 for several signs of good and inadequate nutrition

15. Nursing measures appropriate for each nursing diagnosis: see appropriate subsection in Coping with Nutritional-Related Discomforts of Pregnancy section
    A. *Imbalance nutrition: less than body requirements related to inadequate intake associated with nausea and vomiting:* see Nausea and Vomiting section for several relief measures
    B. *Constipation related to decreased intestinal motility associated with effects of increased progesterone and enlarging uterus:* see Constipation section; include adequate fluid and roughage/fiber intake, exercise

and activity, regular time for elimination

C. *Acute pain related to reflux of gastric contents associated with progesterone effect on gastric motility:* see Pyrosis section; small frequent meals, drink fluids between not with meals, avoid spicy foods, remain upright after eating

16. *Determining BMI and recommended pregnancy weight gain pattern:* see Fig. 15-2 or use formula in text to calculate BMI; see Weight Gain and Pattern of Weight Gain sections to determine weight gain patterns based on each woman's BMI; keep in mind that each woman should gain 1 to 2.5 kg in the first trimester; weight gain per week is recommended for the second and third trimester
    - June: BMI 22 (normal); total 11.5 to 16 kg; 0.4 kg/week
    - Alice: BMI 29 (overweight); total 7 to 11.5 kg; 0.3 kg/week
    - Ann: BMI 16 (underweight); total 12.5 to 18 kg; 0.5 kg/week

17. T, 18. F, 19. T, 20. T, 21. F, 22. F, 23. T, 24. T, 25. T, 26. F, 27. F, 28. T, 29. F, 30. T, 31. F, 32. F, 33. T, 34. F, 35. T, 36. T, 37. F

38. *Nutrition guidelines for lactation* (see Nutrient Needs during Lactation section): adequate calcium intake and other nutrients (e.g., protein, vitamins, minerals), at least 1800 (about 500 kcal above nonpregnant intake) kcal/day, adequate fluid intake (should not experience thirst), and avoid tobacco, alcohol, and excessive caffeine

39. *Factors that increase nutrient need during pregnancy* (see Table 15-3): growth and development of uterine-placental-fetal unit, expansion of maternal blood volume and RBCs, mammary changes, increased BMR; explain consequences to mother and fetus/newborn of inadequate intake of nutrients

40. D is correct; bran, tea, coffee, milk, oxalates, and egg yolks all decrease iron absorption; tomatoes and strawberries contain vitamin C which enhances iron absorption; meats contain heme iron, which also enhances absorption; ideally, iron is best absorbed on an empty stomach and should be taken between not with meals.

41. B is correct; BMI indicates woman is at a normal weight; total gain should be 11.5 to 16 kg representing a gain of 0.4 kg/week and 1.6 kg/month during the 2nd and 3rd trimesters.

42. C is correct; small, frequent meals are better tolerated than large meals that distend the stomach; hunger can worsen nausea therefore meals should not be skipped; dry starchy foods should be eaten in morning and at other times during the day when nausea occurs; fried, fatty, and spicy foods should be avoided; a bedtime snack is recommended.

43. B is correct; legumes are a good source of folic acid as are green leafy vegetables, whole grains and fortified cereals, papaya, asparagus, and liver; A and D are not good sources of folic acid though they do supply other important nutrients for pregnancy; corn does contain folate but not at a high level.

44. A is correct; only 6 ounces from the meat, poultry, fish, dry beans, eggs, and nut group are required during pregnancy; B, C, and D are all appropriate for pregnancy; orange juice contains Vitamin C, which will enhance iron absorption

Critical Thinking Exercises

1. Nutrition and weight gain concerns during pregnancy

A. *Concern regarding amount of recommended weight gain during pregnancy:*
- Identify components of maternal weight gain; use Fig. 15-3 to illustrate how the weight gain is distributed.
- Discuss impact of maternal weight gain on fetal growth and development; associate inadequate maternal weight gain and low birth weight, preterm birth, and infant mortality.
- Discuss weight gain total and pattern recommended for a woman with a normal BMI of 20.

B. *Eating for two during pregnancy:*
- Emphasis on quality of food that meets nutritional requirements, not on the quantity of food.
- Discuss expected weight gain total and pattern for a woman with a normal BMI of 21.
- Excessive weight gain during pregnancy may be difficult to lose after pregnancy and could lead to chronic obesity; excessive fetal size and childbirth problems could also result.

C. *Vitamin supplementation during pregnancy:* determine what and how much she takes; compare to recommendations for pregnancy; discuss potential problems with toxicity, especially with overuse of fat-soluble vitamins

D. *Heartburn (pyrosis):* recommend relief measures such as small frequent meals, fluids between not with meals, avoiding spicy, fatty foods, and remaining upright after meals

E. *Weight-reduction diets during pregnancy:*
- BMI indicates overweight status; a gain of 7 to 11.5 kg should occur during pregnancy.
- Discuss hazards of inadequate caloric intake during pregnancy in terms of growth and development of fetus and pregnancy-related structures; impact of ketoacidosis.
- Discuss quality foods and development of good nutritional habits to be used during the postpartum period as part of a sensible weight loss program.
- Discuss importance of exercise and activity during pregnancy.

F. *Reduction of water intake:* discuss importance of fluid to meet demands of pregnancy-related changes, regulate temperature, prevent constipation and UTIs; consider possible association between dehydration and preterm labor and oligohydramnios

G. *Lactose intolerance:* discuss basis for problem; reduce lactose intake by using lactose-free products, nondairy sources of calcium and calcium supplements; take lactase supplements; see Box 15-3 for additional calcium sources if milk is not tolerated

H. *Weight loss lactation:* discuss weight loss patterns with lactation; emphasize that fat stores from pregnancy are used during the lactation process with a resultant weight loss; inform her of increased need for nutrients, calories, and fluids, which are used up with lactogenesis

2. *Taking iron supplements effectively:* see Iron and Counseling about Iron Supplementation sections, Table 15-1 for iron sources, and Teaching for Self-Care Box—Iron Supplementation
- Discuss importance of iron.
- Emphasize importance of vitamin C for iron absorption; discuss food sources high in iron and vitamin C.
- Identify food sources that can interfere with iron absorption such as egg yolks, bran, and milk.
- Discuss ways to take iron supplements to enhance absorption and minimize side effects including GI upset and constipation.

3. Native American woman—meeting nutritional needs
   A. *Counseling approach:*
      - Assess her current nutritional status and habits; obtain a diet history.
      - Analyze current patterns as a basis for menu planning.
      - Discuss weight gain pattern for an underweight woman.
      - Use a variety of teaching methods; keep woman actively involved.
      - Emphasize importance of good nutrition for herself and her newborn.
   B. *Menu plan:* use Table 15-5 for Native American foods and Table 15-4 for servings of required nutrients for a 1-day menu; distribute throughout day—meals/snacks

CHAPTER 16: NURSING CARE DURING PREGNANCY

Chapter Review Activities

1. Presumptive, probable, positive

2. Nägele's, estimated date of birth (EDB), 3 months, 7 days, 1 year, last menstrual period (LMP), trimesters, 38, 40

3. Supine hypotension, vena cava, aorta, pallor, dizziness, faintness, breathlessness, tachycardia, nausea, clammy (damp, cool) skin, sweating

4. Fundal height, pinch

5. Fetal heart tones, fetal movement, fundal height, abnormal maternal or fetal symptoms, gestational age

6. Developmental, accepting pregnancy, identifying with role of parent, reordering personal relationships, establishing relationship with fetus, preparing for childbirth

7. Biologic fact of pregnancy, "I am pregnant," growing fetus as distinct from herself, "I am going to have a baby," birth, parenting of the child, "I am going to be a mother"

8. Emotional lability, hormonal, finances, changed lifestyle, ambivalence

9. Announcement, biologic fact of pregnancy, moratorium, accept the pregnancy, focusing, negotiate, labor, parenthood

10. Couvade, couvade syndrome
11. Prescriptions, proscriptions, taboos

12. Triple screen, Down syndrome, 16, 18, alpha-fetoprotein, human chorionic gonadotropin, unconjugated estriol

13. Calculate expected date of birth: use Nägele's rule: subtract 3 months and add 7 days, and 1 year (if appropriate) to the first day of the last menstrual period
    A. February 12, 2004
    B. October 21, 2003
    C. June 11, 2003

14. Cultural beliefs and practices: see Cultural Influences section of Variations in Prenatal Care
    A. *Describe how cultural beliefs affect participation in prenatal care:* consider the following factors: beliefs that conflict with typical Western prenatal practices, lack of money and transportation, communication difficulties, concern regarding modesty and gender of health care provider, fear of invasive procedures, view of pregnancy as a healthy state whereas health care providers imply illness, view pregnancy problems as a normal part of pregnancy
    B. *Prescriptions and proscriptions:* see specific subsections for emotional responses, clothing, physical activity and rest, sexual activity, diet

15. *Complete table regarding components of initial and follow-up visits*; see Initial Visit and Follow-up Visits sections to complete the table

16. *Components of fetal assessment* (see Follow-up Visits section): measurement of fundal height, determination of gestational age, assessment of health status of the fetus including FHR pattern, fetal movements, and unusual or abnormal maternal or fetal signs and symptoms; teach woman how to do daily fetal movement counts beginning at approximately 27 weeks' gestation

17. Warning signs of potential complications during pregnancy
    A. *List signs of complications:* see Signs of Potential Complications Box, which lists signs according to the first, second, and third trimesters
    B. *Nursing approach when discussing signs of complications with pregnant woman and her family:*
       • Discuss the signs, possible causes, when and to whom to report.
       • Present the signs verbally and in written form.
       • Provide time to answer questions and discuss concerns; make follow-up phone calls.
       • Gather full information of signs that are reported; use information as a basis for action.
       • Document all assessments, actions, and responses including the date(s) that information regarding these signs was given, the methodology used, and the woman's reaction to the information.

18. F, 19. F, 20. T, 21. T, 22. T, 23. F, 24. F, 25. F, 26. F, 27. F, 28. T, 29. T, 30. T, 31. F, 32. F, 33. T, 34. T, 35. T, 36. F, 37. T, 38. T, 39. T, 40. F, 41. T, 42. T, 43. F, 44. F, 45. T, 46. T

47. *Protocol for fundal measurement:* consider woman's position, type of measuring tape used, measurement method (Fig. 16-7), and conditions of the examination such as an empty bladder and relaxed or contracted uterus

48. *Factors used to estimate gestational age:* menstrual history, contraceptive history, pregnancy test result, and specific findings related to the maternal-fetal unit, for example time of appearance of the specific signs of pregnancy, uterine size, FHT

49. Prevention of injury:
    A. *Principles of body mechanics:* see Figs. 16-12 and 16-14, and Teaching for Self-Care Box—Posture and Body Mechanics
    B. *Safety Guidelines:* see Teaching for Self-Care Box—Safety During Pregnancy and the prevention measures identified in Education for Self-Care section

50. *Contraindications for breastfeeding:* deep-seated aversion to breastfeeding by woman or partner, need to take certain medications that can be harmful to the newborn, medical disorders such as active TB, newly diagnosed breast cancer, and HIV-positive status (in developed countries)

51. *Male styles of involvement in pregnancy:* see Accepting the Pregnancy subsection of Paternal Adaptation section for a full description of each involvement style listed: observer, expressive, instrumental

52. B is correct; A and C are probable signs and D is a positive sign, diagnostic of pregnancy

53. C is correct; use Nägele's rule by subtracting 3 months and adding 7 days and one year (if appropriate) to the first day of the last menstrual period, which in this case is November 9, 2003

54. D is correct; supine hypotension related to compression of aorta and vena cava is being experienced; the first action is to remove the cause of the problem by turning the woman on her side; this should alleviate the symptoms being experienced including nausea; assessment of vital signs can occur after the woman's position is changed

55. C is correct; during this normal quiet period a woman focuses on her fantasy child; sexual desire is decreased during the 1st and 3rd trimesters and increased in the 2nd; ambivalence is a common response when preparing for a new role; safe passage and birth preparation is a concern during the 3rd trimester

56. A is correct; intake of at least 2 to 3 liters per day is recommended; B, C, and D are all accepted methods of preventing UTIs along with frequent, regular urination, good genital hygiene, and avoiding wearing tight-fitting jeans for long periods

Critical Thinking Exercises

1. Health history interview: see Initial Visit and Follow-up Visits sections
   A. *Purpose of the health history interview:*
      - Establish therapeutic relationship with the pregnant woman and her family.
      - Planned time for purposeful communication to gather baseline data related to the woman's subjective appraisal of her health status and to gather objective information based on observation of the woman's affect, posture, body language, skin color, and other physical and emotional signs.
      - Update information and compare with baseline information during follow-up interviews.
   B. *Write for each component of initial health history interview:* be sure questions reflect principles of effective questioning; consider the need to ask follow-up questions to clarify and gather further information when a problem is identified
   C. *Write four questions for the follow-up health history interviews:* focus on updating baseline information and asking questions related to anticipated events and changes for the woman's gestational age at the time of the visit

2. *Care of woman at initial visit who is anxious and unsure about prenatal care:* answer should emphasize
   - Establishing a therapeutic, trusting relationship so woman will feel comfortable continuing with prenatal care
   - Teaching the woman about the importance of prenatal care for her health and that of her baby; determine if barriers are present that may limit participation in prenatal care
   - Involving her boyfriend in the care process so he will encourage her participation in prenatal care; consider that the father of the baby is often considered to be the most significant person
   - Following guidelines for health history interview, physical examination, and laboratory testing; ensure privacy and comfort during the examination and teach her about how her body is changing and will continue to change with pregnancy
   - Evaluating the desire for this pregnancy and the need for community agency support

3. Couple during first trimester—concerns and questions
   A. *Accuracy of EDB:* reliability depends on the accuracy of date used and the regularity of her menstrual cycles; most women give birth within 1 week before and 1 week after the expected date of birth

B. *Kegel exercises:* pelvic muscle exercises to maintain muscle tone and ability to support pelvic organs; see Kegel Exercises section of Education for Self-Care (see Chapter 5: Teaching for Self-Care Box—Kegel Exercises)

C. *Effect of pregnancy on sexuality:* see Teaching for Self-Care Box—Sexuality in Pregnancy and Fig. 16-19; emphasize that intercourse is safe as long as pregnancy is progressing normally and it is comfortable for the woman; sexual expression should be in tune with the woman's changing needs and emotions; inform that spotting can normally occur related to the fragility of the vaginal mucosa and cervix and that changes in positions and activities may be helpful as pregnancy progresses

D. *Morning sickness:* see Table 16-2 (first trimester section) and Box 16-5; fully assess what she is experiencing, then discuss why it happens, how long it will likely last, and relief measures that are safe and effective including complementary and alterative approaches (also see Nutritional Discomforts section of Chapter 15)

4. *Physical activity and exercise in pregnancy:* see Physical Activity section of Education for Self-Care and Teaching for Self-Care Box—Exercise Tips for Pregnant Women; assess her usual pattern of exercise and activity and consider their safety during pregnancy; discuss precautions and guidelines for safe, effective exercise; emphasize that moderate physical activity benefits her and her baby and will prepare her for the work of labor and birth; caution her to take note of the effects of exercise in terms of temperature, heart rate, and feeling of well-being

5. Nursing diagnoses, expected outcomes and nursing measures for women in various situations during pregnancy:

A. *Risk for urinary tract infection related to lack of knowledge regarding changes of the renal system during pregnancy*
   - Woman will drink at least 2 to 3 liters of fluids per day; will empty bladder at first urge.
   - Explain changes that occur in the renal system during pregnancy; increase fluid intake, use acid-ash forming fluids, void frequently including before going to bed to keep bladder empty, perform good perineal hygiene and wear appropriate clothing, use lateral position to enhance renal perfusion and urine formation.

B. *Acute pain in lower back related to neuromuscular changes associated with pregnancy at 23 weeks' gestation*
   - Woman will experience lessening of lower back pain following implementation of suggested relief measures.
   - Explain basis for lower back pain and relief measures including back massage, pelvic rock, and posture changes (see Table 16-2 and Fig. 16-11); encourage woman to change her footwear for better stability and safety.

C. *Anxiety related to lack of knowledge concerning the process of labor and birth and appropriate measures to cope with the pain and discomfort*
   - Couple will enroll in a childbirth education program in the 7th month of pregnancy.
   - Explain the childbirth process and describe the many nonpharmacologic and pharmacologic measures to relieve pain; discuss role of coach and possibility of hiring a doula; make a referral to a childbirth education program and assist with the preparation of a birth plan; discuss childbirth options and prebirth preparations.

6. Woman in the second trimester—questions and concerns
   A. *Purpose of fundal height measurement:* indirect assessment of how her fetus is growing
   B. *Determining fetal health status:* discuss FHR (let her listen) and fetal movement assessments (tell her how)
   C. *Clothing choices during pregnancy:* consider safety and comfort in terms of low-heeled shoe and nonrestrictive clothing
   D. *Gas and constipation:* see Table 16-2 (second trimester section); assess problem and lifestyle factors that may be contributing to the problem; discuss why it occurs and appropriate relief measures (fluids, roughage, activity)
   E. *Itchiness:* if the woman is experiencing noninflammatory pruritus use Table 16-2 (second trimester section) for basis of discomfort and relief measures; be sure to rule out rashes related to infection or allergic reactions
   F. *Travel during pregnancy:* see Travel section of Education for Self-Care; tell her that she may travel if her pregnancy is progressing normally; emphasize importance of staying hydrated, wearing seat belt and shoulder harness, doing breathing and lower extremities exercises, ambulating every hour for 15 minutes, and voiding every 2 hours

7. Woman experiencing supine hypotension syndrome (see Emergency Box—Supine Hypotension)
   A. *Explanation of assessment findings:* supine hypotension
   B. *Immediate action:* turn her on her side and maintain the position until vital signs stabilize and signs and symptoms diminish; place wedge to maintain a lateral tilt then continue the assessment; when completed, help her to rise slowly to an upright position—observe for signs of postural hypotension

8. Woman during third trimester—questions and concerns
   A. *Nipple condition for breastfeeding:* perform pinch test to see if nipples will evert; if they do not, the woman can be taught to use a nipple shell to help her nipples to protrude; no special exercises are recommended because they could stimulate preterm labor in susceptible women as a result of secretion of oxytocin; keep nipples and areola clean and dry
   B. *Ankle edema:* see Table 16-2 (third trimester section); discuss basis of the edema and encourage use of lower extremities exercises and elevation of legs periodically during the day (Fig. 16-15); emphasize importance of fluid intake
   C. *Leg cramps:* see Table 16-2 (third trimester section); discuss basis of leg cramps then demonstrate relief measures such as pressing weight onto foot when standing or dorsiflexing the foot while lying in bed; avoid pointing the toes; ensure adequate intake of calcium

9. Woman concerned about preterm labor
   A. *Nursing diagnosis:* anxiety related to perceived risk for preterm labor and birth; woman will identify signs suggestive of preterm labor and the action to take if they occur
   B. *Signs of preterm labor:* see Teaching for Self-Care Box—How to Recognize Preterm Labor and Fig. 16-18; emphasize that signs are vague so she must be alert for even subtle changes; teach her how to palpate her abdomen to detect uterine contractions
   C. *Action if signs are detected:* empty bladder, drink three to four glasses of water, assume a side-lying position, and count contractions for another hour; if

contractions continue call health care provider

10. *Sibling reactions to mother's pregnancy*: see Sibling Adaptation section of Preparing for Childbirth and Box 17-4 in Chapter 17, which provides tips for sibling preparation; emphasize importance of considering each child's developmental level; prepare children for prenatal events, time during hospitalization, and the homecoming of the new baby; refer to sibling classes and encourage sibling visitation after birth; suggest books and videos that parents could use to prepare their children for birth

11. Expectant father concerned about wife's mood swings
    A. *Nursing diagnoses*: deficient knowledge related to pregnant spouse's mood changes; Tom will explain basis for wife's mood swings and strategies that he can use to cope with these changes and support his spouse
    B. *Nurse's response*: see Maternal Adaptation section and Table 16-2 (first trimester section); discuss the basis for the mood swings and experiences during the first trimester including ambivalence; identify measures he can use to support her

12. *Woman experiencing introspection*: see Reordering Personal Relationships section; explain that she is concentrating on having a baby and forming a relationship with the fetus; emphasize her partner's important role as a caregiver and nurturer

CHAPTER 17: CHILDBIRTH AND PERINATAL EDUCATION

Chapter Review Activities

1. Preconception education and care, 17, 56
2. Grantly Dick-Read, fear-tension-pain, relaxation

3. Lamaze, controlled muscle relaxation, breathing
4. Bradley, breath control, abdominal breathing, general body relaxation, darkness, solitude, quiet
5. Intellectually, emotionally, physically, wellness, lifestyle behaviors
6. Birth plan
7. Obstetrician
8. Nurse-midwife
9. Direct entry midwives, certified professional midwives
10. Doula, physical, emotional, informational
11. Labor-delivery-recovery (LDR)
12. Labor-delivery-recovery-postpartum (LDRP)
13. Free standing birth

14. F, 15. F, 16. T, 17. F, 18. F, 19. T, 20. F, 21. T, 22. T, 23. F

24. *Nursing role in preconception education and care* (see Preconception Education and Care section and Box 17-1)
    • Convince persons of childbearing age of the importance of preconception education and care for positive pregnancy outcomes.
    • Conduct an assessment as outlined in Box 17-2 focusing on identifying risk factors and evaluating general health status through a health history interview, physical examination, and laboratory testing as indicated.
    • Based on assessment findings
      • Reinforce health-promoting behaviors (e.g., balanced nutrition, exercise, relaxation, immunizations, regular health care).
      • Teach related to changing behaviors that can adversely influence health in general and when pregnant (e.g., inadequate nutrition, inappropriate weight, environmental hazards, substance abuse, stress).

- Help them to determine best time for pregnancy and to use effective birth control measures until then.
  - Treat and modify risk behaviors including appropriate referrals.
- Advocate for healthy environment and funding for preconception education and care.

25. *Explain specific tension-reducing and pain relief measures of childbirth education methods:* see Childbirth Education—Early Methods section for a discussion of Grantly Dick-Read, Lamaze, and Bradley methods

26. *Components of the Philosophy of Birth:* see Childbirth Education—Current Practices section for a description of this philosophy

27. *Nonpharmacologic pain relief methods* (see Pain Management section): brief description of each method is included; also, consult Chapter 19

28. *Role of childbirth education in reducing rate of cesarean births and increasing rate of VBACs* (see Cesarean Birth section):
    - Inform regarding measures to reduce necessity of cesarean birth by emphasizing natural approaches to childbirth, avoiding epidurals, increasing quality labor support.
    - Encourage couples to be proactive in determining cesarean section rates of their health care provider and birth setting and degree of support they offer for natural, nonpharmacologic approaches.
    - Discuss risks for cesarean birth compared to vaginal births and differences in postpartum recovery.

29. D is correct; the Bradley method emphasizes the importance of darkness, solitude, and quiet to facilitate working in harmony with the body.

30. C is correct; remaining in bed for labor and birth will need to be modified because changing upright positions, remaining upright, ambulating, and using water therapy all enhance the labor and birth process; A, B, and D are all appropriate and realistic options.

31. D is correct; continuous support is critical and involves praise, encouragement, reassurance, comfort measures, physical contact, as well as explanations; the doula does not get involved in clinical tasks; she is not a substitute for the father but rather encourages his participation as a partner with her in supporting the laboring woman.

32. C is correct; a pain-free childbirth is not realistic; rather the woman will use what she needs recognizing that the childbirth techniques often decrease her need for pharmacologic interventions—pain will be present but she will be in control of the pain not the pain in control of her; presence of family members is not an outcome of childbirth education—it is the woman's choice to have them present or not

Critical Thinking Exercises

1. Woman planning for pregnancy with her husband (see Preconception Education and Care section)
   A. *Explain importance of participation:* review importance by including purposes of preconception care and anticipated outcome of preconception on pregnancy; focus on importance of day 17 to day 56 of a pregnancy when the woman may not even realize she is pregnant
   B. *Process to follow with preconception care:* use Boxes 17-1 and 17-2 and Role of the Nurse as an Early Pregnancy Educator section when outlining the process of preconception care for the couple and the development

interventions related to assessment findings

2. Birth plan development (see Birth Plan section)
   A. *Purpose of birth plan:* means of open communication about the childbirth process between the woman and her partner and with the health care providers in an effort to have a childbirth experience that meets their expectations and wishes as closely as possible; it is a tool that couples can use to stay in control
   B. *Guidelines for formation of birth plan:* begin discussion early in pregnancy so full consideration can be given to each option; identify components that should be included in the plan; facilitate decision making concerning the options available; recognize risk status implications for care options
   C. *Topics for discussion/decision-making:* partner's role during childbirth and who will be present; setting for the birth; labor management measures including pain control, comfort measures, positions, events at the birth, newborn, and postpartum care (e.g., celebratory activities, breastfeeding, mother-baby care)

3. *Decision making regarding birth setting:* see Birth Setting Choices section; answer should include
   • Descriptions of each option along with the criteria for use and the advantages and disadvantages.
   • Onsite visits and interaction with health care providers responsible for care at each site should be encouraged.
   • Speak to couples who gave birth in these setting to get their impressions.
   • Emphasize that the decision is theirs and that they should choose what is comfortable for them; a decision should

be made on the basis of a full understanding of each option.

4. Doulas (see Doula section)
   A. *Role of doula:* describe what a doula is, what they do; cite research that illustrates the benefits of using a doula for labor support; emphasize that the doula's role is to provide physical, emotional, and informational care and that her role does not involve the performance of clinical tasks
   B. *Finding a doula:* community contacts, other health care professions especially those involved in childbirth care or education, organizations such as DONA, persons who have used a doula; emphasize the importance of starting early so that there is time to make the right choice
   C. *Questions to ask during an interview with a prospective doula:* use Box 17-3 for question ideas; discuss these questions with the woman and put them in writing so that the woman will have them to refer to during the interview

5. Home birth (see Home Birth section)
   A. *Discuss decision-making process:*
      • Fully review advantages and disadvantages of home birth so an informed decision can be made and appropriate arrangements can be devised to enhance the advantages and offset the disadvantages.
      • Speak to couples who have experienced a home birth.
   B. *Preparation measures:*
      • Preparation of home including obtaining supplies and equipment, arranging for medical backup and transportation in the event of an emergency; measures to increase safety should be emphasized.
      • Choosing and preparing the persons who will be attending including children and grandparents.

6. Concerns of couples at a childbirth education class (see Parenting, Infant Stimulation and Massage, and Family Adjustments to Parenthood sections):
    A. *Crying infant*: discuss why babies cry and the influence of parental emotions on baby; emphasize that infants cannot be spoiled by having needs met and being held because they are learning to trust; teach parents how to interact with a newborn and how to use techniques such as massage for comfort
    B. *Sibling preparation*: see Box 17-4—Tips for Sibling Preparation and Sibling Classes section

CHAPTER 18: LABOR AND BIRTH PROCESSES

Chapter Review Activities

1. Passenger, passageway, powers, maternal position, psychologic response
2. Membrane-filled spaces, sutures
3. Overlapping, bones, head
4. Part, inlet, cephalic, breech, shoulder
5. First felt by the examining finger, vaginal examination, occiput, chin, sacrum, scapula
6. Flexed, occiput
7. Spine (long axis), spine (long axis), spines are parallel, spines are at right angles
8. Fetal body parts to one another, general flexion
9. Transverse, anteroposterior, flexion
10. Presenting part, four quadrants of the maternal pelvis
11. Largest transverse diameter, pelvic brim or inlet, true pelvis, ischial spines
12. Presenting part, ischial spines, centimeters (cm), ischial spines, descent
13. Shortening, thinning, cervix, first, percentages
14. Enlargement, widening, cervical opening (os), cervical canal, centimeters (cm), 1, 10
15. Presenting part, true pelvis, 2 weeks, onset of true labor
16. Uterine contractions, bearing down efforts, pushing
17. Brownish or blood tinged cervical mucoid, mucous plug, ripens
18. Turns, adjustments, fetal head, pelvis, cardinal movements, engagement, descent, flexion, internal rotation, extension, external rotation (restitution), expulsion
19. Valsalva, breath, abdominal muscles, intrathoracic pressure, venous return, venous pressure, cardiac output, blood pressure, pulse, hypoxia
20. Ferguson, bear down, perineal floor, oxytocin
21. Regular uterine contractions, dilation of cervix, latent, active, transition
22. Cervix is fully dilated, birth of the fetus, latent, active
23. Birth of the fetus, placenta is delivered
24. Recovery following birth, homeostasis, 2 hours
25. Position, blood pressure, uterine contractions, umbilical cord blood flow
26. *Describe five factors and how they affect the process of childbirth*: see separate sections for each of the five factors in Factors of Labor section; consider the factors of passenger, passage, powers, position of mother, psychologic response of mother
27. *Explain how the cardinal movements of labor facilitate birth*: see Mechanism of Labor section in Process of Labor and Fig. 18-14; describe engagement and descent, flexion, internal rotation, extension, external rotation and restitution, expulsion
28. Label illustrations:
    Fetal skull: A. mentum (chin); B. occipitofrontal diameter; C. frontal bone (sinciput); D. suboccipitobregmatic diameter; E. parietal bone (vertex); F. occipitomental diameter; G. occiput; H. sagittal suture; I. lambdoid suture;

J. posterior fontanel; K. biparietal diameter;
L. coronal suture; M. frontal suture;
N. anterior fontanel (bregma)
Maternal pelvis: A. symphysis pubis;
B. anteroposterior diameter of inlet;
C. transverse diameter of the inlet;
D. sacral promontory; E. sacrum;
F. sacroiliac joint; G. ischial spine; H. pubic
bone; I. sacrotuberous ligament; J. pubic
arch; K. ischial tuberosity; L. coccyx;
M. sacroiliac joint

29. *Indicate presentation, presenting part, position,*
    lie, and attitude represented by each illustration
    A. Cephalic (vertex), occiput, LOA,
       longitudinal, flexion
    B. Cephalic (vertex), occiput, LOT,
       longitudinal, flexion
    C. Cephalic (vertex), occiput, LOP,
       longitudinal, flexion
    D. Cephalic (vertex), occiput, ROA,
       longitudinal, flexion
    E. Cephalic (vertex), occiput, ROT,
       longitudinal, flexion
    F. Cephalic (vertex), occiput, ROP,
       longitudinal, flexion
    G. Cephalic (face), mentum, LMA,
       longitudinal, extension
    H. Cephalic (face), mentum, RMP,
       longitudinal, extension
    I. Cephalic (face), mentum, RMA,
       longitudinal, extension
    J. Breech, sacrum, LSA, longitudinal,
       flexion
    K. Breech, sacrum, LSP, longitudinal,
       flexion
    L. Shoulder, scapula, ScA, transverse,
       flexion

30. F, 31. T, 32. F, 33. F, 34. T, 35. T, 36. F,
    37. T, 38. F, 39. F, 40. T, 41. T, 42. F,
    43. T, 44. T, 45. T, 46. F, 47. F

48. B is correct; attitude is extension of head
    and neck as indicated by the mentum
    (chin) as the presenting part; the lie is
    longitudinal as indicated by the cephalic
    presentation.

49. C is correct; systolic blood pressure
    increases with uterine contractions in the
    first stage while both systolic and diastolic
    blood pressure increase during a
    contraction in the second stage; white
    blood cell count increases, gastric
    motility decreases and can lead to
    nausea and vomiting especially during
    the transition phase of the first stage of
    labor.

50. A is correct; the second stage of labor lasts
    an average of 50 minutes or longer and up
    to 2 to 3 hours especially in nulliparous
    labors or if an epidural was used; third stage
    of labor averages 3 to 5 minutes up to
    1 hour; fourth stage lasts approximately
    2 hours.

51. D is correct; quickening refers to the
    woman's first perception of fetal movement
    at 16 to 20 weeks' gestation; urinary
    frequency, lightening, weight loss of
    0.5 to 1.0 kg occur to signal that the
    onset of labor is near; backache, stronger
    Braxton Hicks and bloody show are also
    noted.

Critical Thinking Exercises

1. *Analysis of vaginal examinations:*
   Exam I: ROP (right occiput posterior,
   cephalic [vertex] presentation, longitudinal
   lie, flexed attitude),—1 (station at one
   centimeter above the
   ischial spines), 50% effaced, 3 cm
   dilated
   Exam II: RMA (right mentum anterior,
   cephalic [face] presentation, longitudinal
   lie, extended attitude), 0 (station at the
   ischial spines, engaged), 25% effaced, 2 cm
   dilated
   Exam III: LST (left sacrum transverse,
   breech presentation, longitudinal lie, flexed
   attitude), +1 (station at one centimeter

below the ischial spines), 75% effaced,
6 cm dilated

Exam IV: OA (occiput anterior, cephalic
[vertex] presentation, longitudinal lie,
flexed attitude), +3 (station at 3
centimeters below the ischial spines near or
on the perineum), 100% effaced, 10 cm
(fully dilated)

2. Woman with questions and concerns about
process of labor
  A. *Onset of labor:* see Onset of Labor
     subsection of the Process of Labor
     section; explain in simple terms the
     interaction of maternal and fetal
     hormones, uterine distention,
     placental aging, fetal fibronectin,
     prostaglandins
  B. *Signs of prodromal labor:* see Box 18-1
     for the signs that occur prior to the
     onset of labor including lightening,
     urinary frequency, backache, Braxton
     Hicks contractions, weight loss, energy
     surge, bloody show, possible rupture of
     the membranes; health care provider
     would detect cervical changes such
     as ripening, effacement, and
     dilation
  C. *Duration of labor:* see Stages of Labor
     section for approximate times for each
     stage; give woman ranges rather than
     absolute numbers especially because
     this will be her first labor; discuss her
     role in facilitating the progress of labor
  D. *Position changes during labor:*
     • Emphasize that the position of
       the woman is one of the 5 Ps of labor.
     • Discuss each position and describe its
       effect (Fig. 18-12).
     • Demonstrate each position and have
       her practice each of them with her
       partner.
     • Emphasize the beneficial effects of
       ambulation and changing positions
       on fetus, circulation, comfort, and
       progress.

CHAPTER 19: MANAGEMENT OF DISCOMFORT

Chapter Review Activities

1. B, 2. F, 3. H, 4. A, 5. G, 6. J, 7. M, 8. D,
   9. I, 10. L, 11. C, 12. E, 13. K

14. Visceral, cervical, lower uterine segment,
    ischemia, lower portion

15. Somatic, perineal tissues, pelvic floor,
    peritoneum, uterocervical supports,
    lacerations of soft tissues

16. Referred, uterus, abdominal wall, back, iliac
    crests, gluteal area, thighs

17. Gate control, massage, stroking, music,
    focal points, imagery, cognitive, breathing,
    relaxation

18. Endorphins
19. Walk, talk, slow-paced abdominal, half
20. Modified-paced, more shallow, twice
21. Deep cleansing breath

22. Patterned-paced, transition,
    hyperventilation, respiratory alkalosis,
    lightheadedness, dizziness, tingling of
    fingers, circumoral numbness, breathe into
    a paper bag held tightly around her nose
    and mouth, carbon dioxide, bicarbonate
    ion, twice

23. Effleurage, counterpressure, heel, fist, gate
    control

24. Water (hydrotherapy) therapy, active

25. Transcutaneous electrical nerve stimulation
    (TENS), thoracic, sacral, placebo,
    endogenous opiates (endorphins)

26. Acupressure
27. Biofeedback
28. Aromatherapy

29. Intradermal water block, counter-irritation, gate control, endogenous opiates (endorphins)

30. *Factors influencing nursing diagnosis of acute pain:* major factors include endorphin level, anxiety and fear, culture, previous experience, knowledge and expectations, childbirth preparation, available support and comfort, physical condition of the woman at the onset of labor, history of substance abuse or sexual abuse, environmental factors

31. *Theoretical basis for effectiveness of massage, stroking, music, and imagery in reducing sensation of pain:* discuss the gate-control theory of pain (see Childbirth Preparation section)

32. *Complete table related to analgesic and anesthetic methods:* see appropriate sections in Pharmacologic Management of Discomfort for each method cited in the table

33. Systemic analgesics affect on fetus (see Systemic Analgesics section of Pharmacologic Management of Discomfort)
    A. *Factors influencing effect of systemic analgesics on fetus:* maternal dosage, characteristics of the specific drug, route, time when administered during labor
    B. *Fetal/newborn effects:* CNS depression as a result of the direct effect of the drug when it crosses the placenta and/or the indirect effect of maternal hypotension and hypoventilation resulting from the drug's action on maternal function; CNS depression slows the FHR and decreases variability and leads to respiratory depression and hypoxia; decreased alertness and delayed sucking

34. *Complete table related to medications used during labor:* see specific sections in

Pharmacologic Management of Discomfort for each medication cited in the table

35. *Intravenous administration of systemic analgesics as the preferred route* (see Administration of Medication section): onset of action is faster and more reliable and predictable when administered intravenously

36. T, 37. F, 38. T, 39. T, 40. T, 41. T, 42. T, 43. F, 44. T, 45. F, 46. T, 47. F, 48. T, 49. F, 50. F, 51. T

52. D is correct; maternal temperature must be monitored because an elevation can increase the FHR; woman can and should change her position while in the bath, using lateral and hand-and-knees when indicated; as long as amniotic fluid is clear or only slightly meconium tinged, a whirlpool can continue; there is no limit to the time she can spend in the water—she can stay as long as they wish.

53. B is correct; Narcan is an opioid antagonist; Stadol is an opioid agonist-antagonist analgesic; Sublimaze is an opioid agonist analgesic.

54. D is correct; onset of effect is within 30 to 60 seconds of IV injection; a 25-mg dose is appropriate for IV administration; this medication is a potent opioid agonist analgesic, therefore respiratory depression is a concern.

55. C is correct; as an opioid antagonistic it will reverse the effects of the opioid agonist analgesic administered for pain; maternal side effects include hypotension/ hypertension, tachycardia, nausea, and vomiting; Narcan is administered parenterally at a dose of 0.1 to 0.2 mg; it may be repeated in 2 to 3 minutes if needed for adequate reversal.

56. A is correct; position with a curved back separates the vertebrae and facilitates administration of the anesthetic; alternating lateral positions after administration will prevent supine hypotension; she should be encouraged to empty her bladder every 2 hours; because the dura is not punctured there is no leakage of cerebrospinal fluid that could cause a spinal headache.

Critical Thinking Exercises

1. *Explaining basis of childbirth pain to expectant fathers:* see Neurologic Origins of Pain section in Discomfort During Labor; describe why pain occurs and its very real basis; discuss how women experience the pain and factors that influence the experience; identify measures they can use to help their partners reduce and cope with the pain.

2. Nurse sensitivity to client's pain experience (see Expression of Pain section of Discomforts During Labor and Nonpharmacologic Management of Discomfort section)
   A. *Effects of and responses to pain in labor:*
      - Physiologic effects: alteration in vital signs and skin color, diaphoresis, nausea and vomiting, stress responses decreasing placental perfusion and uterine activity
      - Sensory responses: describes pain as prickling, stabbing, burning, itching, bursting, aching, heaving, pulling, throbbing, sharp, stinging, cramping
      - Emotional responses: tiring, exhausting, annoying, sickening, nauseating
      - Affective expressions: anxiety, writhing, crying, groaning, gesturing, muscular movements; keep in mind that expressions of pain vary according to a woman's cultural background

   B. *Measures to alter perception of pain:* consider the specific factors influencing each woman's response when determining measures to use

3. *Working with couple with unrealistic, inaccurate views regarding pain and pain relief during labor*
   - Inform couple regarding the basis of pain and its potentially adverse effects on the maternal-fetal unit and the progress of labor.
   - Discuss a variety of nonpharmacologic and pharmacologic measures that are safe and effective to use during labor and can have beneficial effects on the maternal-fetal unit and can enhance the progress of labor.
   - Emphasize that the mother and fetus will be thoroughly assessed before, during, and after use of any measure to ensure safety.

4. *Benefits of water therapy:*
   - Describe the beneficial effects of water therapy and how it can facilitate the labor process by promoting relaxation, decreasing the stress response, relieving discomfort and tension, and enhancing oxytocin release, shortening the duration of labor, thereby decreasing the possibility of cesarean birth; use research findings to substantiate these claims.
   - Describe the successful experiences of other agencies that have implemented water therapy; state how it has affected the number of births.
   - Use favorable reports of women who have used water therapy; consider how this could affect other women preparing for childbirth.
   - Prepare a cost-benefit analysis.

5. Occurrence of hypotension after administration of epidural block during labor (see Emergency Box—Maternal Hypotension with Decreased Placental Perfusion)

A. *What is being experienced by this woman:* maternal hypotension related to effect of epidural anesthesia/analgesia (block), which can cause a rapid vasodilation thereby decreasing placental perfusion; results in an alteration in fetal oxygen level, reflected in nonreassuring changes in FHR pattern

B. *Nursing diagnosis:* ineffective tissue perfusion to placenta related to maternal hypotension associated with epidural block anesthesia

C. *Immediate nursing actions:* turn on her side or put a wedge under her hip to displace the uterus and enhance cardiac output; maintain circulating volume by continuing or increasing rate of IV infusion; administer oxygen via mask; elevate legs from hip; assess effects of actions taken on maternal-fetal unit; notify primary health care provider for further instruction including the possible administration of a vasopressor such as ephedrine; document all assessment findings, actions taken, and client responses

6. Woman receiving an epidural block: (see Epidural Analgesia/Anesthesia [Block] section of Pharmacologic Management of Discomfort and Care Management section)

A. *Assessment prior to induction of block:* status of maternal-fetal unit, progress of labor in terms of phase, contraindications to use

B. *Preparation measures:* answer should reflect actions related to explanation of procedures used, informed consent, hydration, bladder condition

C. *Positions for induction:* lateral (modified Sims with back curved forward) or sitting with back curved forward to separate vertebrae; assist her with assuming and maintaining the position without movement during the induction

D. *Nursing management during the epidural block:* assess the response on the maternal-fetal unit and progress of labor; maintain hydration; assist with bladder emptying and positioning of legs safely; change position frequently from side to side and assist with activity according to the degree of strength and sensation in lower extremities; maintain site to prevent infection; consider postpartum recovery care measures

CHAPTER 20: FETAL ASSESSMENT DURING LABOR

Chapter Review Activities

1. I, 2. J, 3. H, 4. G, 5. K, 6. F, 7. C, 8. B, 9. D, 10. E, 11. A, 12. L

13. Reassuring, nonreassuring, compromise, hypoxemia, hypoxia

14. Auscultation, fetoscope, ultrasound device

15. Electronic fetal monitoring (EFM), ultrasound transducer, tocotransducer, spiral electrode, intrauterine pressure catheter (IUPC)

16. Oligohydramnios, variable deceleration, amnioinfusion, saline, lactated Ringers

17. Tocolytic, tocolysis, blood flow, placenta, uterine contractions

18. Factors that affect fetal oxygen supply and expected characteristics of FHR and uterine activity (see Fetal Response section)

A. *Factors that can reduce fetal oxygen supply:* reduction in blood flow through maternal vessels, reduction in oxygen content of maternal blood, alterations in fetal circulation, and reduction in placental perfusion

B. *Characteristics of reassuring FHR patterns:* baseline rate of 110 to 160 beats per minute, no periodic changes, moderate baseline variability, accelerations with fetal movement

   C. *Characteristics of normal uterine activity:* frequency every 2 to 5 minutes, duration less than 90 seconds, intensity less than 100 mm Hg, rest period of at least 30 seconds with an average IUP of 15 mm Hg or less

19. *Characteristics of nonreassuring FHR pattern:* see Fetal Compromise section of Basis for Fetal Monitoring; characteristics are fully identified in terms of changes in baseline rate, variability, and the occurrence of periodic and episodic changes

20. 20
21. 30 minutes, 15 minutes
22. 15 minutes, 5 minutes

23. Intermittent auscultation to assess fetal status during labor (see Intermittent Auscultation section and Box 20-3)
   A. *State advantages and disadvantages:*
     • Advantages: high touch/low tech approach, natural method facilitating activity, comfortable, noninvasive
     • Disadvantages: inconvenient and time consuming, increased anxiety if nurse has difficulty locating PMI, less information about FHR pattern is obtained, less accurate
   B. *Guidelines to follow:* cite the six specific guidelines that should be used

24. *Legal responsibilities related to fetal monitoring during childbirth:* see Legal Tip—Fetal Monitoring Standards in Plan of Care and Interventions section; evaluate FHR pattern at frequency that reflects professional standards, agency policy, and condition of maternal-fetal unit; consider the correct interpretation of FHR pattern as reassuring or nonreassuring; take appropriate action; evaluate response to actions taken; notify primary health care provider in a timely fashion; know the chain of command if a dispute about interpretation occurs; document assessment findings, actions, and responses

25. T, 26. F, 27. T, 28. F, 29. T, 30. T, 31. T, 32. F, 33. F, 34. T, 35. F, 36. T, 37. F, 38. T, 39. T

40. *Nonreassuring pattern noted upon evaluation of a monitor tracing:* see Box 20-3 and Tables for each individual nonreassuring pattern to determine appropriate actions which most often involve repositioning the mother, administering oxygen, altering rate of IV, discontinuing Pitocin, assessing for possible causes, notify primary health care provider, prepare for emergency treatment such as operative vaginal birth, cesarean birth, amnioinfusion, tocolysis

41. *Nursing care measures for woman being monitored externally:* see Boxes 20-3 and 20-4 for a detailed outline related to teaching and explanations, assessing tracings and maternal responses, and caring for woman in terms of comfort, changing position, and transducer placement and site care

42. D is correct; the resting pressure should be 15 mm Hg or less; A, B, and C are all findings within the expected ranges.

43. B is correct; Leopold maneuvers are used to locate the PMI for correct placement of the ultrasound transducer; the tocotransducer is always placed over the fundus; reposition the ultrasound transducer every 2 hours and the tocotransducer every hour; it is not the nurse's role to apply a spiral electrode.

44. A is correct; the baseline rate should be 110 to 160 beats per minute; accelerations should occur with fetal movement; no late deceleration pattern of any magnitude is reassuring especially if it is repetitive or uncorrectable.

45. C is correct; the FHR increases as the maternal core body temperature elevates; therefore, tachycardia would be the pattern exhibited; it is often a clue of intrauterine infection because maternal fever is often the first sign.

46. B is correct; the pattern described is an early deceleration pattern which is considered to be benign, requiring no action other than documentation of the finding; changing a woman's position and notifying the physician would be appropriate if nonreassuring signs such as late or variable decelerations were occurring; prolapse of cord is associated with variable decelerations as a result of cord compression.

Critical Thinking Exercises

1. *Woman concerned about use of external monitoring to assess her fetus and labor:* see Box 20-4 for client/family teaching when electronic fetal monitoring is used
   - Discuss how fetus responds to labor and how the monitor will assess these responses.
   - Explain the advantages of monitoring.
   - Show her a monitor strip and explain what it reveals; tell her how to use the strip to help her with breathing techniques.

2. Woman whose labor is being induced and monitored externally (see Table 20-5 and Fig. 20-7)
   A. *Pattern described and causative factors:* late deceleration patterns as a result of uteroplacental insufficiency associated with intense uterine contractions, supine position (supine hypotension), and placental aging related to postterm gestation of 43 weeks
   B. *Nursing interventions:* discontinue Pitocin to stop stimulation of contractions but continue primary infusion; change to lateral position and elevate legs to enhance uteroplacental perfusion; administer oxygen via mask to increase oxygen availability to fetus; assess response to actions and notify primary health care provider regarding assessment findings, actions taken, and responses; document

3. Analyze monitor tracings:
   A. *Reassuring FHR pattern with normal uterine activity:* see Fetal Response section in Basis for Monitoring; compare the criteria of a reassuring FHR pattern and normal uterine activity with monitor tracing
   B. *Late deceleration pattern with minimal variability:* see Figs. 20-5 and 20-7, B and Tables 20-3 and 20-5
   C. *Bradycardia with minimal variability:* average FHR is 90 beats per minute; see Fig. 20-5 and Tables 20-2 and 20-3
   D. *Early deceleration:* recognize this as reassuring pattern; see Fig. 20-7, A and Table 20-4
   E. *Tachycardia:* average FHR is 210 beats per minute; see Table 20-2
   F. *Variable deceleration pattern:* see Fig. 20-7, C and Tables 20-5

Chapter 21: Nursing Care During Labor

Chapter Review Activities

1. F, 2. G, 3. J, 4. H, 5. B, 6. M, 7. A, 8. E, 9. K, 10. N, 11. D, 12. C, 13. I, 14. L, 15. TL, 16. FL, 17. FL, 18. TL, 19. TL, 20. FL, 21. TL, 22. FL, 23. TL, 24. TL, 25. TL

26. Regular uterine contractions, dilation, effacement, mucous plug

27. 0, 3, 6, 8, 4, 7, 3, 6, 20, 40, 8, 10

28. Infant is born, cervical dilation, effacement, baby's birth, sweat on upper lip,

vomiting, increased show, shaking of extremities, restlessness, involuntary bearing down efforts, latent, descent, transition, powers, analgesia/anesthesia, physical and emotional, position, activity, parity, pelvic size, presentation and position, support

29. Baby is born, placental is expelled, separation, firmly contracted fundus, discoid, globular or ovoid, gush of dark blood, lengthening of umbilical cord, vaginal fullness

30. Uterine contractions
31. Increment
32. Acme
33. Decrement
34. Frequency
35. Intensity
36. Duration
37. Resting tone
38. Interval
39. Bearing down effort

40. Characteristics of uterine contractions (see Fig. 21-9 and Assessment of Uterine Contraction section):
    A. *Label illustration:* A. beginning (onset of a contraction); B. duration; C. frequency; D. relaxation (interval between contractions); E. intensity; 1. increment; 2. acme; 3. decrement
    B. *Method of assessment:* place hand on fundus and determine changes in tone for several contractions and rest periods; press finger into fundus at acme (peak) of contraction to determine intensity

41. Admission of woman in labor (see Assessment and Nursing Diagnoses section of Care Management—First Stage of Labor)
    A. *Information from prenatal record:* see Prenatal Data subsection; include such information as age, weight gain, health status and medical problems during pregnancy, past and present obstetric history (gravida, para) including outcomes and problems encountered, laboratory and diagnostic test results, EDB, baseline data from pregnancy including vital signs and FHR
    B. *Information regarding status of labor:* factors distinguishing false from true labor, uterine contractions (onset, characteristics), show, status of membranes, fetal movement, discomfort (location, characteristics), any other signs of the onset of labor experienced
    C. *Information regarding current health status:* health problems, respiratory status, allergies, character and time of last oral intake, emotional status

42. F, 43. F, 44. T, 45. F, 46. T, 47. F, 48. T, 49. T, 50. T, 51. T, 52. F, 53. F, 54. F, 55. F, 56. T, 57. F, 58. F, 59. F, 60. T

61. *Complete table regarding labor stressors and support measures:* see Stress in Labor, Support of Father or Partner, Culture and Father Participation sections; Tables 21-1 and 21-7, Box 21-7, and Care Paths; answer should reflect physical and emotional stressors as well as the changing nature of stressors as labor progresses; support measures identified should reflect the changing nature of the stressors; a couple's Birth Plan often identifies the type of support measures they are most likely to respond to in a positive manner

62. *Signs of potential complications:* see Signs of Potential Complications Box—Labor for a full list of signs to consider throughout labor

63. *Complete table regarding labor positions and their advantages:* see Box 21-5 and Ambulation and Positioning section of Plan of Care and Interventions—First Stage of Labor

64. *Critical maternal-fetal factors to assess during labor*: see Care Paths for first and second/third stages of labor;
    - *Maternal factors*: vital signs, uterine activity, cervical changes, show/bleeding/amniotic fluid, behavior, appearance, mood, energy level, bearing down effort, use of childbirth preparation methods
    - *Fetal factors*: FHR pattern, activity level, progress in cardinal movements of labor, passage of meconium

65. *Laboratory and diagnostic tests during labor*: see Laboratory and Diagnostic Tests section of Assessment and Nursing Diagnosis—First Stage of Labor; CBC, blood type and Rh factor, analysis of urine, dipstick for protein, glucose, acetone, nitrazine and ferning tests for amniotic fluid; additional tests may be done depending on state laws and maternal condition such as HIV or drug screening, vaginal cultures

66. *Complete table for events/behaviors and support measures for second stage of labor*: see Second Stage of Labor section, Table 21-7, and Care Path to complete table

67. *Second stage positions*: see Preparing for Birth—Maternal Position section and Figs. 21-18, 21-19, 21-20; describe squatting, side-lying, semirecumbent, standing, hands-and-knees

68. A is correct; although B, C, and D are all important questions, the first question should gather information regarding whether or not the woman is in labor.

69. C is correct; pH of amniotic fluid is 6.5 or higher, ferning is noted when examining fluid with a microscope, and the fluid is relatively odorless; a strong odor is strongly suggestive of infection.

70. C is correct; O or occiput indicates a vertex presentation with the neck fully flexed and the occiput in the transverse section (T) of the woman's pelvis; the station is 2 cm below the ischial spines (+2); the woman is in the active phase of labor; the lie is longitudinal because the head (cephalic/vertex) is presenting.

71. B is correct; maternal BP, pulse, and respirations should be assessed every 30 minutes; temperature should be assessed every 2 hours once the membranes rupture; vaginal examinations are performed as indicated by labor events and not on a regular basis.

72. B is correct; research has indicated that enemas are not needed during labor; according to research findings A, C, and D have all been found to be beneficial and safe during pregnancy.

Critical Thinking Exercises

1. Woman thinking she is in labor calls nurse (see Teaching for Self-Care Box—How to Distinguish True Labor from False Labor and Box 21-1)
    A. *Nursing approach*: determine the status of her labor, asking her to describe what she is experiencing and comparing her description to the characteristics of true and false labor
    B. *Write questions*: questions should be clear, concise, open-ended, and directed toward distinguishing her labor status and determining the basis for action
    C. *Instructions for home care of woman in latent labor*: discuss comfort measures, distracting activities, measures to reduce anxiety, and measures to enhance the labor process; inform regarding assessment measures to determine progress and identify signs of problems, when and whom to call, and when to come to the hospital; nurse can make follow-up call to determine how the woman is progressing

2. Women in first stage of labor at various phases:
   A. *Identify phase of labor:* see Table 21-3 to determine phase; Denise (active); Teresa (transition); Danielle (latent)
   B. *Describe behavior and appearance:* see Tables 21-1 and 21-3 for descriptions; consider the phase of the woman's labor when formulating your answer
   C. *Specify physical care and emotional support required:* see Care Path—low risk woman in first stage of labor and Tables 21-1 and 21-5 for care measures required by each woman according to her phase of labor

3. *Procedure for locating PMI prior to auscultation of FHR or application of ultrasound transducer:* realize that presentation and position affect location of PMI (see Procedure Box—Leopold Maneuvers and Figs. 21-7 and 21-8) and that Leopold maneuvers will facilitate location of this point; the PMI will change as the fetus progresses through the birth canal

4. Woman experiencing difficulty with vaginal examinations during labor (see Vaginal Examination section of Physical Examination)
   A. *Nurse's response to concerns:* explain purpose of the examination and the information that will be obtained during each examination in terms of the progress of labor and the status of the fetus; compare findings obtained from a vaginal examination with information on the monitor tracing
   B. *Measures to enhance comfort and safety:* deep breathing and gentleness during the examination; limit frequency and explain why each examination is needed, what you are doing, and the results you are obtaining; acknowledge her feelings and ensure her privacy; use infection control measures such as

perineal care before, sterile gloves and lubricant to perform; never perform when active bleeding is present

5. *Actions and rationale when membranes rupture:* immediate assessment of the FHR and pattern (prolapse of the cord could have occurred, compressing the cord and leading to hypoxia, loss of variability and variable deceleration patterns); vaginal examination (status of cervix, check for cord prolapse); assess fluid, document findings and notify primary health care provider; strict infection control measures after rupture since risk for infection increases

6. *Nursing diagnosis:* anxiety related to lack of knowledge and experience regarding the process of childbirth
   Expected outcome: couple will cooperate with measures to enhance progress of labor as their anxiety level decreases
   Nursing measures: provide full, simple explanations about each aspect of labor and care measures required as they occur; demonstrate and assist with simple breathing and relaxation techniques; make use of phases of labor to tailor health teaching (doing more during latent phase and less as labor progresses); model coaching and comfort measures father can perform

7. Cultural and religious beliefs and practices during labor:
   A. *Questions to determine cultural and religious preferences:* see Callister (1995) topics for questions in Cultural Factors section of Assessment and Nursing Diagnoses—First Stage of Labor
   B. *Importance of determining cultural preferences:* see Cultural Considerations Box and Table 21-2; consider preferences so couple can act in ways that are comfortable to enhance the progress of labor and their view of

health care providers; such an approach demonstrates respect, concern, and caring

8. *Couple surprised by changes in approaches to facilitate the labor process:*
   - Discuss advantages of new approaches: internal locus of control (listening to her own body); maternal positions that enhance circulation to the placenta and apply the principle of gravity to facilitate and even shorten labor; new bearing down efforts are safer (better oxygenation for fetus) and more effective (less tiring while applying effective force to facilitate descent).
   - Use illustrations, model, and video to help couple learn techniques.
   - Demonstrate positions; help them to try.

9. Home birth (see Mechanism of Birth Vertex Presentation and Immediate Assessment and Care of Newborn sections and Box 21-8)
   A. *Measures to reassure and comfort:* use eye contact; assume a relaxed, calm, and confident manner; explain what is happening and what you are going to be doing to help her give birth; inform her and her husband about what they will need to do
   B. *Crowning* (guideline 6): break membranes, tell her to pant or blow to reduce force, use Ritgen's maneuver to control delivery of the head without trauma to fetus or to maternal soft tissues
   C. *Actions after appearance of head* (guideline 7): check for cord around neck, support head during external rotation and restitution, and ease shoulders out one at a time with anterior first then posterior
   D. *Prevention of neonatal heat loss* (guideline 11 and 12); dry baby, wrap up with mother, cover head
   E. *Infection control* (Box 21-3): use standard precautions during childbirth

adapting to the home setting; use handwashing, clean materials, wear gloves if available
   F. *Prevention of bleeding* (guideline 17): breastfeed, assess fundus and massage prn, expel clots if present once fundus is firm, assess bladder and encourage voiding, allow placenta to separate naturally
   G. *Documentation* (guideline 20, items a-i): include date, time, assessment of mother and newborn, family present, events, blood loss, Apgar

10. *Criteria of effective pushing:* see Bearing Down Efforts section of Second Stage of Labor—Plan of Care and Interventions and Care Path; cleansing breaths to begin and end each contraction; open glottis pushing with no breath holds longer than 5 to 7 seconds; frequent catch breaths; strong expiratory grunt; upright or lateral position

11. *Second stage of labor with reluctance to bear down and give birth* (see Bearing Down Efforts section of Second Stage of Labor—Plan of Care and Interventions)
    A. *Reasons for reluctance:* many are listed in the subsection and can include not feeling ready to become a mother, waiting for someone to come, embarrassment about pushing and what happens during bearing down effort including passage of feces, fear for self and baby, giving up, previous negative experience with birth
    B. *Nursing interventions:* recognize and acknowledge her feelings, identify her reason for not continuing, address her concerns and help her to continue

12. *Is an episiotomy needed?* see Perineal Trauma related to Childbirth section; compare episiotomies with spontaneous lacerations in terms of tissue affected, long-term sequelae, healing process, discomfort; compare reasons given for performing an

episiotomy with what research findings demonstrate to be true

13. *Siblings at childbirth:* include research findings regarding effect of sibling participation on family and on the sibling; consider the developmental readiness of the child and use developmental principles to prepare him or her for the experience; offer family and sibling classes to prepare them for participation in the birth process; evaluate parental comfort with this option; arrange for a support person to remain with the child during the entire childbirth process

14. Primipara exhibiting disinterest in newborn during the fourth stage of labor (see Family-Newborn Relationships section of Plan of Care and Interventions—third stage of labor)
   A. *Factors accounting for the behavior:* exhaustion, discomfort, cultural beliefs, disappointment, difficult labor and birth, taking in stage of recovery
   B. *Nursing measures:* continue to assess response to newborn, provide time for close contact with newborn when she is more comfortable and rested, help her to meet her needs during the taking in stage in terms of comfort, rest, and desire to review what happened during the process of labor and birth; document findings related to family interactions with newborn, actions taken, and responses of the family and newborn

CHAPTER 22: POSTPARTUM PHYSIOLOGY

Chapter Review Activities

1. T, 2. F, 3. F, 4. F, 5. T, 6. T, 7. T, 8. T, 9. F, 10. F, 11. F, 12. T, 13. F, 14. T, 15. T, 16. F, 17. F, 18. F, 19. T, 20. T

21. Assessing the bladder for distention (see Urinary System section)
   A. *Risk for bladder distention:* birth-induced trauma to urethra and bladder; edematous urethra; increased bladder capacity and diuresis; diminished sensation of bladder fullness related to use of spinal block (conduction anesthesia); pelvic soreness, lacerations, and episiotomy
   B. *Implications of bladder distention:*
      • Bladder pushes uterus up and to side, inhibiting uterine contraction, leads to excessive bleeding
      • Overdistention can lead to stasis of urine, increasing risk for UTI and impeding resumption of normal voiding

22. *Factors interfering with bowel elimination:* see Gastrointestinal section; decreased muscle tone, effect of progesterone on peristalsis, prelabor diarrhea, limited oral intake and dehydration from labor, anticipated discomfort related to hemorrhoids and perineal trauma leads to resisting urge to defecate

23. *Hypovolemic shock is less likely:* see Cardiovascular system section; pregnancy-induced hypervolemia allows most women to tolerate a considerable blood loss; size of maternal vascular bed decreases with expulsion of placenta, loss of stimulus for vasodilation, and extravascular water stores of pregnancy are mobilized back into vascular system for excretion

24. *Risk for thrombophlebitis:* see Blood Components section; increase in clotting factors and fibrinogen levels during pregnancy continues into the immediate postpartum period; hypercoagulable state combined with vessel damage during childbirth and decreased activity level of the postpartum period increase risk for thrombus formation

25. *Compare and contrast lochial and nonlochial bleeding*: see Table 22-1 for the information to complete your answer

26. D is correct; fundus should be at midline; deviation from midline could indicate a full bladder; full saturation of a pad in 1 hour or less would be a concern; edema and erythema are common shortly after repair of a wound; decreased abdominal muscle tone and enlarged uterus results in abdominal protrusion; separation of the abdominal muscle walls, diastasis rectus abdominis, is common during pregnancy and the postpartum period.

27. B is correct; the woman is describing the normal finding of postpartum diaphoresis, which is the body's attempt to excrete fluid retained during pregnancy; documentation is important but not the first nursing action; infection assessment and physician notification are not needed at this time.

28. D is correct; afterpains are most likely to occur in the following circumstances: multiparity, overdistention of the uterus (macrosomia, multifetal pregnancy), breastfeeding (endogenous oxytocin secretion), and administration of an oxytocic.

Critical Thinking Exercises

1. Postpartum women express questions and concerns:
   A. *Afterpains*: breastfeeding with newborn sucking causes posterior pituitary to secrete oxytocin stimulating the let-down reflex; uterine contraction is also stimulated leading to afterpains, which will occur for the first few days postpartum
   B. *Length of time fundus can be palpated*: within 2 weeks the uterus will be in the true pelvis; she will not be able to palpate it
   C. *Stages and duration of lochia*: see Lochia section; discuss characteristics of rubra, serosa, and alba lochia in terms of color, consistency, amount, odor, and duration
   D. *Protruding abdomen*: see Abdomen section; enlarged uterus along with stretched abdominal muscles with diminished tone create a still-pregnant appearance for the first few weeks after birth; by six weeks the abdominal wall will return to approximately its prepregnant state: skin will regain most of its elasticity and striae will fade but remain; discuss exercise and a sensible weight-loss program to facilitate the return of tone and diminish protrusion
   E. *Diaphoresis and diuresis*: see Urinary System section; discuss normalcy of these processes designed to rid the body of fluid retained during pregnancy
   F. *Breastfeeding as a reliable contraceptive method*: see Pituitary Hormones and Ovarian Function section; emphasize that breastfeeding is not a reliable method because return of ovulation is unpredictable partly related to breastfeeding patterns and may precede menstruation; discuss appropriate contraceptive methods for a breastfeeding woman, taking care to avoid hormonal based methods until lactation is well established
   G. *Lactation suppression in bottle-feeding woman*: see Breast section; milk production begins when estrogen and progesterone levels fall with expulsion of the placenta; by second or third day engorgement occurs related to congestion of veins and lymphatics and formation of some milk; prolactin levels fall because if milk is not removed the cycle will shut down and the milk will be absorbed into the circulatory system; she will need to support her breasts with a snug bra/binder and avoid warmth on her breasts and expressing any of the milk; ice pack application and mild analgesics can be used for discomfort

H. *Sexuality during the postpartum period of breastfeeding women:* see Reproductive System and Associated Structures section; discuss role of prolactin in suppressing estrogen secretion thereby inhibiting vaginal lubrication and resulting in vaginal dryness and dyspareunia that will persist until ovulation resumes; use of water-soluble lubricant or the spermicide used with a condom for birth control can reduce discomfort; trauma to soft tissues increases discomfort until healing is complete

Chapter 23: Nursing Care of the Postpartum Woman

Chapter Review Activities

1. Fourth stage of labor
2. Couplet care, mother-baby, single room maternity
3. Early postpartum discharge, shortened hospital stay, 1-day maternity stay
4. Oxytocic
5. Uterine atony, excessive bleeding/hemorrhage
6. Sitz bath
7. Afterpains (after-birth pains)
8. Splanchnic engorgement, orthostatic hypotension
9. Homans sign
10. Kegel
11. Engorgement
12. Rubella
13. RhoGAM (Rh Immune Globulin), Kleihauer-Betke

14. *Reasons for breastfeeding in fourth stage of labor:* takes advantage of the infant's alert state during the first period of reactivity and readiness to nurse, aids in contraction of the uterus to prevent hemorrhage, good opportunity to instruct mother and assess breasts, facilitates the bonding/attachment process because infant is ready to feed and success is likely, stimulates infant peristalsis facilitating excretion of bilirubin in the meconium; reduces the risk for hypoglycemia and hyperbilirubinemia; offers immunologic benefits

15. *Measures to assist with voiding:* see Prevention of Bladder Distention section in Plan of Care and Interventions; help her to assume an upright position on bedpan or in bathroom, listen to running water, put hands in warm water, pour water over vulva with peri bottle, stand in a shower, or sit in a sitz bath, provide analgesics

16. *Measures to prevent thrombophlebitis:* see Ambulation section of Plan of Care and Interventions; exercise legs with active ROM of knees, ankles, feet, and toes, ambulate, wear support hose (if varicosities are present), keep well hydrated

17. *Postanesthesia recovery:* see Postanesthesia Recovery section of Assessment and Nursing Diagnoses—Fourth Stage of Labor
    A. *Components of PAR score:* activity, respirations, blood pressure, level of consciousness, color
    B. *Criteria to determine recovery from anesthesia:*
       General Anesthesia: LOC/alertness, orientation, vital signs, oxygen saturation of at least 95%, deep breaths, color, keep her on her side until fully oriented and gag reflex returns to prevent aspiration
       Epidural or spinal anesthesia: return of movement and sensation in lower extremities, decrease in numbness, tingling/prickly sensation in legs, ability to feel bladder and to void

18. *Measures for bottle-feeding mother to suppress lactation and relieve discomfort of engorgement:* see Breastfeeding Promotion and Lactation Suppression section of Plan

of Care and Interventions; wear supportive bra or a breast binder 24 hours a day for at least the first 72 hours postpartum, avoid stimulating breasts (no warm water during shower, no infant sucking, no pumping or removal of milk), apply ice packs intermittently to relieve soreness and use fresh cabbage leaves

19. *Two interventions to prevent postpartum hemorrhage in early postpartum period:* see Prevention of Excessive Bleeding section
    - Maintain uterine tone: massage fundus if boggy, expel clots when fundus is firm, administer oxytocic medications, breastfeed or stimulate nipples.
    - Prevent bladder distention.

20. T, 21. F, 22. T, 23. T, 24. F, 25. F, 26. T, 27. F, 28. F, 29. T, 30. F, 31. T, 32. T, 33. F

34. Performing a postpartum assessment (see Box 23-1)
    A. *Position for fundal palpation:* supine, head and shoulder flat, arms at sides, knees slightly flexed
    B. *Fundal characteristics to assess:* consistency (firm or boggy), height (cm/fingerbreadths above, at, below umbilicus), location (midline or deviated to the right or left)
    C. *Position for assessment of perineum:* lateral or modified Sims position flexing upper leg on hip
    D. *Episiotomy characteristics to assess:* REEDA (redness, edema, ecchymosis, drainage, approximation), presence of hematoma or hemorrhoids, adequacy of hygiene including cleanliness, presence of odor, method used to cleanse perineum and apply topical preparations
    E. *Characteristics of lochia to assess:* stage, amount, odor, clots

35. *Recovery room nurse report:* see Table 23-1 for outline of essential information that should be reported regarding the woman, the baby, and the significant events and findings from her prenatal and childbirth periods

36. Infection control measures (see Prevention of Infection section of Plan of Care and Interventions and Box 23-3)
    A. *Measures to prevent transmission of infection from person to person:* clean environment, handwashing, use of standard precautions, proper care and use of equipment
    B. *Infection prevention measures to teach the woman:* avoid walking barefoot, handwashing, hygiene measures (general, breast, perineal), proper breastfeeding techniques, prevention of bladder infection, measures to enhance resistance to infection including nutrition, rest, and stress reduction

37. *Signs of postpartum complications during postpartum period:* see Signs of Potential Complications Boxes—Physiologic Problems and Psychosocial Needs

38. D is correct; these tremors are not related to infection; theories include sudden release of pressure on pelvic nerves after birth, response from a fetus to maternal transfusion at placental separation, or reaction to increased maternal adrenaline production or epidural anesthesia; they are self limiting, lasting only a short period of time.

39. C is correct; the woman should be assisted into a supine position with head and shoulders flat, arms at sides, and knees flexed.

40. A is correct; Methergine is an oxytocic that contracts the uterus thereby preventing excessive blood loss; lochia will therefore reflect expected characteristics.

41. B is correct; a direct and indirect Coombs must be negative, indicating that antibodies have not been formed and maternal sensitization has not occurred, before RhoGAM can be given; it must be given within 72 hours of birth; the newborn needs to be Rh positive; it is often given in the third trimester and then again after birth.

42. D is correct; this is a medical aseptic procedure therefore clean, not sterile, equipment is used, the water should be warm at 38° to 40.6° C; it is often used two to three times a day for 20 minutes each time.

Critical Thinking Exercises

1. *Pain relief for a postpartum breastfeeding mother:* see Comfort section of Plan of Care and Interventions; assess characteristics of pain (severity, location, relief measures already tried and effectiveness); use a combination of pharmacologic and nonpharmacologic measures as indicated by the nature of the pain being experienced; if breastfeeding, administer a systemic analgesic at time of or just after a feeding session; make sure she is not allergic to the medication and that the medication is not contraindicated for breastfeeding women

2. Woman exhibiting signs of hemorrhage and shock (see Prevention of Excessive Bleeding section of Plan of Care and Interventions and Emergency Box—Hypovolemic Shock)
   A. *Criteria to determine if flow is excessive and signs of shock are exhibited:* note length of time pad was worn and the degree to which it was saturated with blood; check the bed to determine if lochia has pooled under buttocks; pad saturation in less than 1 hour indicates a profuse flow; take note of other symptoms such as weakness, anxiety, lightheadedness, pallor, cool/clammy skin, increasing pulse and decreasing blood pressure; signs may be delayed related to hypervolemic state of pregnancy
   B. *Priority action:* assess fundus and massage if boggy; once firm, express clots, check bladder for distention and assist to empty, and administer oxytocics if ordered
   C. *Nurse's legal responsibility:* remain with woman and call for help; leaving her alone in an emergency could lead to a charge of abandonment
   D. *Additional interventions:* see list of measures identified in Emergency Box—Hypovolemic Shock

3. *Administering rubella vaccine to a postpartum woman:* see Health Promotion of Future Pregnancies and Children section; recheck titer results and order; determine if woman or any household members are immunocompromised; check allergies (duck eggs); inform her of side effects and emphasize that she must not become pregnant for at least 2 to 3 months after the immunization

4. *Administering RhoGAM to a postpartum woman:* see Health Promotion of Future Pregnancies and Children section and Medication Guide; check woman's and newborn's Rh status and Coombs test results; obtain RhoGAM and check all identification data; administer intramuscularly into deltoid or gluteal muscle; woman must be Rh and indirect Coombs negative; newborn must be Rh positive and direct Coombs negative

5. *Sexual changes after pregnancy and childbirth:* see Sexual Activity and Contraception section of Discharge Teaching and Teaching for Self-Care Box—Resumption of Sexual Intercourse; identify changes that may occur; discuss physical and emotional readiness of the woman; stress importance

of open communication; discuss how to prevent discomfort in terms of position and lubrication; emphasize the importance of birth control because return of ovulation cannot be predicted with accuracy

6. Postpartum women—nursing diagnoses, expected outcomes, and nursing management
   A. *Nursing diagnosis:* risk for infection of episiotomy related to ineffective perineal hygiene measures
      Expected outcome: Episiotomy will heal without infection
      Nursing management: see Prevention of Infection section of Plan of Care and Interventions and Box 23-3 for full identification of measures to enhance healing and prevent infection; teach woman how to assess perineum for progress of healing
   B. *Nursing diagnosis:* constipation related to inactivity and deficient knowledge regarding measures to enhance bowel elimination
      Expected outcome: woman will have soft formed bowel movement
      Nursing management: see Promotion of Normal Bladder and Bowel Patterns section; determine usual elimination patterns and measures used to enhance elimination; encourage activity, roughage, fluids; obtain order for mild combination stool softener-laxative
   C. *Nursing diagnosis:* acute pain related to episiotomy and hemorrhoids
      Expected outcome: woman will experience a reduction in pain following implementation of suggested relief measures
      Nursing management: see Promotion of Comfort section and Box 23-3; emphasize nonpharmacologic relief measures such as perineal care, sitz bath, topicals (e.g., Tucks), side-lying position, Kegel exercises, measures to enhance bowel and bladder

elimination; use pharmacologic measures if local measures are ineffective or pain is severe

7. Fundus above umbilicus and to the right of midline
   A. *Most likely basis for finding:* bladder distention; confirm by palpating the bladder and asking the woman to describe the last time she voided
   B. *Nursing action:* assist woman to empty bladder; measure amount voided and assess characteristics of the urine; palpate bladder and fundus again to determine response; catheterization may be required if she is unable to empty her bladder fully because a distended bladder can lead to uterine atony with excessive bleeding and UTIs

8. *Resumption of physical activity after giving birth:* see Postanesthesia Recovery section and Ambulation section of Plan of Care and Interventions
   - Assess postanesthesia recovery and physical stability especially with regard to return of sensation and strength in lower extremities.
   - Assist and supervise first few times out of bed because orthostatic hypotension can cause her to be dizzy and fall.
   - Show her where the call light is and what to do if she is alone and begins to feel dizzy or lightheaded.

9. *Resumption of full oral intake after giving birth:* see Fourth Stage of Labor section and Promotion of Nutrition section of Plan of Care and Interventions section; assess woman for physiologic stability (VS, fundus, lochia, perineum) before resuming full diet; determine type of anesthesia used for birth—if general anesthesia was used, make sure woman is fully alert and gag reflex has returned

10. Woman preparing for early discharge
    A. *Nurse's legal responsibility:* assess woman, newborn, and family to confirm that criteria for discharge are fully met; notify primary health care provider if criteria are not met; document all assessment findings, actions, and responses; recognize that current laws allow for a minimum hospital stay of 48 hours after vaginal birth
    B. *Criteria for discharge—maternal, newborn, general:* see Box 23-2
    C. *Outline essential content that must be taught prior to discharge:* see Discharge Teaching section; include information regarding self- and newborn care, signs of complications, prescribed medications; arrange for first postpartum check-up and for a follow-up telephone call or home visit usually within 1 to 2 days after discharge

11. Cultural beliefs and practices (see Plan of Care and Interventions—Psychosocial Needs section and Cultural Considerations Box)
    A. *Importance of using a culturally sensitive approach:* recognition of cultural beliefs and practices is essential to meet her individual needs; such an approach demonstrates respect, caring, and concern and enhances a woman's participation in and decision making regarding her own care; care must be taken not to stereotype
    B. *Korean-American woman—heat and cold balance:* ask woman the substances and practices that she identifies to be hot and cold, then intervene appropriately; provide her with warm substances to eat and drink
    C. *Muslim woman in postpartum period:* emphasize diet modification, gender issues, and modesty when planning care

CHAPTER 24: TRANSITION TO PARENTHOOD

Chapter Review Activities

1. *Complete table related to maternal adjustment:* see Table 24-4 and specific subsections for each phase in the Maternal Adjustment section.

2. *Complete table related to paternal adjustment:* see Table 24-5 and the Paternal Adjustment section.

3. Attachment of newborn to parents and parents to newborn (see Parental Attachment, Bonding, and Acquaintance section)
   A. *Define attachment and bonding:*
      • Attachment: parents come to love and accept child and child comes to love and accept parents
      • Bonding: sensitive period after birth when parents have close contact with their infant
   B. *Critical attributes of attachment:* discuss influence of proximity, reciprocity, and commitment
   C. *Conditions that facilitate attachment:* emotionally healthy parents, competent in communication and caregiving; parent and newborn fit in terms of state, temperament, and gender; parental proximity to infant; adequate social support system
   D. *Acquaintance process:* parents use eye contact, touch, talking, and exploring to get to know their newborn; claiming or identification in terms of likeness, differences, and uniqueness is part of this process
   E. *Assessment of process of attachment:* see Assessment of Attachment Behaviors section and Teaching for Self-Care Box—Assessment of Attachment Behavior for specific behaviors indicating the quality of the

attachment that is developing; it is critical that nurses provide opportunities for parent and infant contact and to be present during these contacts to observe the interaction that is taking place

4. *Parental tasks:* see Parental Tasks and Responsibilities subsection of Parental Role after Childbirth section for a full description of each of the required tasks

5. *Parent-infant contact:* see specific subsections for each form of contact in Parent-Infant Contact section
   - Early contact: important to provide time for parents to see, touch, and hold their newborn as soon as possible after birth; stress that attachment is an ongoing process; interference with this early contact because of maternal and/or newborn problems should not have a long-term effect as long at it is balanced by opportunities for close contact as soon as possible after birth as appropriate for maternal and/or newborn condition
   - Extended contact: family-centered care, mother-baby care, and use of LDRP/LDR rooms to facilitate this type of contact

6. *Components of the parenting process:* see Parenting Process section; parenting is a process of role attainment and transition that begins during pregnancy and ends when the parent is comfortable and confident in the parenting role; nurse should teach, demonstrate, provide time for practice and feedback, arrange for follow-up phone call, and refer to community agencies and parenting support groups
   - Skill/knowledge component: feeding, holding, clothing, bathing, protecting their newborn are skills that must be learned; parents need a desire to succeed and obtain support from others
   - Affective component: tenderness, awareness, concern for infant's needs and desires; affects manner in which child

care is performed and emotional response of child to the care

7. *Periods of parental role attainment during the fourth trimester:* see Parental Role after Childbirth section
   - Early period: parents need time to reorganize their lives to include their newborn; focus is on caregiving activities and meeting needs of infants for shelter, nourishment, protection, socialization; characterized by intense learning and need for nurturing
   - Consolidation period: drawing together and uniting of family unit, negotiation of roles, stabilization of tasks, and coming to terms with commitments; becoming more attuned to infant behaviors; competence is growing in performance of care activities

8. Transition, meanings, expectations, level of knowledge, environment, level of planning, emotional, physical well-being, subjective well-being, role mastery, well-being of interpersonal relationships

9. Attachment, bonding, proximity, reciprocity, commitment

10. Mutuality, crying, smiling, cooing, rooting, grasping, postural adjustments

11. Acquaintance, eye contact, touching, talking, exploring

12. En face, face to face, positioning mom and baby together after birth, dimming lights so baby can open eyes, delaying eye prophylaxis

13. Claiming, likeness, differences, uniqueness

14. Entrainment, waving arms, lifting head, kicking legs, dancing in tune

15. Biorhythmicity, loving care, alert, responsive, social interactions, learning

16. Reciprocity, synchrony

17. Rhythm, behavioral repertoires, responsivity

18. Rhythm, alert

19. Repertoire, gazing, vocalizing, facial expressions, looking, response, infantilize, facial expressions, communicate

20. Responsivity, smiling, cooing, eye contact, en face

21. Engrossment, touch, eye-to-eye contact

22. *Complete table regarding infant/parent facilitating and inhibiting behaviors:* see Table 24-1, which covers infant behaviors affecting parent attachment and Table 24-2, which covers parental behaviors affecting infant attachment to complete this table

23. *Factors influencing parental responses to the birth of their child:* see subsection for each factor in the Factors Influencing Parental Responses section

24. D is correct; A reflects the first phase of identifying likenesses; B reflects the second phase of identifying differences; C reflects a negative reaction of claiming the infant in terms of pain and discomfort; D reflects the third or final stage of identifying uniqueness.

25. B is correct; early close contact is recommended to initiate and enhance the attachment process.

26. A is correct; engrossment refers to a father's absorption, preoccupation, and interest in his infant; B represents the claiming process phase I identifying likeness; C represents reciprocity; D represents en face or face-to-face position with mutual gazing.

27. B is correct; taking in is the first 24 hours but may range from 1 to 2 days of recovery

following birth; other behaviors exhibited include reliance on others to help her meet needs, being excited and talkative, and focusing on self and meeting basic needs

28. C is correct; approximately 50% to 80% of women experience postpartum blues; new parents should be reassured that their skills as parents develop gradually and they should seek help to develop these skills; postpartum blues that are self limiting and short lived do not require psychotropic medications; support and care of the postpartum woman and her newborn by her partner and family is the most effective prevention and coping strategy; feelings of fatigue from childbirth and meeting demands of newborn can accentuate feelings of depression.

Critical Thinking Exercises

1. Teaching parents communication skills with their newborns (see Communication between Parent and Infant section)
   A. *Communication techniques:* discuss touch, eye contact, voice, and odor; demonstrate techniques, have parents try, and point out newborn response in terms of quieting, alerting, making eye contact, gazing; help parents interpret cues
   B. *Newborn's communication:* point out infant responses; discuss processes of entrainment, biorhythmicity, reciprocity, synchrony, and repertoire of behaviors

2. *Woman following emergency cesarean birth: disappointment with lack of immediate bonding time with newborn:*
   - Discuss concepts of early and extended contact.
   - Emphasize that the parent-infant attachment process is ongoing—her emotional bond with her baby will not be weaker.

- Help her to meet her own physical and emotional needs so that she develops readiness to met her newborn's need.
- Help her to get to know her baby, interact with and care for him; point out newborn characteristics including how the baby is responding to her efforts.
- Show her how to communicate with her newborn and how her newborn communicates with her.
- Arrange for follow-up after discharge to assess how attachment is progressing.

3. *Sibling adaptation to newborn:* see Sibling Adaptation section and Box 24-2, which identifies strategies parents can use to help their other children adapt; caution her that adjustment takes time and is strongly related to the developmental level and life experiences of the sibling(s)

4. Parents unsure and anxious about caring for their newborn (see Table 24-3)
   A. *Nursing diagnosis:* risk for impaired parent-infant attachment related to lack of knowledge and feeling of incompetence regarding infant care
   B. *Nursing measures to facilitate attachment:*
      - Perform newborn assessment with parents present, pointing out newborn characteristics and encouraging parents to participate and ask questions.
      - Demonstrate newborn care measures and provide time for parents to practice and obtain feedback.
      - Provide extended contact time with newborn until discharge; encourage parents to hold infant; show them how to interact with their newborn and point out how newborn responds.
      - Make referral for follow-up with telephone contacts and home visits; refer to parenting classes and support groups, lactation consultant and La Leche.

- Recommend books, magazines, and videos that discuss newborns and their care.
- Advocate for care management approaches that facilitate contact time with newborn and continuity of care (e.g., rooming-in, mother-baby or couplet care, LDR and LDRP rooms, extended visiting hours for members of maternal support group).

5. *Parental disappointment with newborn's gender and appearance:* see Parental Tasks and Responsibilities section; foster attachment and claiming; help parents to get acquainted with the infant and to reconcile the real child with the fantasy child; discuss the basis of molding, caput succedaneum, and forceps marks and how they will be resolved; be alert for problems with attachment and care so follow-up can be arranged

6. *Grandparent adjustment:* see Grandparent Adaptation section; observe interaction between grandparents and parents taking note of signs of effective interaction and conflict; involve grandparents in teaching sessions as appropriate for this family; spend time with grandparents to help them to be supportive without "taking over" or being critical; help the new parents to recognize the unique role grandparents can play as parenting role models, nurturers, and providers of respite care

7. *Woman experiencing postpartum blues:*
   - *Nursing diagnosis:* Ineffective maternal coping related to hormonal changes and increased responsibilities following birth
   - *Expected outcome:* Woman will report feeling more content with her role as mother following the use of recommended coping strategies
   - *Nursing management:* see Teaching for Self Care Box—Coping with Postpartum Blues; involve both Jane and her

husband in the teaching session and in the development of a plan for coping with the blues; this must occur early to prevent development of postpartum depression

Chapter 25: Physiologic and Behavioral Adaptations of the Newborn

Chapter Review Activities

1. K, 2. F, 3. B, 4. J, 5. D, 6. I, 7. H, 8. A, 9. E, 10. G, 11. C, 12. P, 13. N, 14. N, 15. P, 16. N, 17. P, 18. N, 19. N, 20. N, 21. N, 22. N, 23. N, 24. P, 25. N, 26. N, 27. N, 28. P, 29. N, 30. N, 31. N, 32. P, 33. N, 34. N

35. *Factors initiating breathing after birth*: reflex to breathe is triggered by such environmental factors as pressure changes, chilling, noise, light, and other sensations associated with birth; chemoreceptor activation of respiratory center by lowered oxygen level, higher carbon dioxide level, and lower pH

36. Thermoregulation, hypothermia, thermogenesis, brown fat, metabolic activity

37. Thermal insulation, blood vessels, body surface to body weight (mass) ratio, flexed

38. Cry, restless, muscular activity, respiratory rate

39. Convection, wrap, 24° C

40. Radiation, nursery cribs, examination tables, outside windows

41. Evaporation, dry, too slow drying

42. Conduction, warmed crib

43. *Two measures to prevent or limit physiologic hyperbilirubinemia*: see Physiologic Jaundice section

- Early feeding stimulates gastrocolic reflex, leading to passage of meconium, which contains bilirubin that would otherwise be absorbed into the circulatory system.
- Prevent cold stress because acidosis frees bilirubin.

44. Sleep-wake
45. Deep, light
46. Drowsy, quiet alert, active alert, crying, quiet alert

47. 17, increasing
48. Habituation, respond, inhibit responding
49. Orientation

50. *Factors influencing newborn's behavior*: see section for each factor listed in Behavioral Characteristics; each factor is described in terms of its influence on newborn behavior

51. *Complete table related to phases of newborn transition period to extrauterine life*: see Transition Period section at beginning of chapter for identification of each phase and description of timing/duration and typical newborn behaviors for each phase

52. T, 53. F, 54. F, 55. F, 56. T, 57. F, 58. T, 59. T, 60. F, 61. T, 62. F, 63. T, 64. T, 65. T, 66. F, 67. F, 68. F

69. D is correct; the newborn at 5 hours old is in the 2nd period of reactivity during which tachycardia, tachypnea, increased muscle tone, skin color changes, mucus production, and passage of meconium occur; although a newborn can have periods of apnea they should not exceed 15 seconds; the average heart rate of a newborn when awake is 120 to 160 beats per minute.

70. A is correct; the rash described is erythema toxicum; it is an inflammatory response that has no clinical significance and requires no treatment because it will disappear spontaneously.

71. B is correct; physiologic jaundice does not appear until 24 hours after birth; further investigation would be needed if it appears during the first 24 hours because this is consistent with pathologic jaundice; A, C, and D are findings within the normal range for a newborn 12 hours old.

72. D is correct; B and C are common newborn reflexes used to assess integrity of neuromuscular system; measurement of legs is not a method for assessing hip dysplasia.

73. C is correct; telangiectatic nevi are also known as stork bites or angel kisses and can also appear on the upper eyelids and lip; milia are plugged sebaceous glands and appear like white pimples; nevus vasculosus or a strawberry mark is a raised, sharply demarcated, bright or dark red swelling; nevus flammeus is a port wine, flat red to purple lesion that does not blanch with pressure.

Critical Thinking Exercises

1. Newborn—risk for cold stress (see Thermogenic System section and Fig. 25-4)
   A. *Dangers of cold stress:* metabolic and physiologic demands are placed on the newborn → increased oxygen need and consumption → oxygen and energy are diverted from brain cell and cardiac function and growth → decreased oxygen leads to vasoconstriction, respiratory distress, and reopening of the ductus arteriosus → acidosis occurs increasing the level of bilirubin → risk for kernicterus increases
   B. *Nursing diagnosis:* risk for imbalanced body temperature—hypothermia related to immature thermoregulation associated with newborn status; *expected outcome:* newborn's temperature will stabilize between 36.5° and 37.2° C within 8 to 10 hours of birth
   C. *Measures to stabilize newborn temperature and prevent cold stress:* see Thermogenic

System section; implement measures that reflect application of heat loss mechanisms of convection, radiation, evaporation and conduction:
   - Dry infant and cover with warmed blankets or wrap with mother.
   - Cover head and feet; double wrap.
   - Use radiant warmer to stabilize temperature, assess newborn, and perform procedures.
   - Adjust environment in terms of temperature and drafts (nursery and mother's room).
   - Place bassinet away from drafts and outside windows.
   - Maintain adequate nutrition (caloric intake).

2. *Parental concern regarding head variations:* see Caput Succedaneum and Signs of Risk for Integumentary Problems sections; discuss each finding in terms of cause, significance for the newborn's health status and adjustment, and how/when it will be resolved; refer to Figs. 25-5 and 25-9 to facilitate parental understanding

3. *Parental concern about weight loss:* see Renal System section; determine percentage of weight loss making sure it does not exceed 10%; explain that their newborn's weight loss of 6% is within the expected range for weight loss during the first 3 to 5 days after birth; discuss the cause of the loss and feeding measures, and inform them that the birth weight should be regained within 2 weeks

4. Parental interest in newborn's sensory capabilities (see Behavioral Characteristics section)
   A. *What nurse should tell parents:* discuss and demonstrate newborn's capability regarding vision, hearing, touch, taste, and smell
   B. *Stimuli parents can provide to facilitate newborn development:* face to face/eye to eye contact, objects (bright or have

Answer Key   459

black and white patterns), sound (talking to infant, music, heart beat simulator), touch (infant massage, cuddling)

5. *Parental concern regarding "bruises" on newborn's back and buttocks:* discuss the characteristics and cause of Mongolian spots (see Integumentary System section and Fig. 25-6)

CHAPTER 26: NURSING CARE OF THE NEWBORN

Chapter Review Activities

1. Tetracycline, erythromycin, gonorrhea, chlamydia, 1 to 2 cm, lower conjunctiva, 1 to 2 hours

2. Vitamin K, 0.5 to 1 mg, 25, 5/8
3. 2, 12, neuromuscular, physical
4. Preterm, premature
5. Term
6. Postterm, postdate
7. Postmature
8. Large for gestational age (LGA)
9. Appropriate for gestational age (AGA)
10. Small for gestational age (SGA)
11. Intrauterine growth restriction (IUGR)

12. Low birth weight (LBW), less than expected rate of intrauterine growth, shortened gestational period, preterm birth, LBW, very low birth weight (VLBW)

13. F, 14. T, 15. F, 16. F, 17. F, 18. F, 19. T, 20. T, 21. T, 22. F, 23. T, 24. T, 25. T, 26. F, 27. T, 28. F, 29. F, 30. F, 31. T, 32. F, 33. F

34. *Creation of a protective environment in terms of infection control and safety:* see Protective Environment section of Plan of Care and Interventions
    - *Environment:* adequate lighting, ventilation, warmth, and humidity;

elimination of fire hazards; ensure safety of electrical equipment
    - *Infection control:* use Standard Precautions with an emphasis on handwashing, provide adequate spacing of bassinets (60 cm), separate areas for cleaning and storing equipment and supplies, keep persons with infections away or use appropriate precautions
    - *Safety:* security precautions, identification measures, instruction for parents

35. *Complete table related to hypoglycemia and hypocalcemia:* see Physiologic Problems section of Assessment of Common Problems in the Newborn for a full description of each electrolyte imbalance in terms of signs, risk factors, and management

36. *Guidelines for weighing and measuring newborn:* (see Table 26-2 and Baseline Measurements of Physical Growth section); wear gloves if performed before first bath
    Weight: balance scale, cover scale with clean scale paper, place undressed infant on scale, keep hand hovering over infant, never turn away
    Head circumference: measure the widest part of head just above ears and eyebrow; repeat if molding is present at birth
    Chest circumference: measure across nipple line
    Abdominal circumference: measure at level of umbilicus
    Length: measure from crown to rump, then rump to heels

37. Maintaining a patent airway and supporting respirations
    A. *Four conditions essential for maintaining an adequate oxygen supply:* removal of lung fluid, synchronous expansion of chest and abdomen, patent airway, and sufficient surfactant

B. *Signs of respiratory distress:* see Signs of Potential Complications Box—Abnormal Newborn Breathing; signs include nasal flaring, retractions and increased use of intercostal muscles, chin tug, grunting with expiration, seesaw respirations, rate of ≤25 or ≥60 breaths per minute at rest, apnea periods lasting longer than 15 seconds, adventitious breath sounds; note that some of these signs may normally be present during the first period of reactivity following birth

C. *Three methods of relieving airway obstruction:* see Emergency Box—Relieving Airway Obstruction found in Chapter 28; methods include back blows, turning infant, chest thrusts; also suctioning can be used to relieve obstruction caused by excessive mucus

38. D is correct; thinning of lanugo with bald spots is consistent with full-term status; pulse and weight are not part of the Ballard scale; the popliteal angle for a full-term newborn would be 90 degrees or less.

39. D is correct; the hemoglobin should be 14 to 24 g/dl; hematocrit should be 44% to 64%; glucose should be 40 to 60 mg/dl; total bilirubin should not be higher than 6 to 8 mg/dl at 1 day of age.

40. B is correct; signs of hypoglycemia include cyanosis along with apnea, jitteriness/twitching, irregular respirations, high-pitched cry, difficulty feeding, hunger, lethargy, eye rolling, and seizures; C and D are consistent with hypocalcemia.

41. A is correct; the control panel should be set between 36° to 37° C; the probe should be placed in the right upper quadrant of the abdomen below the intercostal margin—never over a rib; axillary not rectal temperatures should be taken every hour.

42. B is correct; the infant formula should be withheld for up to 4 hours to prevent vomiting and aspiration but a breastfed infant may nurse right up until the procedure is done; the site should be checked every hour for 12 hours; only warm water should be used to cleanse the site; diaper wipes should not be used on the site because they contain alcohol, which would delay healing and cause discomfort; the yellow exudate is a protective film that forms in 24 hours and it should not be removed.

Critical Thinking Exercises

1. *Apgar scoring:*
   - **Baby boy:** heart rate: 160 (2); respiratory effort: good, crying (2); muscle tone: flexion, active movement (2); reflex irritability: cry with stimulus (2); color: acrocyanosis (1); score is 9; interpretation: score of 7 to 10 indicates that the infant will have no difficulty adjusting to extrauterine life
   - **Baby girl:** heart rate: 102 (2); respiratory effort: slow, irregular, weak cry (1); muscle tone: some flexion (1); reflex irritability: grimace with stimulus (1); color: pale (0); score is 5; interpretation: score of 4 to 6 indicates moderate difficulty adjusting to extrauterine life

2. Assessment of newborn girl
   A. *Protocol for assessment during first two hours:* see Table 26-1 (Apgar score) and Box 26-1 (Initial Physical Assessment by Body System), and Initial Assessment and Nursing Diagnoses section to prepare your outline
   B. *Nurse's responsibility for newborn identification at birth:* see Identification section of Immediate Interventions; complete the identification process before mother and newborn are separated; attach matching ID bands (name, gender, date and time of birth, identification number) to both

immediately after birth; take newborn's footprint and mother's fingerprint(s) and place on appropriate form

C. *Priority nursing diagnoses for immediate postbirth period:* consider nursing diagnoses related to breathing (ineffective airway clearance, impaired gas exchange, ineffective breathing pattern), thermoregulation (risk for hypothermia)

D. *Priority nursing care measures:* discuss each of these areas
- Stabilization of respiration and airway patency
- Maintenance of body temperature
- Immediate interventions in terms of identification, prophylactic medications, promotion of bonding/attachment
- Fulfill routine admission orders (Box 26-2)

3. Performing a physical examination of newborn before discharge (see Physical Assessment section):
A. *Actions to ensure safety and accuracy:* well-lighted, warm, and draft free environment; undress as needed; place on firm surface with constant supervision; progress in a systematic manner form cleanest to dirtiest area (head to toe)
B. *Major areas assessed:* see Table 26-2; areas to include general appearance and behavior; vital signs and weight; integument; head and neck; abdomen and back; genitalia and anus; elimination patterns; extremities; neurologic system including reflexes
C. *Rationale for presence of parents:* chance to observe parent-infant interactions and to identify and meet learning needs; foster active involvement in assessment and care of their newborn; encourage discussion of concerns and asking of questions; chance to explain

and demonstrate newborn characteristics and capabilities

4. Newborn with mucus in airway (see Stabilization and Resuscitation section)
A. *Nursing diagnosis:* impaired gas exchange related to upper airway obstruction with mucus
B. *Steps using bulb syringe* (see Procedure Box—Suctioning with a Bulb Syringe and Fig. 26-2): suction mouth first then nose; compress prior to insertion; insert tip along side of mouth not over tongue, which could stimulate the gag reflex and sucking; release compression slowly; suction nostrils one at a time; continue till breathing sounds clear; teach parents how to use bulb syringe
C. *Guidelines for use of mechanical suction* (see Procedure Box—Suctioning with a Nasopharyngeal Catheter with Mechanical Suction Apparatus): suction for 5 seconds or less per insertion; use <80 mm Hg setting; lubricate catheter with sterile water; insert along base of tongue and up and back into nares; repeat until breathing sounds clear

5. Care of circumcision:
A. *Nursing diagnosis:* risk for infection related to removal of foreskin
B. *Expected outcome:* circumcision site will heal without infection
C. *Teaching about care:* see Teaching for Self-Care Box—Circumcision; emphasize importance of assessing site for infection and progress of healing; discuss measures to keep area clean and dry and to enhance comfort; teach parents how to assess circumcision site for bleeding and what to do if it occurs and emphasize importance of assessing urination and

what to do if the newborn has difficulty voiding

6. Newborn with hyperbilirubinemia (see Physiologic Jaundice and Therapy for Hyperbilirubinemia sections, and Teaching for Self-Care Box—Hyperbilirubinemia)

   A. *Responding to parental concerns:* tell parents in simple terms that their newborn is exhibiting physiologic jaundice, explaining why it occurs, what impact it will have on their newborn's health, and how it will be resolved; emphasize that their newborn's form of jaundice is a common and naturally occurring physiologic process as the newborn adjusts to extrauterine life

   B. *Blanch test:* apply pressure with finger over a bony area (nose, forehead, sternum) for several seconds to empty capillaries at the spot; if jaundice is present the blanched area will appear yellow before the capillaries fill

   C. *Expected findings of physiologic hyperbilirubinemia:* jaundice (cephalocaudal, proximodistal progression), watery greenish stools, sleepiness, alteration in bilirubin levels that follows a specific pattern and degree of elevation (see Chapter 25)

   D. *Precautions and care measures during phototherapy:* Increase fluids and feed at least every 3 hours; cover eyes (removing periodically to assess condition and allow for interaction with parents); monitor temperature for increases or decreases; cleanse stools promptly; do not put lotions on skin; place undressed under lights and change position periodically to expose as much skin to the lights as possible; remove from under lights for feeding, cuddling, and interaction with parents

7. Newborn scheduled for circumcision—pain concerns (see Pain in Neonates section, Table 26-3, and Fig. 26-17)

   A. *Common behavioral responses to pain:* body movements (withdrawal of upper and lower limbs), vocalization (cry that is high-pitched and shrill), cry face and other facial expressions, fussy, irritable, listless

   B. *Changes in vital signs and integument:* increase or decrease in heart rate and blood pressure, rapid, shallow respirations; pale, flushed, moist integument

   C. *CRIES Tool* (see Table 26-3)

   D. *Nursing diagnosis:* acute pain related to effects of circumcision

   E. *Nonpharmacologic and pharmacologic relief measures:*
   - *Nonpharmacologic:* swaddle afterwards, nonnutritive sucking, take to mother to be fed and comforted, distract (older infant), apply Vaseline/ointment to site; change diaper frequently; position on side or back
   - *Pharmacologic:* local anesthesia, topical preparations

CHAPTER 27: NEWBORN NUTRITION AND FEEDING

Chapter Review Activities

1. Daily fluid and calorie requirements during infancy

   A. *Fill in the blanks:* 110, 100, 95, 100, 67, 20, 110 to 140

   B. *Calculation of daily energy requirements*
   - **Jim** (1 month—110 kcal/kg/day): 110 kcal × 4 kg = 440 kcal/day
   - **Sue** (4 months—100 kcal/kg/day): 100 kcal × 6 kg = 600 kcal/day
   - **Sam** (7 months—95 kcal/kg/day): 95 kcal × 7.5 kg = 712.5 kcal/day

- **Jean** (10 months—100 kcal/kg/day): 100 kcal × 10.5 kg = 1,050 kcal/day

2. Lactation structures:
   A. *Label:* A. alveolus; B. ductule; C. duct; D. lactiferous duct; E. lactiferous sinus; F. nipple pore; G. ampulla; H. areola
   B. *Fill in the blanks:*
      1. Lobes (milk glands)
      2. Alveoli
      3. Ductule
      4. Lactiferous duct
      5. Lactiferous sinuses, ampullae
      6. Myoepithelial
      7. Areola

3. *Teaching group of women about breastfeeding:* see Benefits of Breastfeeding section; emphasize the importance and benefits of breastfeeding for infants, mothers, and family/society

4. *Four breastfeeding positions:* see Positioning section of Plan of Care and Interventions and Fig. 27-4; describe the positions of football hold, cradle (traditional), modified cradle (cross over or across the lap), and side-lying

5. Feeding readiness cues (see Feeding Readiness section)
   A. *Cues:* hand-to-mouth or hand-to-hand movements, sucking motions, strong rooting reflex, mouthing
   B. *Rationale for feeding according to these cues:* if cues are missed, baby may cry vigorously, become distraught, or withdraw into sleep; these behaviors will make feeding more difficult or impossible; feeding when the infant exhibits readiness enhances the chance of success

6. *Differences between foremilk and hindmilk:* see Uniqueness of Human Milk section;
   - *Foremilk:* bluish-white, part skim and part whole milk providing primarily lactose, protein, water-soluble vitamins

- *Hindmilk:* cream is "let down" into the feeding; denser in calories from fat to ensure optimal growth and contentment between feedings

7. *Label illustrations of lactation reflexes:*
   - *Milk production reflex:* A. sucking stimulus; B. hypothalamus; C. anterior pituitary gland (prolactin); D. milk production
   - *Let-down reflex:* A. sucking stimulus; B. hypothalamus; C. posterior pituitary gland (oxytocin); D. let-down reflex

8. *Stages of lactogenesis:* see Uniqueness of Human Milk section
   - *Stage I:* begins in pregnancy when breasts are prepared for milk production and colostrum is formed in the breasts
   - *Stage II:* colostrum changes to mature milk; "milk coming in" on the 3rd to 5th day after birth; onset of copious milk production
   - *Stage III:* milk changes over about 10 days when the mature milk is established

9. Proper latch-on (see Latching On section of Plan of Care and Interventions)
   A. *Steps to ensure proper latch-on:* apply colostrum/milk to areola/nipple (lubricate and entice), support the breast (Fig. 27-5), hold baby close and tickle baby's lower lip with the breast to stimulate the rooting reflex and extrusion of tongue; pull baby onto nipple and areola
   B. *Signs of proper latch-on:* see Fig. 27-6; firm, tugging sensation on the nipple but no pinching or pain; baby's cheeks are rounded and jaw glides smoothly with sucking; swallow is audible
   C. *Removal of baby from breast:* see Fig. 27-7; break suction by inserting finger inside of baby's mouth between gums and leaving the finger in until nipple is completely out of the baby's mouth

10. *Calming a fussy baby:* see Special Considerations section and Box 27-4; mother can try holding close perhaps with skin-to-skin contact, swaddling, gently moving and talking soothingly; reducing environmental stimuli; allowing baby to suck on mother's finger

11. *Complete table related to assessment of infant and mother regarding breastfeeding;* see Infant and Mother Assessment and Nursing Diagnoses section and Box 27-2 for information to complete the table

12. Mastitis
13. Massage
14. Lactogenesis, lactation
15. Confusion
16. Lactation consultant
17. Engorgement
18. Feeding readiness cues
19. Weaning
20. Everted, inverted, shell, nipple erection
21. Colostrum
22. Prolactin, oxytocin
23. Crying, shut down
24. Growth spurt
25. Monilia (yeast infection)
26. Football, cradle (traditional)
27. Let-down, milk ejection
28. Rooting, extrusion
29. Latch-on

30. F, 31. F, 32. T, 33. T, 34. F, 35. T, 36. F, 37. F, 38. T, 39. T, 40. F, 41. T, 42. F, 43. T, 44. T, 45. T, 46. F, 47. F

48. B is correct; birth weight is regained in 10 to 14 days; 6 to 8 wet diapers are expected at this time; should be fed every 2 to 3 hours for a total of 8 to 12 times per day.

49. A is correct; swaddling is recommended; removing some clothing might help waken a sleepy baby; B, C, and D are all appropriate actions to calm a fussy baby.

50. D is correct; no soap should be used because it could dry the areola and nipple and increase the risk for irritation; vitamin E should not be used because it is a fat-soluble vitamin that the infant could ingest when breastfeeding; lanolin or colostrum/milk are the preferred substances to be applied to the area; plastic liners can trap moisture and lead to sore nipples.

51. B is correct; a hormonal contraceptive could decrease the milk supply if given before lactation is well established during the first 6 weeks after birth; after 6 weeks a progestin-only contraceptive could be used because it is the least likely hormonal contraceptive to affect lactation; even complete breastfeeding is not considered to be a reliable method because ovulation can occur unexpectedly even before the first menstrual period.

52. C is correct; the baby should be placed on the right side after feeding because it allows air bubbles to come up easily; tap water can be used unless the water supply is unsafe or if otherwise instructed; formula should never be heated in the microwave because it could be overheated or unevenly heated.

Critical Thinking Exercises

1. A. –
   B. +
   C. –
   D. –
   E. +
   F. –
   G. +
   H. +
   I. –
   J. –
   K. +
   L. –

2. *Bottle-feeding mother wishes to give her newborn skim milk to prevent cardiac problems:* see Fat subsection of Nutrient

Needs section; emphasize the importance of fat in the newborn's diet for energy and supplying essential fatty acids for growth and tissue maintenance, cell membranes, and hormone production; at least 15% of calories must come from fat; skim milk and low-fat milk lack essential fatty acids

3. Infant feeding method decision making during prenatal period (see Choosing an Infant Feeding Method section)
    A. *Nursing diagnosis:* decisional conflict related to lack of knowledge and experience with newborn feeding method
    Expected outcome: couple will choose the feeding method for their newborn that is most comfortable for them
    B. *Rationale for couple making the decision together:* both should learn about the pros and cons of feeding methods with an emphasis on the benefits of breastfeeding and how the partner can help with the method; partner support is a major factor in her ability to breastfeed successfully
    C. *Making decision prenatally:* the prenatal period is a less stressful time, allowing for full consideration of options, how feeding methods would be incorporated into life activities (such as work outside the home), and learning about breastfeeding by attending classes and reading
    D. *How the nurse can facilitate decision-making process:* provide information about feeding methods in a nonjudgmental manner while still emphasizing the importance of breastfeeding as the preferred method, dispel myths, address personal concerns of the couple, and make needed referrals to WIC, lactation consultant, breastfeeding classes, and the La Leche League

4. Breastfeeding mother's questions and concerns (see Milk Production section of Overview of Lactation section for A and B)
    A. *Breast size:* discuss development of lactation structures during pregnancy; emphasize the importance of this development and not the breast size for successful lactation
    B. *Let-down reflex:* explain what it is and why it happens (including physical and emotional triggers); emphasize its importance in providing the infant with hindmilk
    C. *Signs that breastfeeding is going well:* see Box 27-2; which identifies maternal and newborn indicators of effective breastfeeding during the first week following birth; put the indicators in writing and go over each one; provide contact person if mother is concerned
    D. *Nipple soreness:* see Special Considerations section of Care of the Mother; discuss and demonstrate measures to prevent and to treat sore nipples including, most importantly, good breastfeeding techniques such as latch-on, removal, and alternating starting breast and positions; discuss breast care measures such as air drying nipples, avoiding soap, and applying colostrum/milk or purified lanolin after feeding; numbing with ice for 2 to 3 minutes
    E. *Engorgement:* see Special Considerations section of Care of the Mother; prevention includes frequency of feeding every 2 to 3 hours with 15 to 20 minutes on each breast; treatment measures include warm packs and massage before feeding, ice afterwards, raw cabbage leaves, supportive bra; use of antiinflammatory analgesics such as ibuprofen; emphasize the temporary, self-limiting nature of engorgement
    F. *Afterpains and increased flow:* explain that oxytocin is released as a result of infant sucking; this triggers the let-

down reflex and stimulates the uterus to contract, causing afterpains for the first 3 to 5 days after birth; oxytocin also reduces excessive bleeding though the contractions can cause flow already in the uterus to be expelled giving the impression of an increased flow

G. *Breastfeeding as a birth control method:* see Effect of Menstruation and Breastfeeding and Contraception sections of Care of Mother; emphasize that breastfeeding is not an effective contraceptive method; although ovulation may be delayed, its return cannot be predicted with accuracy and may occur before the first menstrual period; discuss contraceptive methods that are safe to use with breastfeeding and resuming sexual intercourse during the postpartum period

H. *Weaning:* see Weaning section of Plan of Care and Interventions; emphasize that weaning needs to be a gradual process, eliminating one feeding at a time beginning with the one the baby is most likely to sleep through; discuss the use of bottles and cups; use of formula, cow's milk, and/or solids depends on the age of infant at the time of weaning

5. *Starting solid foods:* see Feeding Readiness and Introduction of Solid Food sections; emphasize importance of waiting to introduce solids at 4 to 6 months of age, when the infant is developmentally ready (e.g., enzymes for digestion of a variety of foods are developed and tongue extrusion reflex disappears); early introduction of solids can lead to allergies, excessive caloric intake, and diminished interest in breastfeeding; there is no evidence that solids encourage the infant to sleep through the night

6. Infrequent feeding of sleeping baby (see Frequency and Duration of Feeding and Special Considerations sections of Plan of Care and Interventions)

A. *Nursing diagnosis:* Imbalanced nutrition: less than body requirements related to infrequent feeding of newborn *Expected outcome:* mother will awaken infant every 2 to 3 hours during the day and every 4 hours at night to feed the infant, achieving approximately 8 to 12 feedings per day

B. *Nursing approach:* discuss feeding readiness cues to facilitate proper timing of feedings; discuss techniques to wake sleeping baby (Box 27-3) and signs indicating adequate intake (Box 27-2)

7. Bottle-feeding mother (see Formula Feeding section and Teaching for Self-Care box—Formula Preparation and Feeding)

A. *Nurse's response to mother's concern:* discuss how the mother can facilitate close contact and socializing with the infant during feeding: sit comfortably, touch, sing, and talk quietly to newborn to make feeding a pleasant time for both; reassure that properly prepared formulas will fully meet her newborn's need for nutrients and fluid

B. *Guidelines for bottle feeding:* include instructions related to choosing a formula type; the amount and frequency of feedings; how to prepare formula (follow directions for dilution exactly), warming formula correctly, discarding left-over formula, and bottle and nipple cleansing; principles of the feeding process including semi-upright position, not propping bottles, fluid filling the nipple to limit air consumption, cues of feeding readiness and satiety, and burping

CHAPTER 28: CARE OF THE NEWBORN AT HOME

Chapter Review Activities

1. F, 2. T, 3. F, 4. T, 5. T, 6. T, 7. F, 8. F, 9. T, 10. T, 11. F, 12. T, 13. F, 14. F, 15. T, 16. T, 17. T, 18. F

19. *Criteria for a protective home environment* (see Protective Environment section and Box 28-2): the criteria that should be met include:
    - Adequate lighting and ventilation
    - Elimination of potential fire and electrical hazards
    - Appropriate temperature and humidity
    - Implementation of infection control and cleanliness measures
    - Safety guidelines met for crib, carriers, car, play items

20. *Helping 2-month old infant to learn* (see Box 28-11 and Table 28-7):
    - Discuss muscular activity, use of auditory and visual stimuli, types of toys that would be appropriate.
    - Emphasize importance of keeping baby with rest of family during activities such as meal times.

21. *Infant massage benefits:* see Box 38-12 for a detailed list of the benefits for both parents and infant

22. *Maneuvers for relieving airway obstruction* (see Emergency Box—Relieving Airway Obstruction); maneuvers include back blows, turning infant, chest thrusts, and opening airway

23. C is correct; warm water will cleanse and the petrolatum will soothe; the circumcision site should be assessed every hour for the first 12 to 24 hours; folded sterile gauze should be used to apply gentle pressure because alcohol will increase bleeding and cause burning; the exudate forms as a protective barrier in 24 hours and should not be removed.

24. D is correct; powder if used should be sprinkled into the hand and then gently applied to the dry skin to avoid inhalation of powder particles; A, B, and C are correct actions.

25. A is correct; the crib should not be placed near a window or on an outside wall; the cord could be dangerous as the infant develops the ability to stand and pull on the cord; nothing should be tied around the infant's neck; crib slats should be no more than 2.5 inches apart so infant cannot fit head through.

26. B is correct; the second dose of DPT is due at 4 months; the third dose of HIB is due at 6 months; the first dose of the HBV vaccine should be given before discharge or within 1 to 2 months of age.

27. C is correct; the newborn should void at least 6 times each day during this time; regurgitation is common among newborns related to immature sphincter between stomach and esophagus; axillary temperature should be greater than 97° F and less than 100° F; loose, greenish stools are expected as the newborn excretes excess bilirubin.

Critical Thinking Exercises

1. *Concerns of first-time parents during first week at home* (see section for each concern in Plan of Care and Interventions—First Days at Home section):
    - Emphasize need for using "time savers," being assertive in limiting visitors, taking care of themselves as well as the baby.
    - Provide phone numbers of warm lines.
    - Make referrals for follow-up call, home visits, lactation consultant, parenting classes and groups.

2. Questions of new mother prior to discharge (see Plan of Care and Interventions for First Days at Home section, Teaching for Self Care Box—Sponge Bathing)
   A. *Care of Cord:* discuss keeping the cord dry and the area around the cord clean; specify when the cord will fall off; describe signs of infection
   B. *Use of topicals on skin:* discuss acid mantle of skin as a protection against infection, danger of inhaling powder if not used properly, and danger of irritation/allergy to product components; emphasize that all that is needed is warm water and perhaps a small amount of mild soap in soiled areas such as the genitalia
   C. *Keeping baby clean* (see Box 28-1)
      • Discuss principles of bathing— emphasize safety and prevention of infection and chilling.
      • Discuss how to incorporate bath into family routine and how often to bathe.
      • Describe the benefits of bathing.
      • Discuss care of diaper area and importance of frequent changing.
   D. *Care of circumcision* (see Teaching for Self-Care Box—Circumcision); teach about assessing the site for bleeding and infection, checking for voiding, keeping the area clean, and using measures to enhance the infant's comfort
   E. *Prevention of chilling:* discuss environmental modifications, precautions when bathing, clothing choices including use of head covering to reduce heat loss, and how to swaddle (see Box 28-4)

3. *Parental concerns regarding sleep patterns of infant and fussiness* (see Anticipatory Guidance Regarding the Newborn section); emphasize the normalcy of their infant's behavior; offer helpful suggestions to help infant develop a day-night routine such as:

• Bring baby into center of family activity late in the afternoon
• Place baby in crib to sleep only at night
• Bathe at bedtime
• Feed around 11 PM
• Reduce environmental stimuli when caring for infant at night
• Identify stimuli that calm and quiet (see Boxes 28-4 and 28-5)

4. Home care of infant with physiologic jaundice (see Home Phototherapy section)
   A. *Newborn criteria for home versus hospital treatment* (see Box 28-10); identify criteria related to such factors as age, birth weight and current weight, feeding and elimination patterns, and laboratory results
   B. *Parental and home environment criteria:* consider ability of parents to understand and carry out treatment plan, accept home nurse visits, and assess newborn progress; environment must meet basic requirements for telephone access, electricity, and heat
   C. *Reportable newborn behaviors* (see Box 28-11); consider changes in activity level, unstable temperature, poor feeding, vomiting, inadequate voiding

5. *Maternal concerns regarding immunizations:* emphasize that breastfeeding provides only temporary immunity to some infections and that immunizations must be given as recommended in terms of timing and number in order to achieve adequate immunity to what could be life-threatening infections; provide her with written materials to read and a person to call to ask questions and discuss concerns; make referrals in order to address her financial concern

CHAPTER 29: ASSESSMENT FOR RISK FACTORS

Chapter Review Activities

1. High risk pregnancy

2. Fetal compromise, asphyxia, prevent, minimize

3. Daily fetal movement count, kick count, 12 hours, 3 movements within 1 hour, nonstress test, contraction stress test, biophysical profile, sleep cycle, depressant medications, alcohol, smoking a cigarette, decrease

4. Ultrasonography, transabdominally, transvaginally, transabdominal ultrasound, transvaginal ultrasound, vagina, pelvic, intrauterine pregnancy, ectopic, embryo, abnormalities, gestational age

5. Doppler blood flow analysis, hypertension, intrauterine growth restriction, diabetes mellitus, multiple fetuses, preterm labor

6. Biophysical profile, ultrasonography, fetal monitoring, breathing movements, movement, tone, heart rate pattern, nonstress test, amniotic fluid volume, biophysical, central nervous system, hypoxemic

7. Magnetic resonance imaging, ionizing radiation

8. Amniocentesis, transabdominally, amniotic fluid, genetic disorders (congenital anomalies), pulmonary maturity, fetal hemolytic disease

9. Percutaneous umbilical blood sampling, cordocentesis, blood sampling, transfusion, umbilical vessel

10. Chorionic villus sampling, genetic makeup, 10, 12

11. Maternal serum alpha-fetoprotein, 16, 18

12. Triple marker test, 16, 18, maternal serum alpha-fetoprotein, unconjugated estriol, human chorionic gonadotropin, age

13. Nonstress test, accelerate

14. Contraction stress, late deceleration, nipple-stimulated contraction stress, oxytocin-stimulated contraction stress

15. *Factors placing a pregnant woman and her fetus/newborn at risk:* see Box 29-1, which describes several risk factors in each category listed

16. *Role of nurse when caring for high risk pregnant women undergoing antepartal testing:* see Nursing Role in Antepartal Assessment for Risk section; answer should emphasize education, support measures as well as assisting with or performing the test

17. Woman scheduled for vaginal ultrasound (see Ultrasonography section)
    A. *Cite reason for test for this woman:* to determine location of gestational sac because PID could have resulted in narrowing of fallopian tube and increasing risk for ectopic pregnancy
    B. *Preparation for the test:* explain purpose of test, how it will be performed, and how it will feel; assist her into a lithotomy position or supine position with hips elevated on a pillow; point out structures on monitor as test is performed; emphasize that bladder does not need to be full for this method of ultrasonography

18. *Nurse's role in abdominal ultrasound for monitoring fetal growth:* see Ultrasonography section; instruct woman to come for test with full bladder if appropriate; explain purpose of test and method of examination; assist her into a supine position with head and shoulders elevated on pillow and hip slightly tilted to right or left side; observe for supine hypotension during test and

orthostatic hypotension when rising to upright position after test; indicate how the fetus is being measured and point out fetus and its movements

19. *Risk factors for pregnancy-related problems:* see Box 29-3, which lists risk factors for each pregnancy-related problem identified

20. F, 21. T, 22. F, 23. T, 24. T, 25. T, 26. F, 27. F, 28. F, 29. T, 30. T, 31. F, 32. F, 33. T, 34. F, 35. T, 36. F, 37. F, 38. T, 39. F

40. D is correct; an amniocentesis with analysis of amniotic fluid for the L/S ratio and presence of phosphatidylglycerol (Pg) is used to determine pulmonary maturity; B refers to a contraction stress test; C refers to serial measurements of fetal growth using ultrasound.

41. C is correct; oral intake is not restricted prior to the test; the test will evaluate the response of the FHR to fetal movement—acceleration is expected; external not internal monitoring is used.

42. B is correct; the Triple Marker test is used to screen the older pregnant woman for the possibility that her fetus has Down syndrome; serum levels of AFP, unconjugated estriol, and hCG are measured; maternal serum alpha-fetoprotein alone is the screening test for open neural tube defects such as spina bifida; a 1-hour, 50-g glucose test is used to screen for gestational diabetes; an antibody titer or amniocentesis would determine problems related to her Rh negative status.

43. C is correct; a suspicious result is recorded when late decelerations occur with less than 50% of the contractions; a negative test result is recorded when no late decelerations occur during at least three uterine contractions lasting 40 to 60 seconds each, within a 10-minute period; a

positive test is recorded when there are persistent late decelerations with more than 50% of the contractions; unsatisfactory is the result recorded when there was a failure to achieve adequate uterine contractions or the tracing was too poor to interpret.

44. A is correct; a supine position with hips elevated enhances the view of the uterus; a lithotomy position may also be used; a full bladder is not required for the vaginal ultrasound but would be needed for most abdominal ultrasounds; during the test the woman may experience some pressure but medication for pain prior to the test is not required; contact gel is used with the abdominal ultrasound; water-soluble lubricant may be used to ease insertion of the vaginal probe.

Critical Thinking Exercises

1. Woman having Biophysical Profile (see Table 29-4 for identification of variables tested; scoring)
   A. *Nursing diagnosis:* anxiety related to unexpected need to undergo a biophysical profile
   B. *Nurse's response to woman's concern about the test:* describe how the test will be performed using ultrasound and external electronic fetal monitoring; explain that the purpose of the test is to view the fetus within its environment, to determine the amount of amniotic fluid, and assess the FHR response to fetal activity; show her how her baby moves in utero and discuss meaning of the results
   C. *Meaning of score obtained:* a score of 8 to 10 is a normal result

2. Amniocentesis (see Amniocentesis section and Nursing Role in Antepartal Assessment for Risk sections)
   A. *Preparing woman:* explain procedure, witness informed consent, assess

maternal vital signs and general health status and FHR prior to the test; ensure that ultrasound is performed to locate placenta and fetus prior to the test

B. *Supporting woman during the procedure:* explain what is happening and what she will be feeling; help her to relax; encourage her to ask questions and voice concerns and feelings; assess her reactions

C. *Postprocedure care and instructions:* monitor maternal vital signs and status and FHR; tell her when test results should be available and who to call; administer RhoGAM because she is Rh negative; teach her to assess herself for signs of infection, bleeding, rupture of membranes, and uterine contractions; make a follow-up phone call to check her status

3. Nonstress test (see Nonstress test section of Electronic Fetal Monitoring)
    A. *Tell woman about purpose of test:* response of FHR to fetal activity to determine adequacy of placental perfusion and fetal oxygenation
    B. *Preparation of woman for test:* tell her that she does not need to fast prior to the test; schedule test at a time of day that fetus is usually active; assist woman into a seated position or semi-recumbent position with a slight tilt to the side
    C. *Indicate how test is conducted:* attach tocotransducer to fundus and ultrasound transducer at site of PMI; instruct woman to indicate when fetus moves if movements are not apparent on the tracing; assess change, if any, in FHR following the movement
    D. *Analyze the results:* see Table 29-6 for the criteria to determine the test result to document; see Fig. 29-8 for a typical monitor tracing
        1) Tracing indicates a reactive result: good variability and normal baseline with accelerations following fetal movement that meet criteria for a reactive result
        2) Tracing indicates a nonreactive result: no accelerations with movement and limited variability

4. Contraction stress test (see Contraction Stress Test section of Electronic Fetal Monitoring)
    A. *Tell woman about purpose of test:* the test is a way of determining how her fetus will react to the stress of uterine contractions as they would occur during labor; uterine contractions decrease perfusion through placenta leading to fetal hypoxia; late decelerations during this test could be interpreted as an early warning of fetal compromise
    B. *Preparation:* assess woman's vital signs, general health status, and contraindications for the test; attach external electronic fetal monitor and assess FHR and uterine activity; assist her into the same position as for NST
    C. *Indicate how the test is performed:* see Nipple Stimulation Contraction Stress Test section; stimulate nipple(s) according to protocol until three uterine contractions of good quality occur within a 10-minute period; make sure that contractions subside after the test and assess maternal and fetal responses
    D. *Use of oxytocin to stimulate contractions:* see Oxytocin Stimulated Contraction Stress Test section; administer Pitocin intravenously (similar to induction of labor but with lower dosages) according to protocol, increasing rate until uterine contractions meet criteria indicated for a Nipple Stimulated Contraction Stress test; monitor woman, fetus, and contractions during the test and afterwards until contractions subside
    E. *Analyze the results:* see Table 29-7 for criteria used to interpret the test results

1. Tracing indicates a negative result (see Fig. 29-9, A): no late decelerations are noted
2. Tracing indicates a positive result (see Fig. 29-9, B): late decelerations with the appropriate number of contractions, limited variability

CHAPTER 30: HYPERTENSIVE DISORDERS IN PREGNANCY

Chapter Review Activities

1. E, 2. C, 3. B, 4. A, 5. D

6. Gestational hypertension, chronic hypertension

7. Preeclampsia, 20 weeks, hypertension, proteinuria, mild, severe

8. Hypertension, 140 mm Hg, 90 mm Hg, 105 mm Hg, 2, 4 to 6
9. Proteinuria, 0.1, 1+ to 2+, 2, 6
10. Pathologic edema, 12, 2 kg

11. Severe preeclampsia, 160 mm Hg, 110 mm Hg, 4+, oliguria, cerebral, visual, hepatic, thrombocytopenia, 100,000/ mm^3, pulmonary, cardiac, creatinine, growth restriction

12. Eclampsia
13. HELLP, hepatic, hemolysis (H), elevated liver enzymes (EL), low platelets (LP)
14. Arteriolar vasospasm, placental perfusion, IUGR, glomerular, oliguria

15. *Complete table related to expected physiologic adaptations and ineffective responses related to hypertensive disorders during pregnancy;* see Box 30-3 for a description of normal physiologic adaptations to pregnancy in terms of cardiovascular, hematologic, renal, and endocrine adaptations, and Pathophysiology section in Hypertension in Pregnancy, Fig. 30-1, and Fig. 30-2 for an explanation of ineffective adaptations that lead to hypertensive disorders

16. *Principles for ensuring accurate blood pressure measurement:* see Box 30-1; emphasize consistency in position of woman and her arm, the arm used, proper size of cuff, and provision of a rest period prior to the measurement

17. F, 18. T, 19. F, 20. T, 21. T, 22. F, 23. T, 24. F, 25. T, 26. F, 27. T, 28. F, 29. F, 30. F, 31. T, 32. T, 33. T, 34. F, 35. F, 36. F

37. *Risk factors associated with development of preeclampsia:* see Box 30-2 for a list of factors including renal and hypertensive disease, family history of PIH, multiple gestation, first pregnancy, maternal age, diabetes mellitus, and Rh incompatibility

38. *Assessment techniques to determine findings associated with PIH:* see specific sections for each assessment technique in Physical Examination
   - *Hyperreflexia and ankle clonus:* see Table 30-4, which grades DTR responses and Fig. 30-5, A, B, C for illustrations depicting performance of DTRs
   - *Proteinuria:* describe dipstick and 24-hour urine collection methods to determine level of protein in urine
   - *Pitting edema:* see Fig. 30-3, which illustrates assessment of pitting edema and classifications

39. Preeclampsia and eclampsia: effect on fetal well-being
   A. *Describe effect:* see Significance and Incidence and Pathophysiology sections, Figs. 30-1, and 30-2; major effects on fetus relate to insufficient uteroplacental circulation leading to IUGR, intrauterine fetal death, or perinatal mortality (especially if abruptio placentae occurs); preterm labor and birth, acute hypoxia and abruption can occur with a convulsion

B. *Fetal surveillance measures:* see Mild Preeclampsia and Home Care section in Plan of Care and Interventions; measures can include serial ultrasounds to evaluate fetal growth, NST, BPP, and daily fetal movement counts by the mother

40. A is correct; the woman should rest for at least 5 minutes after assuming her position, and the cuff should cover 80% of the upper arm; the (left) dependent arm should be used for measurement.

41. A is correct; with severe preeclampsia the edema should be generalized with noticeable puffiness of the eyes, face, and fingers, the DTRs should be ≥3+ with possible ankle clonus, and the BP should be ≥160/110.

42. D is correct; a respiratory rate of 12 breaths per minute indicates dangerous CNS depression by the magnesium sulfate; the solution should be 40 g in 1000 ml of Ringers lactate, assessment should occur every 15 to 30 minutes, and the maintenance dose should be 1 to 3 g/hour.

43. B is correct; magnesium sulfate is a CNS depressant given to prevent seizures.

44. D is correct; the woman should weigh herself in the morning, after voiding, before breakfast using the same scale and wearing the same clothing; a clean catch, midstream urine specimen should be used to assess urine for protein using a dipstick; fluid intake should be 6 to 8 glasses a day along with roughage to prevent constipation; gentle exercise improves circulation and helps to preserve muscle tone and a sense of well-being.

Critical Thinking Exercises

1. Woman with mild preeclampsia: home care
   A. *Signs and symptoms:* see Table 30-2, which differentiates between mild and severe preeclampsia in terms of maternal and fetal effects; Table 30-3 lists the changes in laboratory values
   B. *Three priority nursing diagnoses:* nursing diagnoses should consider physiologic effects of preeclampsia such as ineffective tissue perfusion—placenta, risk for injury to mother or fetus; psychosocial effects: anxiety, ineffective individual/family coping, powerlessness, ineffective role performance, interrupted family processes; assessment findings should guide the choice and priority of nursing diagnoses especially with regard to those that apply to psychosocial impact
   C. *Organization of home care:* see Mild Preeclampsia and Home Care section and Plan of Care; help couple mobilize their support system, make referrals to home care if needed, discuss frequency of prenatal visits and antepartal testing
   D. *Teaching regarding assessment of status and signs of a worsening condition:* see Table 30-2 and Teaching for Self-Care Box—Assessing and Reporting Clinical Signs of Preeclampsia; discuss signs and put them in writing so couple can refer to them at home; have woman keep a daily diary of her findings, feelings, and concerns; teach woman and family to take BP, weigh accurately, assess urine, and whom to call if problems or concerns arise
   E. *Instructions about nutrition and fluid intake:* see Diet section and Teaching for Self-Care Box—Nutrition; emphasize the importance of protein, calcium, balance of roughage and fluids, and avoiding foods/fluids that are high in salt or contain alcohol or caffeine; explain rationale for dietary recommendations
   F. *Coping with bed rest:* see Activity section Teaching for Self-Care Box—Coping with Bed Rest, and the Plan of Care; explain rationale for bed rest and

activity restrictions; clarify what this restriction means, for example how long she can be out of bed in a day and what type of activity is okay; discuss importance of lateral position when in bed, relaxation exercises, and nonstressful, calming diversional activities

G. *Risk for constipation:* see Teaching for Self-Care Boxes—Nutrition and Coping with Bed Rest; roughage (whole grains, bran, raw fruits and vegetables), 6 to 8 glasses of fluid each day, keep fruit and fluids nearby

2. Woman with severe preeclampsia—hospital care

A. *Signs and symptoms:* see Table 30-2, which differentiates between mild and severe preeclampsia in terms of maternal and fetal effects; Table 30-3 lists changes in laboratory values

B. *Three priority nursing diagnoses:* impaired tissue perfusion, risk for impaired gas exchange, and injury take priority as the physiologic nursing diagnoses because her condition is worsening and the safety of the maternal-fetal unit is jeopardized; anxiety or fear would be the priority psychosocial nursing diagnosis

C. *Precautionary measures:* see Box 30-4, which lists precautionary measures in terms of environmental modifications, seizure precautions, and readiness of emergency medications and equipment

D. *Administration of magnesium sulfate:* for numbers 1, 3, and 4 see Box 30-5; for numbers 5 and 6 use Nurse Alert in Magnesium Sulfate subsection of Severe Preeclampsia and HELLP Syndrome section

1) *Guidelines:* list the guidelines for preparing and administering the medication solution safety including dosage, IV solution, and infusion rate; identify essential assessment measures that must be completed and documented before and during the infusion

2) *Nursing diagnosis:* Risk for ineffective breathing pattern related to the central nervous system depressant effects of magnesium sulfate infusion

3) *Explain expected therapeutic effect:* discuss that this medication is used for its CNS depressant effects to prevent convulsions; describe how it will be given, how she will feel, and what will be done while she is receiving the infusion

4) *Maternal-fetal assessments:* VS, FHR pattern, intake and output, urine for protein, DTRs and ankle clonus, signs of improvement or worsening condition including signs of an imminent seizure

5) *Signs of magnesium sulfate toxicity:* hyporeflexia, respiratory depression, oliguria, diminished LOC

6) *Immediate action:* discontinue the magnesium sulfate infusion, administer calcium gluconate slowly IV push according to protocol

E. *Seizure occurs:* see Eclampsia subsection and Emergency Box—Eclampsia

1) *Emergency measures at onset of convulsion and immediately following:*
   - Emphasize importance of maintaining a patent airway, preventing injury, and calling for help.
   - Observe effect of seizure on mother and fetus.
   - Document the event and care measures implemented during and after seizure.
   - Provide comfort and reassurance after the convulsion; orient to what happened; never leave alone because another seizure could occur or signs of complications can begin; inform family.

2) *List potential complications that can occur:* rupture of membranes, preterm labor and birth, altered LOC, abruptio placentae, fetal distress

F. *Postpartum period recovering from eclampsia:* see Postpartum Nursing Care section
  - Provide close and comprehensive assessment with emphasis on signs of hemorrhage (low platelets, DIC, effect of magnesium sulfate), impending seizures, and status of preeclampsia.
  - Continue hospital precautionary measures.
  - Continue magnesium sulfate, antihypertensive medications; Pitocin is oxytocic of choice because Methergine could elevate BP even further especially if given parenterally.
  - Provide emotional and psychosocial support for woman and her family; provide time for them to be together and with their baby but be careful to keep environmental stimuli at a low level until the danger of seizures passes.
  - Discuss how her recovery is progressing and the prognosis for the rest of the postpartum period and for future pregnancies.

CHAPTER 31: ANTEPARTAL HEMORRHAGIC DISORDERS

Chapter Review Activities

1. Spontaneous/miscarriage (abortion), incompetent cervix, ectopic pregnancy, hydatidiform mole (molar pregnancy)

2. Placenta previa, abruptio placentae, cord insertion, placenta

3. Abortion, survive in an extrauterine environment, 20, 500 g, spontaneous abortion, threatened, inevitable, incomplete, complete, missed

4. hCG, gestational sac, ultrasonography

5. Recurrent premature dilation of the cervix, variable, length, composition, stress, lifestyle, short labors, recurring loss, cerclage, 10 to 12, bed rest, hydration, tocolysis

6. Ectopic pregnancy, fertilized ovum, ampulla, tube, Cullen sign, hematoperitoneum

7. Hydatidiform mole, molar pregnancy, complete (classic), partial

8. Placenta previa, internal cervical os, internal os, entirely, incomplete, internal os, edge, internal os, os, dilates, low-lying placenta, internal os, lower uterine segment, contract, placenta previa, cesarean birth, induced abortion, multiple, closely spaced, maternal age, African, Asian, smoking, cocaine

9. Premature separation of the placenta, detachment, part, all, implantation, Couvelaire uterus, clotting defects (e.g., DIC), hypertension, cocaine, external abdominal, smoking, poor nutrition

10. Velamentous insertion of the cord, vasa previa, rupture of membranes, traction on the cord, Battledore placenta, succenturiate placenta

11. Disseminated intravascular coagulation (DIC), external bleeding, internal bleeding

12. F, 13. F, 14. T, 15. F, 16. T, 17. F, 18. T, 19. F, 20. T, 21. T, 22. F, 23. F, 24. F, 25. F, 26. T, 27. T, 28. T, 29. T, 30. F, 31. F, 32. T, 33. T, 34. T, 35. F, 36. T, 37. F, 38. T

39. *Clotting disorders in pregnancy* (see Clotting Disorders in Pregnancy section)
  A. *Predisposing conditions:* abruptio placentae, hemorrhage, severe preeclampsia, HELLP syndrome,

retained dead fetus, amniotic fluid embolism, gram-negative sepsis

B. *Pathophysiology of DIC:* pathologic diffuse clotting that consumes large amounts of clotting factors, leading to widespread external and/or internal bleeding

C. *Clinical manifestations:* unusual and/or excessive bleeding, abnormal results on clotting tests

D. *Priority nursing care measures:* careful and thorough assessment including signs of bleeding, renal function, and fetal well-being, lateral position, administration of blood/blood products and oxygen as ordered, education and emotional support of woman and family

40. *Positive effects of maternal hypervolemic state during pregnancy:* answer should include: meets the metabolic demands of maternal/fetal unit; protection against effect of impaired venous return by enlarging uterus; safeguard against effects of childbirth blood loss

41. A is correct; the woman is experiencing a threatened miscarriage, therefore a conservative approach is attempted first; B and C reflect management of an inevitable and complete or incomplete abortion; cerclage or suturing of the cervix is done for recurrent, spontaneous miscarriage associated with premature dilatation (incompetent) cervix.

42. C is correct; A, B, and D are appropriate nursing diagnoses, but deficient fluid volume is the most immediate concern, placing the woman's well-being at greatest risk.

43. B is correct; methotrexate destroys rapidly dividing cells, in this case the fetus and placenta, to avoid rupture of tube and need for surgery; follow-up with blood tests is needed for 2 to 8 weeks, vitamins (folic

acid) and alcohol increase the risk for side effects with this medication.

44. C is correct; the clinical manifestations of placenta previa are described; dark red bleeding with pain is characteristic of abruptio placentae; massive bleeding from many sites is associated with DIC; bleeding is not an expected sign of preterm labor.

45. A is correct; hemorrhage is a major potential postpartum complication because the implantation site of the placenta is in the lower uterine segment, which has a limited capacity to contract after birth; infection is another major complication but it is not the immediate focus of care; B and D are also important but not to the same degree as hemorrhage which is life threatening.

Critical Thinking Exercises

1. Woman with ruptured ectopic pregnancy (see Ectopic Pregnancy section)

A. *Risk factors:* see Incidence and Etiology subsection; history of STIs, PID, tubal sterilization and surgical reversal of tubal sterilization; previous history of ectopic pregnancy

B. *Assessment of findings:* see Clinical Manifestations section; findings begin with signs of an unruptured tubal pregnancy (missed period, adnexal fullness and tenderness, dull or colicky pain); these signs are subtle and often missed; signs of rupture are more acute (abnormal bleeding, acute abdominal pain and referred shoulder pain, signs of hemorrhage and shock, Cullen sign) and may be mistaken for other acute abdominal conditions

C. *Differential diagnosis:* see Table 31-2; miscarriage, appendicitis, salpingitis, ruptured ovarian cyst

D. *Major care management problem:* hemorrhage; much of the blood accumulates in the abdominal cavity

E. *Two priority nursing diagnoses:* deficient fluid volume and acute pain as well as fear/anxiety and anticipatory grief

F. *Nursing measures for the preoperative and postoperative period:* see Collaborative Care—Hospital Care section; assessment, general preoperative and postoperative care measures, fluid replacement, major emphasis on emotional support to facilitate grieving, discussion of impact of rupture on future pregnancies, referral for counseling as appropriate, prepare for discharge with instructions for postoperative self-care including self-assessment for complications such as infection, measures to enhance healing, importance of follow-up appointment to assess progress of recovery

2. Woman with signs of miscarriage (see Table 31-1)

A. *Basis for signs and symptoms:* signs indicate the woman is experiencing a threatened miscarriage

B. *Expected care management:* bed rest, sedation, avoidance of stress and orgasm; follow progress with hCG levels and ultrasound to assess integrity of gestational sac; watch for signs of progress to inevitable abortion; caution her to save peri pads and tissue passed

3. Woman with signs of miscarriage (see Box 31-1 and Table 31-1)

A. *Questions:* determine what she means by a lot of bleeding and if she is experiencing any other signs and symptoms related to miscarriage such as pain and cramping; determine the gestational age of her pregnancy and if there is anyone to bring her to the hospital if inevitable miscarriage is suspected

B. *Assessment findings indicative of an incomplete miscarriage:* heavy, profuse bleeding, severe cramping, passage of tissue, cervix is dilated with tissue present

C. *Priority nursing diagnosis at this time:* deficient fluid volume related to blood loss secondary to incomplete abortion

D. *Nursing measures:* prompt termination of pregnancy: assess before and after procedure (e.g., dilation and curettage), explain what will occur, provide emotional support, refer for counseling if needed, prepare for discharge, and arrange for follow-up to assess physical and emotional status

E. *Discharge instructions:* see Home Care section and Teaching for Self-Care Box—Discharge Teaching for the Woman after Early Miscarriage; advise regarding signs and symptoms of complications (bleeding, infection), what to expect regarding progress of healing (pain, discharge), measures to prevent complications (hygiene, nutrition, rest); advise her to take measures to avoid pregnancy for at least 2 months

F. *Nursing measures for anticipatory grieving:* see Home Care section and Teaching for Self-Care Box—Discharge Teaching for the Woman after Early Miscarriage; acknowledge her loss and provide time for her to express her feelings; inform her about how she may feel (mood swings, depression); refer her for grief counseling, support groups, clergy; make follow-up phone calls

4. *Care of woman following cerclage* (see Incompetent Cervix section); answer should include the following care measures:
   - Assessment for uterine contractions, rupture of membranes, infection
   - Explanation of activity restrictions, warning signs including those that would require immediate transfer to the hospital, and treatments including medications

- Discussion of her feelings regarding the pregnancy and her understanding of her health problem and its treatment
- Identification and involvement of support system as appropriate

5. Woman with complete hydatidiform mole (see Hydatidiform Mole section)
   A. *Typical signs and symptoms:* see Clinical Manifestations section; scant to profuse vaginal bleeding (dark brown to bright red), larger or smaller uterus for dates, anemia, hyperemesis gravidarum, signs of preeclampsia before 20 weeks' gestation
   B. *Post-treatment instructions:* see Nursing Care and Home Care section; frequent physical and pelvic examinations, regular measurement of serum hCG levels following protocol for frequency for at least 1 year or longer; emphasize importance of follow-up assessments and strict birth control to prevent pregnancy until hCG levels have been normal for a specified period of time; provide time to discuss knowledge of disorder, treatment, and follow-up and to express feelings; referral to support group may be helpful
   C. Choriocarcinoma, hCG, uterus

6. Comparison of a woman with marginal placenta previa to a woman with abruptio placentae, grade II
   A. *Comparison of findings:* see Placenta Previa and Abruptio Placentae subsections and Table 31-3 to compare findings for each disorder in terms of characteristics of bleeding, uterine tone, pain and tenderness, and ultrasound findings regarding location of placenta and fetal presentation/position, hypertension associations, and fetal effects
   B. *Priority nursing diagnoses:* consider diagnoses related to major physical problems such as deficient fluid volume related to blood loss, ineffective tissue

perfusion (placenta), and risk for fetal injury; major psychosocial nursing diagnoses could include fear/anxiety, interrupted family processes, and anticipatory grieving
   C. *Comparison of care management approaches:* consider home care versus hospital care for woman with placenta previa; hospital care is the safest approach for woman experiencing abruptio placentae; discuss active versus expectant management for each disorder
   D. *Postpartum considerations:* potential complications should be the basis for the special postpartum care requirements; hemorrhage (placenta previa related to limited contraction of lower portion of uterus; abruptio placentae related to Couvelaire uterus and DIC) and infection (lower implantation site, anemia from blood loss) are the major physiologic complications that need to be addressed; emotional and psychosocial support are important related to the high risk nature of the pregnancy, especially if fetal loss, maternal loss, or both was the outcome

CHAPTER 32: ENDOCRINE AND METABOLIC DISORDERS

Chapter Review Activities

1. *Interrelationship of the clinical manifestations of diabetes mellitus:* see Pathogenesis subsection of Diabetes Mellitus section for a full description of each of the clinical manifestations listed in terms of cause and interrelationship with one another

2. Hyperglycemia, insulin secretion, insulin action

3. Polyuria, polydipsia, polyphagia, glycosuria
4. Pregestational, gestational

5. Glucose control, conception, gestational

6. Hypoglycemia, hypoglycemic, nausea, vomiting, cravings, glucose

7. Hyperglycemia, diabetic ketoacidosis (DKA), insulin

8. Phosphatidylglycerol, lecithin, sphingomyelin (L/S)

9. Glycosylated hemoglobin, 65 mg/dl, 95 mg/dl, 130 mg/dl, 120 mg/dl, euglycemia, 65 mg/dl, 130 mg/dl, 60 mg/dl, 200 mg/dl

10. Blood glucose, 30 to 35, 50% to 60%, simple, complex, 12% to 20%, 20% to 30%, 10%, 12 kg

11. Breakfast, lunch, dinner, bedtime, middle of the night, postprandial, second, third, increased, hypoglycemia, hyperglycemia, insulin dose, diet, nausea, vomiting, diarrhea, infection

12. 2/3, before breakfast, longer acting (NPH), short acting (regular), 1/3, before dinner, hypoglycemia, short acting, before dinner, longer acting, bedtime, short acting, longer acting

13. Hyperemesis gravidarum, 5%, dehydration, electrolyte imbalance, ketosis, acetonuria, 20 years old, obese, nonsmokers, multifetal, molar

14. *Maternal and fetal/neonatal risks and complications related to pregestational diabetes:* see Maternal Risks/Complications and Fetal Risks sections
    - *Maternal:* increased rate of childbirth complications, hypertensive disorders, miscarriage and preterm labor/birth, hydramnios, postpartum hemorrhage, infection, hypoglycemia, hyperglycemia, DKA
    - *Fetal/newborn:* congenital anomalies, macrosomia with related birth injuries, IUGR, RDS, neonatal hypoglycemia, hypocalcemia, hyperbilirubinemia

15. *Complete table related to metabolic changes in pregnancy and impact on diabetes:* see Metabolic Changes associated with Pregnancy section of Diabetes Mellitus for a description related to changes associated with pregnancy and the postpartum period.

16. *Recommendations for screening for and diagnosing gestational diabetes:* see Screening for Gestational Diabetes Mellitus subsection of Care Management of Gestational Diabetes Mellitus section
    - Avoid screening low risk women
    - Screen with 50-g, 1-hour glucose test at 24 to 28 weeks' gestation
    - If result is ≥140 mg/dl, follow with a 3-hour, 100-g glucose test
    - Diagnosis of gestational diabetes is made if ≥2 values of the 3-hour glucose test are met or exceeded

17. *State effect of thyroid disorders on reproduction and pregnancy:* see Thyroid Disorders section for a full description of hyperthyroidism and hypothyroidism; consider effects of these disorders on reproductive development, sexuality, fertility in terms of ability to conceive and to sustain a pregnancy to viability, potential fetal/newborn complications related to maternal treatment of her thyroid disorder

18. T, 19. T, 20. F, 21. T, 22. F, 23. F, 24. F, 25. T, 26. T, 27. T, 28. F, 29. F, 30. T, 31. T, 32. F, 33. T, 34. F, 35. F, 36. T, 37. F, 38. F, 39. F, 40. T, 41. F, 42. F, 43. T

44. D is correct; the woman is exhibiting signs of DKA; insulin is the required treatment with the dosage dependent on blood glucose level; intravenous fluids may also be required; A is the treatment for hypoglycemia; B and C, although they may increase the woman's comfort, are not the priority.

45. C is correct; a 2-hour postprandial blood glucose should be less than 120 mg/dl; A, B, and D all fall within the expected normal ranges.

46. B is correct; calories should be increased to 30 to 35 kcal/kg; a minimum of intake of 250 mg of carbohydrates is recommended daily; protein intake should range between 12% and 20%.

47. D is correct; washing hands is important but gloves are not necessary for self-injection; vial should be gently rotated, not shaken; regular insulin should be drawn into the syringe first; because she is obese, a 90-degree angle with skin taut is recommended.

48. A is correct; she should be kept NPO for 24 to 48 hours or until vomiting is controlled; oral hygiene is important when NPO and after vomiting episodes to maintain the integrity of oral mucosa; taking fluids between (not with) meals reduces nausea, thereby increasing tolerance for oral nutrition.

Critical Thinking Exercises

1. *Preconception counseling for a woman with diabetes mellitus:* see Pregestational Counseling section of Pregestational Diabetes Mellitus;
   - Discuss purpose in terms of planning pregnancy for the optimum time when glucose control is established within normal ranges because this will decrease incidence of congenital anomalies; diagnose any vascular problems; emphasize the importance of her health prior to pregnancy helping to ensure a positive outcome.
   - Discuss how her diabetes management will need to be altered during pregnancy; include her husband because his health is important, as is his support during pregnancy.

2. Pregnant woman with pregestational diabetes experiencing hypoglycemia (see Table 32-1, Teaching for Self-Care Box—Treatment for Hypoglycemia, and Metabolic Changes associated with Pregnancy and Pregestational Diabetes Mellitus sections
   A. *Problem:* signs and symptoms suggest hypoglycemia resulting from insufficient caloric intake with no adjustment in insulin dosage
   B. *Action:* check blood glucose level if possible, eat or drink something that contains 10 to 15 g of simple carbohydrate, rest for 15 minutes, recheck blood glucose level, repeat if glucose level remains too low
   C. *Glucose boosters:* unsweetened fruit juice, regular soda, Lifesavers candy, honey, corn syrup, milk, glucose tablets

3. Woman with pregestational diabetes: care management
   A. *Additional antepartal fetal assessments:* see Fetal Surveillance section of Plan of Care and Interventions; tests can include ultrasound examination (growth, congenital anomalies such as spina bifida), maternal serum alpha-fetoprotein, fetal echocardiography (increased risk for cardiac disorders), Doppler blood flow analysis, daily fetal movement counts, NST, BPP, CST
   B. *Stressors facing woman and family:* alteration in daily living including usual diabetes management, need for additional antepartal testing and prenatal visits, financial implications
   C. *Nursing diagnoses:* consider both physiologic and psychosocial concerns; consider areas of deficient knowledge, anxiety/fear, ineffective coping, risk for maternal or fetal injury, imbalanced nutrition
   D. *Activity/exercise recommendations:* see Exercise section of Plan of Care and

Interventions; recommend exercises according to her diabetic status (e.g., presence of vasculopathy); discuss when she should exercise and emphasize the importance of checking blood glucose level before, during, and after taking care to adjust caloric intake and insulin administration accordingly

E. *Complete table related to care management during antepartum, intrapartum, and postpartum periods:* see specific subsections for diet, glucose monitoring, and insulin in Plan of Care and Intervention section and the Teaching for Self-Care Boxes for information regarding interventions and health teaching; the Plan of Care for a Pregnancy complicated by pregestational diabetes may also be helpful in completing the table

F. *Birth control recommendations:* see Postpartum subsection; discuss risks and benefits of methods including their impact on glucose levels (hormone based) and infection (IUD); barrier method is preferred starting with condom and spermicide until diaphragm or cervical cap can be refitted; stress importance of delaying intercourse until healing is complete to prevent infection

4. Hispanic woman with gestational diabetes (see Gestational Diabetes section)

A. *Complication of pregnancy exhibited with validating findings:* gestational diabetes; 50-g glucose test result 152 mg/dl (≥140 mg/dl); 3-hour glucose test reveals three values exceeding the normal range (fasting, 1-hour result, and 2-hour result—see Fig. 32-4)

B. *Risk factors exhibited:* older than 30 years of age, obese, mother with type 2 diabetes, previous birth of baby over 9 pounds

C. *Pathophysiology of gestational diabetes;* pancreas unable to meet demands for increased insulin to compensate for the insulin resistance during the second and third trimesters; cannot maintain euglycemic state

D. *Maternal and fetal/newborn risks:* see Maternal-Fetal Risks section of Gestational Diabetes; similar risks as for pregestational diabetes except for congenital anomalies, which are the same as for the nondiabetic population

E. *Ongoing assessment:* see Antepartum subsection of Interventions section; emphasize importance of monitoring blood glucose levels at recommended times, antepartal fetal surveillance measures, and increased frequency of prenatal visits

F. *Nursing diagnoses:*
   • Anxiety OR deficient knowledge related to ineffective glucose metabolism during pregnancy associated with gestational diabetes
   • Risk for fetal injury related to excessive intrauterine growth associated with gestational diabetes

G. *Dietary changes:* see Diet subsection; woman is placed on a standard diabetic diet for pregnancy at 30 to 35 kcal/kg/day for a total of 2000 to 2500 kcal/24 hours; spaced over three meals and two snacks including one at bedtime

H. *Implications of gestational diabetes mellitus:* see Postpartum subsection; most women return to normal glucose levels, but GDM is likely to recur in subsequent pregnancies; there is an increased risk for developing type 2 diabetes within 5 years of pregnancy; infant is more likely to be obese and have diabetes mellitus in the future; discuss lifestyle changes including weight reduction and a regular exercise program

5. *Woman with type 2 diabetes unable to take oral hypoglycemic agents:* inform her that these agents have teratogenic potential; help her to self-inject insulin through

teaching, demonstration, practice, and support; see Teaching for Self-Care Box— Administration of Insulin

6. Woman with hyperemesis gravidarum (see Hyperemesis Gravidarum section)

A. *Predisposing/etiologic factors:* see Etiology section, which lists physiologic and psychologic factors including the factors present in this situation: primigravida, maternal age less than 20 years, obesity, ambivalence about pregnancy, lifestyle alterations; additional factors include multifetal pregnancy, molar pregnancy, body change concerns

B. *Assessment of physiologic and psychosocial factors upon admission:*
   - *Physiologic:* full description of nausea and vomiting, presence of other GI symptoms, relief measures used, weight including changes, vital signs, signs of fluid, electrolyte, and acid/base imbalances, urine check for ketones (ketonuria) and specific gravity, CBC, serum electrolytes, liver enzymes, bilirubin levels
   - *Psychosocial:* discuss concerns regarding self and pregnancy; assess support system

C. *Priority nursing diagnoses:* deficient fluid volume, risk for fetal and maternal injury, anxiety, powerlessness, ineffective individual or family coping; woman's condition and circumstances will determine the priority with physiologic diagnoses taking precedence in the acute phase

D. *Care measures during hospitalization:*
   - Restore fluid and electrolyte balance with intravenous administration of fluids, electrolytes, and nutrients.
   - Restore ability to tolerate oral nutrition: gradual progression from NPO to full diet.
   - Monitor progress to determine effectiveness of therapeutic regimen, readiness for discharge, and need for

continuing treatment with home care.
   - Provide psychosocial support for woman and her family; make referrals as appropriate.
   - Teach woman and family about the disorder, how it is treated, its effect on pregnancy and fetus.

E. *Home care:*
   - Discuss follow-up care requirements, types of foods to eat and ways to eat (similar to recommendations for morning sickness).
   - Include family in plan of care especially with regard to meal preparation and support and encouragement of the woman.
   - Teach woman how to assess herself in terms of weight, urine for ketones, signs of developing problems that should be reported including weight loss, return of nausea and vomiting, pain, dehydration.

CHAPTER 33: MEDICAL-SURGICAL PROBLEMS IN PREGNANCY

Chapter Review Activities

1. Cardiac decompensation, 28, 32, childbirth, 24, 48

2. Functional classification of organic heart disease, asymptomatic at normal levels of activity, symptomatic with increased activity, symptomatic with ordinary activity, symptomatic at rest

3. Peripartum cardiomyopathy
4. Rheumatic heart disease
5. Mitral valve stenosis, rheumatic heart disease
6. Infective endocarditis
7. Eisenmenger syndrome
8. Mitral valve prolapse

9. Marfan syndrome
10. Pulmonary hypertension

11. Sickle cell hemoglobinopathy, anemia, African-American, Mediterranean
12. Thalassemia (Mediterranean or Cooley anemia)
13. Bronchial asthma, hyperactive airways, breathe, wheezing, cough, sputum, dyspnea

14. Adult respiratory distress syndrome (ARDS), gastric contents, DIC, hypertensive, abruptio placentae, dead fetus, amniotic fluid embolism

15. Cystic fibrosis
16. Epilepsy
17. Systemic lupus erythematosus (SLE)
18. Cholelithiasis
19. Cholecystitis
20. Appendicitis
21. Bell palsy

22. *Maternal and fetal complications related to maternal cardiovascular problems:* see Cardiovascular Disorders section; increased risk for miscarriage, preterm labor and birth, IUGR, maternal mortality, and stillbirth

23. Pregnant women requiring abdominal surgery (see Surgery during Pregnancy section)
    A. *Factors that complicate diagnosis and treatment for abdominal problems:* enlarged uterus and displaced internal organs interfere with palpation, alter position of the affected organ and/or change the usual clinical manifestations associated with a specific disorder
    B. *Major fear expressed by women undergoing surgery:* fear of losing baby, the effects of the procedure and medications on fetal well-being and the course of the pregnancy; women should be encouraged to express their fears, concerns, and questions

C. Fetus, FHR, uterine contractions, lateral tilt, vena caval compression, FHR, uterine monitoring, preterm labor, tocolysis
D. *Discharge planning:* see Home Care section and Box 33-4; teach woman and family about what to watch for, care of incision site, activity and rest considerations, and nutrition guidelines for healing and recovery

24. *Modifications in CPR and Heimlich maneuver when a woman is pregnant:* see Cardiopulmonary Resuscitation of the Pregnant Woman section, Emergency Box—Cardiopulmonary Resuscitation for Pregnant Woman, and Fig. 33-2; modifications include
    - Standard CPR but with uterus displaced laterally
    - Place paddles of defibrillator one rib interspace higher
    - Monitor fetus and prepare for immediate cesarean birth
    - Heimlich: place arms under axilla, across chest with thumb side of fist against middle of sternum, then perform backward chest thrusts

25. T, 26. F, 27. F, 28. F, 29. T, 30. T, 31. T, 32. F, 33. T, 34. F, 35. T, 36. T, 37. F, 38. T, 39. T, 40. F, 41. T, 42. T, 43. T, 44. T, 45. T, 46. F

47. D is correct; other signs of cardiac compensation include moist, productive, frequent cough, crackles at bases of lungs, and orthopnea; supine hypotension is a common finding during pregnancy related to compression of vena cava and aorta, not cardiac decompensation.

48. A is correct; this woman is exhibiting signs of cardiac decompensation; further information regarding her cardiac status is required to determine what further action would be needed.

49. C is correct; furosemide is a diuretic; propranolol is used to manage hypertension and cardiac dysrhythmias; although warfarin is an anticoagulant, it can cross the placenta and affect the fetus (congenital anomalies and hemorrhage) whereas heparin, which is a large molecule, does not.

50. B is correct; bed rest is not required for a woman with a class II designation; she will need to avoid heavy exertion and stop activities that cause fatigue and dyspnea; actions in A, C, and D are all appropriate and recommended for class II.

51. C is correct; fat should be reduced to 40 to 50 g; protein should be limited to 10% to 12% of total calories; fatty/fried foods should be avoided.

Critical Thinking Exercises

1. Pregnant woman with mitral valve stenosis—Class II (see Cardiovascular Disorders section)
   A. *Two nursing diagnoses*: several nursing diagnoses and expected outcomes of care are listed in the Assessment and Nursing Diagnoses subsection; use assessment findings to determine the priority for a specific pregnant woman;
      - Fear/anxiety would be a top priority psychosocial nursing diagnosis for this woman because it is her first pregnancy and she does not really know what to expect; expected outcome would be: woman/couple will openly express concerns and seek information as needed
      - Physiologically, activity intolerance, risk for ineffective tissue perfusion, and decreased cardiac output would be priorities as pregnancy advances and the cardiac workload increases; expected outcome: woman will follow recommended therapeutic regimen to reduce stress on her heart

   B. *Recommended therapeutic plan for a pregnant woman designated as Class II*: see Antepartum section of Plan of Care and Interventions focusing on specific guidelines for Class II; see Teaching for Self-Care Box—Pregnant Woman at Risk for Cardiac Decompensation
      - *Rest/sleep/activity patterns*: avoid heavy exertion, stop if signs of decompensation occur; sleep 8 to 10 hours/night; 30-minute naps after meals; keep a record of the effect of various activities
      - *Prevention of infection*: good hygiene and health habits to maintain resistance; identify early and treat promptly; use of prophylactic antibiotics may be required because she has a valvular problem
      - *Nutrition*: well-balanced diet with iron and folic acid and high in protein, adequate calories, sodium restriction as appropriate for her cardiac condition, need for potassium; keep weight gain at lower end of recommended range for her BMI
      - *Bowel elimination*: prevent constipation to avoid Valsalva maneuver; activity, fluids, and roughage/fiber

   C. *Factors increasing stress*: see Assessment and Nursing Diagnoses subsection
      - *Physiologic stress*: anemia, infection, edema, constipation
      - *Psychosocial stress*: depression, anxiety and fear, financial concerns, anger, impaired social interactions, feelings of inadequacy, cultural expectations, inadequate support system

   D. *Subjective symptoms of cardiac decompensation*: see Signs of Complications Box—Cardiac Decompensation

   E. *Objective signs of cardiac decompensation*: see Signs of Complications Box—Cardiac Decompensation

F. *Care during labor:* see Intrapartum section
- Comprehensive assessment for decompensation
- Decrease fear and anxiety with one-on-one care and support in a calm atmosphere; keep couple informed about what is happening and how woman and fetus are progressing
- Provide pain relief (epidural is recommended); use of comfort measures
- Vaginal birth is the best approach from a lateral position; avoid Valsalva maneuver and use of stirrups; use open glottis pushing with assistance of low forceps/vacuum and episiotomy, oxygen via mask, antibiotic therapy
- Avoid use of ergot products to prevent postpartum bleeding; intravenous Pitocin is recommended for this purpose

G. *Risk for postpartum cardiac decompensation:* problems occur as a result of hemodynamic changes associated with birth of baby and the circulatory and hormonal changes occurring with separation and expulsion of the placenta; cardiac output increases

H. *Nursing Diagnoses for early postpartum period:*
- Risk for excess fluid volume related to extravascular fluid shifts following birth would be the top priority physiologic nursing diagnosis
- Ineffective breastfeeding, risk for impaired mother-infant attachment, OR situational low-self esteem can be priority psychosocial nursing diagnoses related to the woman's need for activity reduction and limited ability to care for newborn on her own

I. *Stress reduction during postpartum period:* see Postpartum section; encourage rest in a lateral position; assist with ADLs and progressive ambulation; provide for pain relief and comfort; emphasize measures to prevent infection and constipation; assist with newborn care while keeping newborn nearby so she can see and touch her baby

J. *Breastfeeding:* breastfeeding is allowed but the woman will need extra support and rest owing to the increased energy demands associated with lactation

K. Discharge plan: emphasize the following:
- Follow-up with health care providers for assessment of postpartum recovery and cardiac status
- Contraception, future pregnancy, and sexuality issues
- Assistance with infant, self, and home care; make referrals as needed
- Importance of balancing rest and activity
- Instruct regarding the healing process, how to assess progress, and prevent complications

2. Pregnant woman with cardiac disorder needs to take heparin (see Antepartum section)
A. *Explain why heparin instead of Coumadin will be used:* discuss importance of taking an anticoagulant to prevent thrombus formation; inform that Coumadin will cross placenta and could cause congenital anomalies and fetal hemorrhage; heparin does not cross the placenta
B. *Information to ensure safe use of heparin:*
- Safe administration; teach subcutaneous injection technique to Allison and family
- Stress importance of routine blood tests to assess clotting ability
- Discuss foods that contain vitamin K, which will inhibit effectiveness of heparin; discuss alternative sources for folic acid

- Review side effects including unusual bleeding and bruising and measures to prevent injury (use soft tooth brush, no razors to shave)

3. *Pregnant woman with epilepsy:* see Epilepsy section of Neurologic Disorders; inform her that effects of pregnancy on epilepsy are unpredictable; convulsions may injure her or her fetus and lead to miscarriage, preterm labor, or separation of the placenta; medications, which will be given in the lowest therapeutic dose, must be taken to prevent convulsions; folic acid supplementation is important because anticonvulsants deplete folic acid stores

CHAPTER 34: OBSTETRIC CRITICAL CARE

Chapter Review Activities

1. Colloid osmotic pressure (COP), capillary, interstitial space, colloids, proteins, COP, hemodilution, proteins, capillary hydrostatic, pulmonary capillary wedge pressure (PCWP)

2. Respiratory alkalosis

3. Hypercoagulable, hemoconcentration, preeclampsia-eclampsia, dehydration

4. Systemic vascular resistance (SVR), ejection, vasodilation, uteroplacental circulation, SVR, pulmonary vascular resistance, decrease

5. Cardiac output, stroke volume, heart rate, increase

6. Heart rate, preload, afterload, contractility

7. T, 8. T, 9. F, 10. F, 11. F, 12. T, 13. T, 14. F, 15. F, 16. F, 17. T, 18. F, 19. T, 20. T, 21. F, 22. T, 23. F, 24. F, 25. F, 26. T, 27. T, 28. F, 29. T

30. *Rationale for obstetric critical care units:*
    - Differences in hemodynamics as a result of changes with pregnancy
    - Health care practitioners have expertise in caring for the unique needs of critically ill pregnant women
    - Ensure optimum outcome for both mother and infant; will enhance swift recognition of problems and prompt initiation of care that is adjusted to the needs of pregnant women
    - Appropriate equipment for care is readily available
    - Increased demand for this care as a result of women surviving childhood illnesses owing to advances in pediatric care; now as adults they are willing to take a chance on pregnancy

31. *Factors responsible for altering cardiac output during labor and the postpartum periods:* see Cardiac Output section of Hemodynamic Monitoring
    - *Labor:* 40% additional increase in cardiac output related to catecholamine release in response to pain and shunting of blood from placental-fetal unit during uterine contractions
    - *Postpartum:* large increase in cardiac output after birth; hemodynamic fluctuations related to net effect of blood loss and autotransfusion with approximately 1000 ml of blood that occurs after uterus is emptied; accumulated 6 to 8 L of extravascular fluid is mobilized into intravascular compartment, remaining for 7 to 10 days until diuresis can decrease it to prepregnant range

32. Techniques used to monitor oxygenation (see specific section in Hemodynamic Monitoring—Oxygenation)
    A. *Arterial blood gas analysis:* reflects dissolved oxygen in plasma, which is 1% to 2% of total oxygen content; requires arterial puncture or an arterial

catheter; see Table 34-3 for normal nonpregnant and pregnant ABG values

B. *Pulse oximeter*: measures blood bound to hemoglobin and available for cellular use; the oxygen saturation of hemoglobin represents 98% to 99% of total oxygen content; values for pregnancy range from 97% to 100%

C. *SvO$_2$ monitoring*: reflects balance between oxygen delivery and oxygen use; requires insertion of a fiberoptic PAC that is connected to a bedside microprocessor for a continuous SvO$_2$ value; normal value is 60% to 80%

33. B is the correct answer; pH ranges from 7.40 to 7.45; PO$_2$ during pregnancy ranges from 104 to 108 mm Hg; PCO$_2$ during pregnancy ranges from 27 to 32 mm Hg; bicarbonate during pregnancy ranges from 18 to 31 mEq/L.

34. A is correct; woman should be assisted into a slight Trendelenburg position with hip wedge; lidocaine hydrochloride should be on hand for arrhythmias; site care should be performed every shift or daily.

35. C is correct; the formula that should be used is:

$$\frac{\text{systolic} + 2(\text{diastolic})}{3}$$

36. B is correct; elevate nondominant hand; tell client to clench and unclench fist to facilitate venous drainage; only release pressure on the ulnar artery—capillary refill should occur in ≤5 seconds

Critical Thinking Exercises

1. Pregnant woman in obstetric critical care unit as a result of trauma
   A. *Insertion of an arterial pressure catheter;* see Arterial Pressure Catheter section of Hemodynamic Monitoring and Box 34-4 (Allen test); perform Allen test on nondominant hand to assess quality of circulation from ulnar artery in case of damage during puncture of radial artery; explain procedure to woman; comfort and support her during the procedure because stress and restlessness alter arterial blood gases and increase risk for arterial damage
   B. *Blood gas analysis:* see Table 34-3; values fall within the normal range for a pregnant woman
   C. *Glasgow Coma Scale:* see Box 34-6; consider ability for spontaneous movement (eyes) and conversation, ability to respond to verbal commands with movement and knowing name, date, time, and place, and respond to painful stimuli
   D. Left ventricle, slight Trendelenburg, hip wedge, engorged (distended), assess knowledge level and explain procedure, obtain and confirm an informed consent, support and encourage throughout procedures, initiate and obtain baseline ECG pattern, arterial pressure, pulse oximeter, cardiac, fluid, pulmonary
   E. *Positions to enhance cardiac output in a pregnant woman:* see Table 34-5 to determine cardiac output in a variety of positions; note that the lateral position supports an appropriate cardiac output
   F. *Supportive care measures for woman and family:* see Family Centered Obstetric Critical Care section; consider components of open visitation, parent-infant interaction and attachment, sibling and family visitation, information, and grief support

2. Trauma during pregnancy (see Trauma during Pregnancy section)
   A. *Significance of problem:* see Significance subsection; 8% incidence during pregnancy making it the leading nonobstetric cause of maternal mortality; risk increases as pregnancy progresses with most injuries occurring

in the third trimester; most common causes are motor vehicle accidents, falls, burns, gunshot wounds, assault

B. *Effects of trauma:* increased risk for miscarriage, preterm labor, abruptio placentae, stillbirth; influenced by gestational, type and severity of the trauma, degree of disruption of uterine and fetal physiologic features

C. *Type of trauma and effect of pregnancy:* see Maternal Physiologic Characteristics section and Table 34-8
- *Location of bladder and uterus:* distended bladder and uterus become abdominal organs, increase risk for injury and rupture
- *Elevation of progesterone levels:* relaxes smooth muscles and gastroesophageal sphincter and decreases gastric motility → increases time for gastric emptying and increases gastric acid production → increases risk for pulmonary trauma with aspiration
- *Changes in hemodynamic function:* always use lateral position or displace uterus laterally with a wedge to prevent supine hypotension; increased tolerance for blood loss related to expanded blood volume

D. *Impact of trauma on fetus:* fetal injury (skull fracture, intracranial hemorrhage, prematurity); death related to maternal death or abruptio placentae

E. *Potential effects of mechanisms of trauma:* see specific subsection for each mechanism in Mechanisms of Trauma section for a full description

F. Resuscitate the woman, stabilize her condition, fetal needs, fetal, maternal

G. *Outline primary and secondary surveys:* see Primary Survey and Secondary Survey sections to highlight the important components of each

CHAPTER 35: MENTAL HEALTH DISORDERS AND SUBSTANCE ABUSE

Chapter Review Activities

1. Mood disorders

2. Anxiety disorders, phobias, panic disorders, obsessive-compulsive disorder, posttraumatic stress disorder

3. Phobias
4. Panic disorder
5. Obsessive-compulsive disorder

6. Posttraumatic stress disorder, traumatic, stimuli, numbing, sleeping, irritability, angry, concentrating, hypervigilance, startle response

7. Sadness, mood swings, 10%, 15%, irritability, significant others, baby, rejection, jealousy, anxiety, panic attacks, crying

8. Depression, delusions, harming herself or her newborn, days, 2 to 3 weeks, 8 weeks, fatigue, insomnia, restlessness, tearfulness, emotional lability, suspiciousness, confusion, incoherence, irrational, obsessive concerns, infant, kill her infant

9. Bipolar disorder, manic, elevated, expansive, irritable
10. Panic attacks

11. F, 12. T, 13. F, 14. T, 15. T, 16. F, 17. T, 18. F, 19. F, 20. T, 21. T, 22. F, 23. T, 24. T, 25. F, 26. T, 27. T, 28. T, 29. F, 30. T, 31. T, 32. T, 33. F, 34. F

35. *Diagnostic criteria for diagnosis of major depression* (see Mood Disorders section); at least five of the following must be present every day: depressed mood, diminished interest, sleep disturbance, weight change,

psychomotor retardation/agitation, fatigue/decreased energy, feeling worthless/guilty, decreased ability to concentrate, suicidal ideation

36. *Risk factors for postpartum depression:* see Etiology and Risk Factors sections of Postpartum Psychologic Complications and Box 35-4; factors include prenatal depression or anxiety, postpartum blues, history of previous depression, child care stress, meager or absent social support, stressful life events, low self-esteem, poor martial/partner relationship, single-parent status, mother or head of household unemployed, difficult infant

37. *Difficulty of diagnosing depression during pregnancy:* see Nurse Alert—Mental Health Disorders during Pregnancy
    - Difficulty: many symptoms of pregnancy mimic depression
    - Cues: presence of psychologic symptoms, suicide plan, major sleep pattern disturbances, presence of risk factors (prior history in self or family, lack of social support, stressful life events, partner discord, history of PMS)

38. *Nursing diagnosis: impaired parent-infant attachment:* see Psychiatric Hospitalization section; reintroduce mother to her baby, help her to meet her baby's needs in a supervised setting, note signs of developing attachment

39. *Measures to prevent postpartum depression:* see Teaching for Self-Care Box—Activities to Prevent Postpartum Depression for several ideas for interventions and areas for teaching

40. CAGE assessment tool
    A. *Purpose for assessment tool:* CAGE questionnaire screen for alcohol use is the most popular test used in primary care; not tested for reliability with pregnant women in order to detect

levels of drinking that are considered harmful during pregnancy
    B. *Questions represented by each letter:* CAGE (Box 35-3)
    C. *Interpretation and scoring:* see Assessment and Nursing Diagnoses section of Substance Abuse during Pregnancy and Box 35-3 to determine scoring; CAGE tool scores yes to even one question as positive for substance abuse

41. *Predisposing factors for cocaine use during pregnancy:* see Cocaine section; polydrug use, poverty, dysfunctional family systems, employment difficulty, stress, anger, poor self-esteem, history of or present abuse (physical, emotional, sexual)

42. *Process of change and readiness for change:* see Plan of Care and Interventions—Substance Abuse during Pregnancy
    - See pregnancy as a window of opportunity for motivation to change.
    - Identify the steps a nurse should follow in order to identify women who are ready for change and the degree of readiness; supportive nursing interventions to facilitate change.
    - Identify problem with abuse and readiness for change (Prochaska-DiClemente model).
    - Use supportive interventions and motivational interviewing.

43. A is correct; Elavil is a commonly used tricyclic antidepressant that is safe to use during lactation especially if administration of medication and breastfeeding are carefully scheduled; Haldol has not been proven safe during lactation; Sinequan can lead to respiratory depression; Eskalith leads to high serum concentrations and is therefore contraindicated.

44. C is correct; the woman needs to avoid being a superwoman and placing unrealistic

expectations on herself; sharing feelings, rest, and some time away from the baby are all adaptive coping mechanisms.

45. A is correct; although the other questions are all appropriate, the potential for harming herself or her baby represents the most serious and very real concern.

46. B is correct; acute onset of labor with long hard uterine contractions and precipitous birth are characteristic of cocaine use; nutritional deficiencies would be characteristic of cocaine use; premature rupture of the membranes is associated with heroin use in pregnancy.

47. D is correct; the nurse should follow a sequence that establishes trust by starting with questions about substances that are least problematic for the woman and her fetus and are therefore the easiest to answer and to progress to questions about substances that are more problematic and therefore more difficult to answer; questions about caffeine, then alcohol, and lastly cocaine would be asked.

Critical Thinking Exercises

1. Woman with postpartum depression
   A. *Signs and symptoms indicative of postpartum depression:* fatigue, concerned about being a good mother but has a low level of self-esteem and self-confidence regarding her effectiveness, expressed jealousy of her husband's seemingly greater enjoyment when spending time with baby than with her, and angry outbursts directed against husband
   B. *Predisposing factors:* prenatal anxiety, meager social support and stressful life events (recent relocation, husband busy with new job), bottle feeding, mother unemployed and inexperienced with newborn care, 35 years of age

   C. *Questions:* see Box 35-4 to formulate questions related to risk factors for postpartum depression and also questions related to common manifestations; be sure to directly ask Mary about contemplating harm to self or baby; use open-ended questions that encourage full expression of feelings and thoughts
   D. *Nursing diagnoses:* several nursing diagnoses are listed in the Assessment and Nursing Diagnosis section; at this point, fatigue, situational low self-esteem, ineffective individual coping, risk for impaired parenting seems to be paramount
   E. *Measures to cope with postpartum depression:* see Plan of Care and Interventions—Home and Community section; include husband in discussions and planning, consider relationship with partner and suggest changes and resources they could seek out from their church and childrearing couples in their community; emphasize safety measures for mother or newborn; referral for psychiatric care with possible use of psychotropic medications if postpartum depression is determined to be moderate to severe; frequent follow-up to check progress is critical

2. Substance abuse during pregnancy (see Substance Abuse during Pregnancy section)
   A. *Profile creation:* see Risk Factors section; low self-esteem, and history of psychiatric illness or abuse are major characteristics of women who abuse substances
   B. *Barriers limiting access to treatment:* see Barriers to Treatment section; knowledge deficit of impact of substance abuse on self, pregnancy, or baby; late entry into prenatal care; expected negative feedback from health care providers; stigma associated with

abuse; denial of or lack of services; inadequate or no health insurance; fear of losing custody of children and criminal prosecution

C. *Approach during first health history interview to screen for substance abuse:* incorporate questions into overall prenatal history; be direct and nonjudgmental; start with questions about over-the-counter medications and gradually proceed to prescription drugs, alcohol, and then to illegal drugs; screen for STIs; use toxicology screens and questionnaires as indicated

D. *Considerations when planning care:*
   - Consider the characteristics of substance abusers including depression related to negative life experiences including violence; substance abuse may serve as a means of relieving loneliness and emptiness; abusers may have grown up in an environment where abuse is normal and have had little opportunity to learn sober living skills.
   - These characteristics can make change and recovery very difficult and interfere with their ability to be caring and nurturing parents; follow-up care is critical for safety of mother and the newborn.
   - Determine readiness for change and use measures that will facilitate change including the window of opportunity for change that pregnancy presents.

E. *Nursing measures:*
   - Assist with decreasing then stopping substance abuse; educate about effects of substances on pregnancy and fetus; be clear and confront if necessary; make referrals for treatment and to help woman deal with negative life experiences that may be contributing to the abuse of substances as a coping mechanism; assess progress and perform toxicology screens as indicated.

   - Recognize that ability to cope with childbirth may be limited; plan for toxicology screens of newborn.
   - Assess progress of maternal-newborn attachment and mother's level of knowledge and skill regarding newborn care; plan for discharge with the safety of the newborn of utmost importance; make arrangements for home visit follow-up and referral to services that will help mother to care for her baby and continue treatment; notify child protective services if indicated.

F. *Complete table related to maternal and fetal/newborn effects of specific substances:* see specific section for each substance to gather the information needed to complete the table

3. *Principles to follow for providing care to women who abuse alcohol or drugs:* see Treatment Programs for Alcohol and Drug Dependent Women section for description of principles to follow; emphasize
   - Family focus
   - Empowerment building
   - A community-based multidisciplinary approach with multiplicity of services; comprehensive, coordinated, holistic treatment
   - Continuum of care with consistent caregiver that allows for development of a trusting nonjudgmental relationship with health care provider and staff

CHAPTER 36: LABOR AND BIRTH COMPLICATIONS

Chapter Review Activities

1. C, 2. B, 3. D, 4. F, 5. A, 6. E, 7. G, 8. E, 9. F, 10. C, 11. D, 12. A, 13. G, 14. B

15. Preterm birth; very preterm birth
16. Preterm labor

17. Length of gestation (<37 weeks' gestation), weight at the time of birth (≤2500 g)

18. Preterm birth, intrauterine growth restriction, hypertensive disorders, poorly nourished

19. Biochemical markers, fetal fibronectin, salivary estriol
20. Fetal fibronectins, 24, 34, high, lower, vaginal
21. Salivary estriol, increase, high, lower

22. Endocervical length, transvaginal ultrasound, cervical length, 30 mm, singleton

23. Premature rupture of membranes (PROM)

24. Preterm premature rupture of membranes (PPROM), infection, infection, chorioamnionitis

25. Dystocia, five factors
26. Dysfunctional labor, cervical dilation, effacement, primary, descent, secondary

27. Hypertonic uterine dysfunction, painful, frequent, cervical dilation, effacement, latent, therapeutic rest

28. Hypotonic uterine dysfunction, weak, inefficient, stop
29. Pelvic dystocia

30. Soft tissue dystocia, placenta previa, leiomyomas (fibroids), ovarian tumors, full bladder, rectum
31. Fetal dystocia, cephalopelvic disproportion (CPD), fetopelvic disproportion (FPD), occipitoposterior position, breech presentation

32. Multifetal pregnancy

33. Cervical dilation, fetal descent, prolonged latent phase, protracted active phase, secondary arrest, protracted descent, arrest of descent, failure of descent, precipitous labor, hypertonic uterine contractions, tetanic

34. External cephalic version (ECV)
35. Trial of labor
36. Induction of labor

37. Bishop score, dilation (cm), effacement (%), station (cm), cervical consistency, cervical position, prostaglandins, ripen

38. Amniotomy, induce, augment
39. Augmentation of labor, oxytocin, amniotomy, nipple
40. Forceps-assisted birth
41. Vacuum-assisted birth, vacuum extraction
42. Cesarean birth
43. Postterm, postdate
44. Shoulder dystocia, excessive fetal size (macrosomia), pelvic abnormalities

45. Prolapse of umbilical cord, long cord, malpresentation (breech), transverse lie, unengaged presenting part, modified Sims, Trendelenburg, knee-chest, presenting part

46. Amniotic fluid embolism (AFE), meconium

47. F, 48. F, 49. T, 50. F, 51. F, 52. T, 53. F, 54. F, 55. T, 56. F, 57. T, 58. T, 59. T, 60. F, 61. T, 62. T, 63. T, 64. T, 65. F, 66. T, 67. T, 68. F, 69. T, 70. F

71. *Identify factors associated with risk categories for preterm labor and birth:* use Boxes 36-1 and 36-2 to complete this activity

72. *Bed rest more harmful than helpful:* see Bed Rest section of Plan of Care and Interventions and Box 36-4
    - Discuss the adverse effects of bed rest in terms of maternal physical and psychosocial effects and the effects on the woman's support system.
    - Cite the fact that there is no research evidence to support the effectiveness of

bed rest in preventing preterm birth or decreasing preterm birth rates.

73. *Five factors that cause dystocia:* see Dystocia section and specific sections for each factor
    - Powers: dysfunctional labor (ineffective uterine contractions or bearing down efforts)
    - Passage: altered pelvic diameters/shape; soft tissue abnormalities
    - Passenger: malpresentation or malposition, anomalies, size, number
    - Psychologic status of mother: past experiences, preparation, culture, support system, stress and anxiety level
    - Position of mother: ability and willingness to assume positions that facilitate uteroplacental perfusion and fetal descent

74. *Therapeutic rest:* see Hypertonic Uterine Dysfunction section
    - Purpose: help woman experiencing hypertonic uterine dysfunction to rest/sleep so active labor can begin usually after a 4- to 6-hour rest period
    - What: use of shower or warm bath for relaxation, comfort measures, administration of analgesics to inhibit contractions, reduce pain, and encourage rest/sleep and relaxation

75. *Complete table related to dysfunctional labor:* see Dysfunctional Labor section and Table 36-2 for information related to each dysfunctional labor pattern in terms of causes, maternal-fetal effects, changes in labor progress, and care management

76. *Amniotic fluid embolism:* see Amniotic fluid embolism section and Emergency Box—Amniotic fluid embolism
    A. *Risk factors:* multiparity, tumultuous labor, abruptio placentae, oxytocin induction, macrosomia, fetal death, meconium passage
    B. *Signs of amniotic fluid embolism:* see Emergency Box—Amniotic Fluid Embolism for a list of signs in terms of respiratory distress, circulatory collapse, hemorrhage
    C. *Recommended care management for amniotic fluid embolism:* see Emergency Box—Amniotic Fluid Embolism; consider interventions related to monitoring status of maternal-fetal unit, oxygenation, maintaining cardiac output, replacing fluid losses, observing for and correcting coagulation failure (DIC), preparing for emergency birth, and providing emotional support

77. *Indications and contraindications for oxytocin induction of labor:* see Oxytocin section of Plan of Care and Interventions—Dystocia; several indicators and contraindications are listed

78. D is correct; women younger than 17 or older than 35 years of age represent a higher risk for preterm labor and birth along with parity of 0 or >4, history of preterm labor or birth, multiple abortions, or short interpregnancy interval; infections of the genitourinary tract including recurrent UTIs and reproductive tract infections such as bacterial vaginosis.

79. A is correct; the woman should count contractions for 1 more hour and drink two to three glasses of water or juice after emptying bladder; conservative measures are tried before coming to the clinic for evaluation; she can resume light activity if contractions subside but should call for further instructions if they do not.

80. B is correct; weight loss, not gain, occurs; sleep disturbances lead to fatigue and emotional changes; lack of weight-bearing activity leads to bone demineralization.

81. C is correct; fluid intake should be limited to 2500 ml per day; increase in heart rate is associated with beta-adrenergic agonist drugs such as ritodrine or terbutaline;

magnesium sulfate is a CNS depressant; woman should alternate lateral positions to decrease pressure on cervix, which could stimulate uterine contractions and to enhance uteroplacental circulation.

82. C is correct; it is inserted into the posterior vaginal fornix; the woman should remain in bed for 2 hours; caution should be used if the woman has asthma, therefore ensure that physician is aware; the insert is removed for severe side effects such as tachysystole or hyperstimulation of the uterus; Cervidil often stimulates contractions and may even induce the onset of labor, eliminating or reducing the need for Pitocin.

83. D is correct; a Bishop score of 9 indicates that the cervix is already sufficiently ripe for successful induction; 10 U of Pitocin are usually mixed in 1000 ml of an electrolyte solution such as Ringers lactate; the Pitocin solution is piggybacked at the proximal port (port nearest the insertion site).

84. A is correct; frequency of uterine contractions should not be less than every 2 minutes to allow for an adequate rest period between contractions; B, C, and D are all expected findings within the normal range.

85. B is correct; at 6 cm the woman is in active labor with progress that is less than 1.5 cm/hr; secondary arrest indicates no progress for ≥2 hours; precipitous labor refers to rapid dilation of 10 cm in 1 hour for a multiparous woman.

86. C is correct; the presentation of this fetus is breech; the soft buttocks are a less efficient dilating wedge than the fetal head, therefore labor may be slower; the ultrasound transducer should be placed to the left of the umbilicus at a level at or above it; passage of meconium is an expected finding as a result of pressure on the abdomen during descent; knee-chest position is most often used for occipitoposterior positions.

Critical Thinking Exercises

1. *Preterm Labor and Birth Prevention Program:* see Predicting Preterm Labor and Birth and Early Recognition and Diagnosis subsections
   - Why: preterm birth is a major factor contributing to perinatal morbidity and mortality; early detection is critical for successful tocolysis and antenatal glucocorticoid therapy
   - Many risk factors for preterm labor have been identified (Boxes 36-1 and 36-2) but risk scoring systems miss 50% of women who go into preterm labor
   - All women should be taught signs of preterm labor and measures to prevent based on risk factors identified that can be manipulated by changes in lifestyle behaviors (see Box 36-3)

2. *Woman with a history of preterm labor and birth*
   A. *Identify signs of preterm labor:* see Box 36-3 as a guide for teaching Sara about preterm labor; see if Sara can retrospectively remember experiencing these vague signs with her first pregnancy
   B. *Implementation of plan to prevent preterm labor:*
      - Evaluate Sara's lifestyle for risky behaviors and health history for risk factors for preterm labor.
      - Discuss how certain factors identified could be changed to reduce her risk especially related to lifestyle (see Lifestyle Modifications section).
      - Consider modification of sexual activity, stress level, activity (work, home), and hygiene (prevent GU tract infections).
   C. *Woman begins to experience uterine contraction:* empty bladder, drink two to

three glasses of water/juice, lie down on left side and count contractions by palpating abdomen for 1 hour; call if contractions continue and progress; resume light activity if they do not

D. *Criteria for use of tocolysis:* assess Sara to make sure that she is indeed in labor and that she does not exhibit contraindications to tocolysis (Box 36-5)

E. *Nursing measures during ritodrine infusion to suppress preterm labor:* see Suppression of Uterine Activity—Tocolytics section including Nurse Alert, Table 36-1: Medication Guide—Tocolytic Therapy for Preterm Labor, and Box 36-6
   - Assessment for labor progress and maternal-fetal responses to ritodrine including adverse reactions
   - Monitor and regulate infusion following protocol for increments in dosage of ritodrine
   - Measure intake and output
   - Provide support and encouragement
   - Maintain bed rest in lateral position

F. *Administration of betamethasone:* see Promotion of Fetal Lung Maturity section
   1. *Purpose:* stimulation of fetal surfactant production
   2. *Protocol:* see Medication Guide Box—Antenatal Glucocorticoid Therapy; assess Sara for signs of infection, explain action and indications for use, administer IM deep into gluteal muscle, 12 mg, twice, 24 hours apart, observe for adverse effects

3. *Woman experiencing preterm labor discharged to home care:* see Suppression of Uterine Activity and Home Care subsections of Preterm Labor Care Management section and Plan of Care for Preterm Labor
   A. *Nursing diagnoses:* Risk for maternal/fetal injury related to effects of terbutaline therapy and bed rest

requirement for the suppression of preterm labor; interrupted family processes related to demands of labor suppression regimen

B. *Instructions for maintaining terbutaline pump* (see Table 36-1): discuss use of pump including signs of problems and site care; site change and adjustment of settings may be done by woman or by home care nurse; identify side effects of terbutaline and whom to call if they should appear; teach her how to assess her vital signs, especially how to count her pulse and assess for changes in her respiratory status

C. *Side effects of terbutaline:* see Table 36-1: Medication Guide, which lists signs that should be taught to the client

D. *Instructions regarding home uterine activity monitor:* see Home Uterine Activity Monitoring subsection; discuss how often to monitor (once or twice a day while lying on side), how to transmit and check results, what to do if contraction patterns indicate resumption of preterm labor; teach her how to palpate abdomen for uterine contractions

E. *Coping with bed rest:* see Teaching for Self-Care Boxes—Suggested Activities for Women on Bed Rest and Activities for Children of Women on Bed Rest; identify members of her support system and include them in discussions of how bed rest will be managed and how they can help; make referrals to home care agencies if needed

4. *Woman with occipitoposterior position and difficulty bearing down* (see Dystocia— Secondary Powers and Fetal Causes— Malposition sections, Table 36-2, and Box 36-7)
   A. *Identifying factors that have a negative effect on bearing down efforts:* amount of analgesia/anesthesia used, exhaustion, maternal position, lack of knowledge

about how to push effectively, lack of sleep, inadequate food and fluid intake

  B. *Measures to facilitate bearing down efforts:* coach her in BDE, help her into an appropriate position, apply counterpressure to sacrum to reduce back pain, demonstrate open glottis pushing and coach her efforts with every contraction, help her to begin pushing when Ferguson reflex is perceived

  C. *Recommended positions:* hands and knees or lateral when the fetus is in an occipitoposterior position can be very effective in facilitating internal rotation and reducing back pain; other positions include squatting, pelvic rocking, stair climbing, or lying on right side

5. *Emergency cesarean birth:* see Cesarean Birth section and Care Path—Cesarean Birth

  A. *Preoperative measures:* implement typical preoperative care measures as for any major surgery in a calm and professional manner explaining the purpose of each measure that must be performed; use a family-centered approach; discuss what will happen; witness an informed consent; assess fetal-maternal unit, insert Foley catheter, start or maintain IV infusion, provide emotional support

  B. *Immediate postoperative measures:* see Immediate Postoperative Care subsection; assess for signs of hemorrhage, pain level, respiratory effort, renal function, circulatory status to extremities, emotional status, and attachment/reaction to newborn; initiate breastfeeding if mother is able and willing

  C. *Ongoing postoperative care measures:* see Postoperative/Postpartum Care section, Care Path, Teaching for Self-Care Boxes; measures include assessment of recovery, pain relief, coughing and deep breathing, leg exercises and assistance

with ambulation, nutrition and fluid intake (oral, IV); provide opportunities for interaction and care of newborn, assisting her as needed; provide emotional support to help her deal with her disappointment and feelings of failure; help her and her family prepare for discharge making referrals a needed

  D. *Nursing diagnosis:* Situational low self-esteem related to inability to reach goal of a vaginal birth secondary to occurrence of fetal distress

- Discuss and review why Anne needed a cesarean birth, how she performed during labor, and that she had no control over the fetal distress that occurred.
- Discuss VBAC and likelihood of it being an option because the reason for her primary cesarean (fetal distress) may not occur again; discuss trial of labor next time to determine her ability to proceed to vaginal birth.
- Use follow-up phone calls to assess progress in accepting cesarean birth.

6. *Fetal position/presentation—RSA:* see Malpresentation section of Dystocia; RSA indicates a breech presentation; consider that descent may be slower, meconium is often expelled increasing danger of meconium aspiration, and risk for cord prolapse is increased; depending on progress of labor and maternal characteristics cesarean or vaginal birth may occur; external cephalic version may be attempted if appropriate

7. *Induction of labor* (see Induction of Labor section and Box 36-8)

  A. *Bishop score:* see Table 36-4 for factors assessed to determine degree of cervical ripening in preparation for labor process and its inducibility; it is used to determine if a cervical ripening method will need to be used to increase the chances of a successful labor induction

B. *Score of 5 for a nulliparous woman:* as a nulliparous woman her score should be 9 or greater to ensure a successful induction; cervical ripening/preparation will be needed prior to her induction

C. *Administration of Cervidil:* see Cervical Ripening Methods section and Medication Guide for dinoprostone (Cervidil)

- Insert into posterior fornix of vagina
- Side effects include headache, nausea and vomiting, fever, diarrhea, hypotension, hyperstimulation of uterine contractions with or without fetal distress
- After administration the woman should remain in bed in a lateral position for approximately 2 hours; she may then be allowed to ambulate
- Monitor vital signs, uterine activity, and FHR pattern

D. *Amniotomy:* see Procedure Box—Assisting with Amniotomy; explain what will happen, how it will feel, and why it is being done; assess maternal-fetal unit including FHR and pattern before and after the procedure; be alert for signs of variable decelerations; assess characteristics of fluid and provide for cleansing and comfort measures; document findings; support woman during procedure, telling her what is happening

E. *Induction protocol:*
1) A
2) A
3) A
4) A
5) NA
6) NA
7) NA
8) A
9) NA
10) A
11) NA

F. *Major side effects of Pitocin induction:* hyperstimulation of the uterus, uterine rupture, nonreassuring FHR patterns, water intoxication

G. *Actions if hyperstimulation occur:* see Box 36-8 and Emergency Box—Uterine Hyperstimulation with Oxytocin, which lists signs related to uterine contractions and nonreassuring FHR patterns as well as immediate interventions such as discontinuing the induction, maintaining the primary infusion of fluid, turning the woman on her side, administering oxygen via mask, monitoring response of maternal-fetal unit to actions, notifying primary health care provider, and preparing for possible administration of terbutaline to suppress contractions

8. *Postterm pregnancy:* see Postterm Pregnancy, Labor, and Birth section

A. *Maternal-fetal risks related to postterm pregnancy:* see Maternal-Fetal Risks section; maternal risk relates to excessive size of fetus and hardness of fetal skull, which increases risk for dystocia and birth trauma, postpartum hemorrhage, and infection; fetal risk relates to postmaturity syndrome as the placenta ages and a stressful labor and birth process including increased risk for hypoxia, birth injury, and neonatal hypoglycemia

B. *Clinical manifestations:* maternal weight loss, decrease in uterine size, meconium in amniotic fluid, advanced fetal bone maturation including the skull

C. *Nursing diagnosis:* Risk for fetal injury related to placental aging and difficult birth associated with prolonged pregnancy

D. *Care measures to insure safety of maternal-fetal unit:* see Collaborative Care section

- Continue prenatal care with more frequent visits

- Antepartal assessments including daily fetal movement counts, NST, amniotic fluid volume assessments, BPP, CST, Doppler blood flow measurements, cervical checks for ripening
- Emotional support; encourage expression of feelings
- Prepare for cervical ripening, induction of labor, monitoring for late and variable deceleration patterns, amnioinfusion, forceps- or vacuum-assisted or cesarean birth

E. *Instructions for self-care at home*: see Teaching for Self-Care Box—Postterm Pregnancy
- Make sure Lora knows how to assess fetal movements and signs of labor.
- Emphasize importance of keeping all appointments for prenatal care and antepartal assessments.
- Identify who to call with concerns, questions, and reports of changing status such as onset of labor or change in fetal movement pattern.

CHAPTER 37: POSTPARTUM COMPLICATIONS

Chapter Review Activities

1. Postpartum hemorrhage (PPH), 10%, hematocrit, erythrocyte transfusion, uterine atony, early (acute, primary) PPH, late (secondary) PPH

2. Uterine atony

3. Pelvic hematoma, vulva hematomas, vaginal hematomas, perineal, rectal, vagina

4. Inversion of the uterus, hemorrhage, shock, pain, fundal, vigorous fundal, excessive traction, uterine atony, leiomyomas (fibroids), placenta tissue

5. Subinvolution, retained placental fragments, pelvic infection
6. Hemorrhagic (hypovolemic) shock

7. Coagulopathy, idiopathic (immune) thrombocytopenic purpura (ITP), Von Willebrand disease, disseminated intravascular coagulation (DIC)

8. Thrombosis, inflammation (thrombophlebitis), obstruction, superficial venous thrombosis, deep venous thrombosis, pulmonary embolism

9. Postpartum or puerperal infection, fever, 2 successive days of the first 10 postpartum days excluding the first 24 hours, uterus, wounds, breasts, urinary tract, respiratory tract

10. Endometritis, placental
11. Mastitis, first-time mothers who are breastfeeding, unilateral, flow of milk

12. F, 13. T, 14. T, 15. T, 16. F, 17. T, 18. F, 19. T, 20. F, 21. F, 22. T, 23. T, 24. F, 25. F, 26. T, 27. F

28. B is correct; although BP should be taken before and after administration of Methergine, the woman's hypertensive status would be a contraindicating factor for its use, therefore the order should be questioned; a more appropriate choice would be Pitocin.

29. D is correct; Hemabate is a powerful prostaglandin that is the third-line medication given to treat excessive uterine blood loss or hemorrhage related to uterine atony; it has no action related to pain, infection, or clotting.

30. A is correct; puerperal infections are infections of the genital tract after birth; pulse will increase not decrease in response to fever; B and C will also occur but are not the first signs exhibited.

31. C is correct; heparin and warfarin are safe for use by breastfeeding women; heparin usually administered intravenously is the anticoagulant of choice during the acute stage of DVT; woman should be fitted for elastic stockings after the acute stage is past when edema subsides.

32. *Twofold focus of management of hemorrhagic shock:* restore circulating blood volume and perfusion and treat the cause of the hemorrhage

33. *Four priority nursing interventions for PPH:* see Nursing Interventions section of Postpartum Hemorrhage; cite interventions related to improving and monitoring tissue perfusion, treating the cause of the hemorrhage, supporting the woman and her family, and fostering maternal-infant attachment as appropriate

34. *Standard of care for bleeding emergencies:* provision should be made for the nurse to implement actions independently—policies, procedures, standing orders or protocols, and clinical guides should be established by the agency and agreed upon by health care providers including nurses; the nurse should never leave the client alone

Critical Thinking Exercises

1. Postpartum woman at risk for postpartum hemorrhage
   A. *Risk factors for early postpartum hemorrhage:* parity (5–1–0–7), vaginal full-term twin birth 1 hour ago, hypotonic uterine dysfunction treated with Pitocin, use of forceps for birth, increased manipulation with birth of twins; increases size and stretch of uterus with a multiple gestation
   B. *Nursing diagnosis:* Risk for deficient fluid volume related to moderate to heavy blood loss associated with vaginal birth of twins
   C. *Nurse's response to excessive blood loss in 15 minutes:* most common cause of the excessive blood loss 1 hour after birth would be uterine atony especially because woman exhibits several risk factors
      • Assess fundus for consistency, height, and location; massage if boggy.
      • Express clots if present once uterus is firm.
      • Check bladder for distention (distended bladder will reduce uterine contraction); check perineum for swelling and ask woman about experiencing perineal pressure (hematoma formation is possible related to use of forceps for birth).
   D. *Guidelines for administering Pitocin IV:* use Table 37-1 in explaining guidelines for administration in terms of dose/route, side effects, nursing management including assessment and maternal support
   E. *Signs of developing hemorrhagic shock:* see Emergency Box—Hemorrhagic Shock, which identifies the priority assessment a nurse should perform and the findings that would indicate progress from hemorrhage to shock; assessment includes VS, skin, urinary output, level of consciousness, and mental status; assessment should be frequent and findings compared to one another to note change
   F. *Nursing measures to support the woman and family:*
      • Explain progress—meaning of findings and need for treatment measures being used including their purpose, and effectiveness
      • Calm, professional, organized approach that incorporates periods of uninterrupted rest
      • Comfort measures
      • Opportunities for interaction with newborn; updates on newborn's status

2. Puerperal infection
   A. *Risk factors:* see Box 37-4; consider preconception, antepartal, and intrapartal factors
   B. *Infection prevention measures:* see Plan of Care and Interventions—Postpartum Infections; emphasize measures to maintain resistance to infection (nutrition, rest, hygiene); use of standard precautions including handwashing, proper use of gloves, and care of equipment; teach woman about prevention measures including genital hygiene and safer sex practices
   C. *Typical signs of endometritis:* see Endometritis subsection; signs include fever, tachycardia, chills, anorexia, nausea, fatigue and lethargy, pelvic pain and uterine tenderness, foul-smelling profuse lochia, leukocytosis, increased RBC sedimentation rate
   D. *Nursing diagnoses:* Acute pain related to effects of infection in uterine tissue; interrupted family process OR anxiety OR ineffective individual or family coping related to unexpected postpartum complication (use assessment findings to determine priority psychosocial nursing diagnoses)
   E. *Nursing measures:* see Plan of Care and Interventions
      • Assess progress of healing.
      • Administer antibiotics as prescribed; teach woman about correct use.
      • Ensure adequate hydration, nutrition, rest to enhance healing.
      • Provide comfort measures and medications for pain relief.
      • Explain health problem, cause, and basis for therapeutic measures implemented.
      • Arrange for newborn interaction and care.
      • Use support measures and teaching to prepare woman for discharge.

3. Woman with mastitis (see Mastitis section)
   A. *Assessment findings associated with mastitis:* unilateral findings well after milk comes in; inflammation and edema with breast engorgement; chills, fever, malaise, localized tenderness, pain, swelling, and redness; axillary adenopathy; an infected nipple fissure may be present
   B. *Nursing diagnoses:* Acute pain related to inflammation of right breast; ineffective breastfeeding OR anxiety related to interruption of breastfeeding while taking antibiotics or related to concerns regarding transmission of infection to newborn
   C. *Treatment measures:* antibiotics, breast support, local heat and cold applications, adequate hydration and nutrition, analgesics; maintain lactation with continued breastfeeding if permitted or with breast pumping
   D. *Measures to prevent recurrence of mastitis:* good breastfeeding technique to preserve nipple and areolar integrity (latch-on and removal, alternating positions and starting breast), frequent feedings (avoid missing feedings, waiting too long, or abrupt weaning), breast care, and early detection and treatment of cracks; cleanliness

4. Woman with deep vein thrombosis (see Thromboembolic Disease section)
   A. *Risk factors:* see Incidence and Etiology subsection; in addition to venous stasis and hypercoagulability of pregnancy continuing into the postpartum period, other risk factors for this woman would be cesarean birth, obesity, age over 35 years, and multiparity
   B. *Signs and symptoms indicative of DVT:* see Clinical Manifestations section; unilateral leg pain and calf tenderness, swelling, redness and warmth, positive Homans' sign; woman may also be

asymptomatic or have few symptoms with a DVT depending on degree of involvement

C. *Nursing diagnosis:* Anxiety related to unexpected development of a postpartum complication

D. *Expected care management:* see Medical Management and Nursing Interventions sections
- Assess for unusual bleeding, signs of pulmonary embolism, circulatory status of lower extremities.
- Administer anticoagulant (usually heparin during the acute phase and warfarin after first few days) as ordered.
- Bed rest with elevation of affected leg; assist to change position; caution not to rub site.
- Pain management using analgesics without aspirin; local application of warm moist heat.
- Fit with elastic support stocking after acute phase.
- Reassure her that she can continue to breastfeed safely.
- Explain disorder and purpose and effectiveness of treatment measures used.
- Assist with care of self and newborn.

E. *Discharge instructions:*
- How to assess leg and for signs of unusual bleeding
- Proper use of elastic/support stockings
- How to take anticoagulant safely and importance of follow-up to assess progress
- Practices to prevent bleeding while taking an anticoagulant and importance of avoiding pregnancy because warfarin is teratogenic

CHAPTER 38: ACQUIRED PROBLEMS OF THE NEWBORN

Chapter Review Activities

1. F, 2. T, 3. T, 4. F, 5. T, 6. F, 7. F, 8. T, 9. T, 10. T, 11. F, 12. F, 13. F, 14. T, 15. F, 16. T, 17. T, 18. T, 19. F, 20. T, 21. T, 22. T, 23. F, 24. F, 25. T, 26. T, 27. T, 28. F, 29. T, 30. F, 31. T, 32. F, 33. T

34. Birth injuries (see Birth Trauma section)
A. *Risk factors for trauma:* macrosomia, CPD, congenital anomalies (e.g., hydrocephalus), abnormal or difficult presentations, prolonged and difficult labor necessitating the use of forceps or vacuum, version, or cesarean birth, precipitous labor, preterm or postterm labor and birth, multiple gestation
B. *Signs of fractured clavicle:* see Skeletal Injuries section; signs include limited motion of arm and absence of Moro reflex on affected side, crepitus over the bone
C. *Treatment:* there is no accepted standard treatment; may be limited to gently handling and supporting shoulder when changing clothes and moving and proper alignment; alert caregivers and parents regarding need for special handling; support and reassure parents

35. Diabetes, obstetric, neonatal, decrease, 2 to 3 times, blood glucose, ketoacidosis, hyperglycemia, glucose, insulin, growth, macrosomia, acidotic, ketoacidosis, carbon dioxide, oxygen, macrosomia, hypoglycemia, polyhydramnios, preterm birth, lung immaturity, glucose

36. *Common congenital anomalies experienced by infants of diabetic mothers:* see Congenital Anomalies section of Infants of Diabetic Mothers for full identification of anomalies in each category

37. Macrosomic infant (see Macrosomia section of Neonatal Complications)
    A. *Characteristics:* round face, chubby body, plethoric/flushed complexion, enlarged organs, increased fat deposits, placenta and cord are larger than average
    B. Hypoglycemia, hypocalcemia, hyperviscosity, hyperbilirubinemia
    C. *Warning signs of potential complications:* see section for each category: birth trauma, perinatal hypoxia, RDS, hypoglycemia, hypocalcemia, hypomagnesemia, cardiomyopathy, hyperbilirubinemia, and polycythemia

38. *Infections represented by TORCH:* see Box 38-1 for infections represented by each letter

39. Sepsis (see Neonatal Infections section)
    A. *Complete table related to modes of transmission of infection:* see Sepsis section for a review of prenatal, perinatal, and postnatal transmission modes
    B. *Risk factors:* see Table 38-2, which lists risk factors according to maternal, intrapartum, and neonatal sources
    C. *Signs of sepsis exhibited by neonate:* see Table 38-3 for a list of signs according to body systems
    D. *Effective nursing measures:* see appropriate sections for Prevention, Cure, and Rehabilitation measures in the Plan of Care and Interventions

40. B is correct; findings are consistent with a bone fracture, in this case the clavicle.

41. C is correct; macrosomic infants are at increased risk for hypoglycemia (e.g., a blood glucose level of 38 mg/dl would be considered hypoglycemia); fracture and trauma are more common in the upper body such as the humerus and clavicle; hypocalcemia is common; the newborn of a pregestational diabetic mother is more likely to experience congenital anomalies such as heart defects; there is no increased risk with gestational diabetes.

42. D is correct; risk for transmission of infection is more likely if membranes rupture more than 4 hours before birth and with preterm birth; elective cesarean birth may be used before rupture of membranes as a protection from HIV transmission.

43. B is correct; isolation is not required nor are gloves for routine care measures; the nurse should be using standard precautions as would be used with all clients; zidovudine treatment begins after birth and continues for 6 weeks following delivery until HIV status is determined.

Critical Thinking Exercises

1. Newborn whose mother is Hepatitis B positive (see Hepatitis B subsection of TORCH Infections section)
    A. *Protocol for newborn care:* Hepatitis B immunoglobulin (HBIG) 0.5 ml intramuscularly as soon as possible within the first 12 hours after birth; administer Hepatitis B vaccine within the first week of birth repeating at 1 month and at 6 months of age
    B. *Safety of breastfeeding:* it is safe to breastfeed after the infant has been cleansed and the vaccine has been administered

2. Newborn whose mother has active herpes at the time of birth (see Herpes Simplex Virus subsection of TORCH Infections section)
    A. *Four modes of transmission:* transplacental; ascending transmission

by way of birth canal; direct contamination during passage through an infected birth canal (mode for this baby); and direct transmission to the newborn by an infected person

B. *Clinical signs of active infection in the newborn:* encephalitis (CNS involvement); disseminated infection involving several body organs especially liver, adrenal glands and lungs; localized infection including vesicles on skin, in oral cavity, in eyes

C. *Recommended nursing measures related to:*
  - *Management after birth, prior to discharge:* wear gloves when handling the newborn; inspect for lesions and obtain cultures from mouth, eyes, and lesions as indicated; delay circumcision; discharge with mother if cultures are negative; breastfeeding is allowed if there are no lesions on the breasts; arrange for follow-up health care
  - *Vidarabine or acyclovir therapy:* Acyclovir is usually administered IV every 8 hours for at least 14 days to treat infection; vidarabine ophthalmic ointment can be used for 5 days to prevent keratoconjunctivitis

3. Newborn whose mother is HIV positive: see HIV/AIDS subsection of TORCH infections section
  A. *Potential for newborn infection:* there is a 25% risk for transmission unless AZT was used during pregnancy, in which case the risk would be reduced to 8%
  B. *Modes of transmission:* prenatal (transplacental); perinatal (exposure to maternal blood and secretions during childbirth process), postpartum (maternal secretions including breast milk)
  C. *Testing protocol:* testing (first 48 hours after birth), at 1 to 2 months of age, and at 3 to 6 months; tests (PCR assays, viral cultures); at least two tests should

be done before a definitive diagnosis is made

  D. *Opportunistic infections:* common AIDS-defining secondary infections can include pneumocystis carinii pneumonia, candidiasis, CMV infection, cryptosporidiosis, herpes simplex or herpes zoster, disseminated varicella

  E. *Care measures:*
  - Standard Precautions; protect infant from further exposure to maternal body fluids; gloves for routine care and isolation are not required
  - Cleanse skin with soap and water and alcohol after birth before invasive procedures are performed
  - Antimicrobials as indicated for treatment and prevention of infection; immunizations except for oral poliovirus and varicella vaccines; treat with AZT for 6 weeks after birth until HIV status is known
  - Arrangements made for counseling, referrals, and follow-up for care and testing as indicated

  F. *Breastfeeding safety:* because breast milk can contain the virus, the newborn should not be breastfed; teach mother how to bottle feed and demonstrate how she can have close contact with her newborn during feeding

4. Infant with thrush (see Fungal Infection section)
  A. *Signs:* white, adherent patches on mucosa, gums, and tongue that bleed when touched
  B. *Modes of transmission:* maternal vaginal infection during birth, person-to-person contact, contaminated hands, bottles, nipples, or other articles
  C. *Management:* infection control measures along with cleanliness and good hygiene to prevent infection and measures to improve resistance to infection; cleanse mouth with sterile water after feeding to wash out residual

milk, then instill nystatin into the mouth with a medicine dropper or swab onto oral mucosa, gums, and tongue; treat mother's breast with topical nystatin

5. Newborn with fetal alcohol syndrome—FAS (see Alcohol subsection of Substance Abuse section)
   A. *Typical characteristics:* see Tables 38-4 and 38-5 and Fig. 38-14 for a full description of the newborn diagnosed with FAS
   B. *Long-term effects:* impaired vasomotor perception and performance, lowered IQ scores, delayed receptive and expressive language, reduced capacity to store and process factual data, poor attention span, disciplinary problems, autism, and social delays (e.g., lack inhibition and stranger anxiety, impaired judgment)
   C. *Nursing measures:* involve parents in care of newborn, encouraging attachment; teach parents what to expect about their child's behavior; help the parents to create a warm and caring home environment that enhances development; make appropriate referrals to community services for the newborn as well as treatment program for the mother to help her with her alcohol abuse problem (father may also need assistance)

6. Effect of maternal substance abuse on the newborn (see Substance Abuse section)
   A. *Signs of withdrawal from heroin and methadone:* see specific subsection for each substance
   B. *Effect of cocaine exposure:* see Box 38-2 for list of neonatal effects in terms of physical and behavioral assessment findings

7. Newborn of mother suspected of abusing drugs during pregnancy
   A. *Signs of neonatal abstinence syndrome:* see Table 38-6 for a list of signs in terms of gastrointestinal, CNS, metabolic, vasomotor, and respiratory function
   B. *Nursing diagnoses:* Deficient fluid volume related to inadequate fluid intake and increased fluid loss related to heroin withdrawal; disorganized infant behavior OR disturbed sleep pattern related to withdrawal from heroin; risk for infection related to risky maternal behaviors associated with drug abuse
   C. *Care management* (see Plan of Care and Teaching for Self-Care Box—Care of Infant Experiencing Withdrawal): encourage parent participation in care of newborn providing education and social support as needed; maintain nutrition, fluid, and electrolyte balance with careful management of feeding; infection control and respiratory care; swaddling and holding; stimuli reduction; pharmacologic treatment as appropriate; discharge planning and referral

CHAPTER 39: HEMOLYTIC DISORDERS AND CONGENITAL ANOMALIES

Chapter Review Activities

1. Inborn errors of metabolism
2. Microcephaly
3. Hypospadias, epispadias, exstrophy of the bladder
4. Hydrocephalus
5. Congenital heart defects
6. Talipes equinovarus
7. Choanal atresia
8. Meningocele
9. Omphalocele, gastroschisis
10. Esophageal atresia
11. Anencephaly

12. Diaphragmatic hernia
13. Myelomeningocele

14. F, 15. T, 16. F, 17. F, 18. T, 19. T, 20. F, 21. T, 22. T, 23. F, 24. F, 25. T, 26. F, 27. F

28. *Physiologic basis for ABO incompatibility:* see ABO subsection of Pathologic Jaundice section; fetal blood is A, B, or AB and mother's blood type is O; naturally occurring anti-A and anti-B antibodies can cross the placenta, resulting in hemolysis of the fetus/newborn's red blood cells; women with blood type O already have anti-A and anti-B antibodies in their blood

29. Congenital anomalies
    A. Genetic, hereditary, congenital, genetic, environmental, multifactorial, genes, environmental, neural tube defects, congenital heart defects, developmental dysplasia of the hip, club foot, cleft lip, palate
    B. *Assessment techniques/considerations guiding prenatal diagnosis:* see Prenatal Diagnosis subsection; analyze history and medical information for factors and exposures associated with congenital disorders; tests: amniocentesis, ultrasound, MsAFP, chorionic villus sampling, percutaneous umbilical blood sampling, gene probes, fetal nuchal translucent screening
    C. *Observations of amount of amniotic fluid:* see Prenatal Diagnosis subsection; hydramnios is commonly associated with congenital anomalies; oligohydramnios often indicates renal/urinary tract anomalies; careful observation at the time of birth is essential so immediate care can be provided as appropriate; take note of color, VS including cardiac and respiratory function, crying, activity level, appearance in terms of structural anomalies such as ears, face, fingers, toes, and feet
    D. *Specific types of postnatal tests for diagnosis of congenital anomalies:* see specific subsections of Postnatal Diagnosis section
       - *Biochemical tests:* testing for inborn errors of metabolism (e.g., PKU, galactosemia, hypothyroidism
       - *Cytologic studies:* chromosomal examination is used to confirm suggestive but not diagnostic clinical appearance
       - *Dermatoglyphics:* study of the pattern of ridges in the skin of the hands, digits, and feet (e.g., simian crease suggestive of Down syndrome)

30. Congenital heart defects (see Cardiovascular System Anomalies section)
    A. *Maternal factors associated with higher risk:* include rubella, alcoholism, diabetes, poor nutrition, age older than 40, ingestion of certain medications, radiation exposure
    B. *Four physiologic classifications; include one example of each* (see Table 39-1 for examples of each classification)
       - Defects that result in increased pulmonary blood flow
       - Defects that involve decreased pulmonary blood flow and typically result in cyanosis
       - Defects that cause obstruction of blood flow out of the heart
       - Complex cardiac anomalies that involve the flow of mixed saturated and desaturated blood in the heart or great vessels
    C. *Signs that could indicate CHD:* weak, muffled, or loud and breathless cry, cyanosis unrelieved by oxygen, cyanosis that increases when newborn is supine or cries, pallor, mottling on exertion, respiratory signs, activity effects, bradycardia or tachycardia, irregular heart rate or murmurs; signs of congestive heart failure

31. B is correct; at 16 mg/dl the serum bilirubin exceeds 15 mg/dl on the second day of life; other signs of pathologic hyperbilirubinemia include serum bilirubin concentration in cord blood >4 mg/dl, increase of ≥5 mg/dl in 24 hours, and appearance of jaundice within the first 24 hours after birth.

32. D is correct; RhoGAM should be administered to the mother within 72 hours of birth; pathologic jaundice is unlikely because Coombs test results indicate that antibodies have not been formed to destroy the newborn's RBCs; RhoGAM is given to prevent formation of antibodies; it would not be given if antibodies have already been formed as indicated by positive Coombs test results.

33. C is correct; newborn should be NPO for 2 to 4 hours prior to the procedure; 75% to 85% of blood is exchanged; hypocalcemia can occur related to preservatives found in donor blood.

34. A is correct; lateral or prone position prevents pressure on the sac that could cause damage; parents can hold newborn if they are supervised regarding how to hold without touching sac; sterile, moist nonadherent dressings are used to protect the cord; Credé's method is used to ensure that all urine is emptied from the bladder to prevent stasis of urine as a result of incomplete emptying because retention is common.

Critical Thinking Exercises

1. Pathologic jaundice (see Hyperbilirubinemia section)
   A. *Complete table regarding difference between pathologic and physiologic jaundice:* see Physiologic and Pathologic sections for information regarding onset, resolution, and serum bilirubin levels to complete the table
   B. Jaundice, kernicterus

C. *Physiologic process that leads to hyperbilirubinemia:* see Hemolytic Disorders in the Newborn section; basically the RBCs are destroyed naturally or as a result of antibodies formed by the mother and transferred to her fetus via the placenta; byproduct of RBC destruction is bilirubin; if too many RBCs are destroyed the liver will be unable to excrete enough bilirubin, resulting in increased serum levels and jaundice

D. *Potential causes for pathologic jaundice:* see Pathologic Jaundice section and Box 39-1
   • *Maternal causes:* Rh and ABO incompatibility; maternal infections and medical conditions such as diabetes; oxytocin administration; maternal ingestion of certain medications
   • *Fetus/newborn:* preterm, hepatic damage hyperthyroidism, polycythemia, intestinal obstruction, pyloric stenosis, biliary atresia, sequestered blood (e.g., cephalhematoma, ecchymosis)

E. *Effective prevention measures:*
   • Identify mother and newborn at risk and institute appropriate measures such as early feeding, prompt care after birth to decrease stress such as cold stress and hypoglycemia.
   • Prevent the occurrence of asphyxia, acidosis, sepsis.
   • Treat woman whose fetus is at risk for hyperbilirubinemia: diabetes, infection, prevent preterm birth.
   • Early identification of Rh-negative woman so RhoGAM can be given to prevent formation of antibodies.

F. *Exchange transfusion:* see Exchange Transfusion section
   1) *Rationale:* reduces serum bilirubin level; removal of RBCs that would be destroyed by maternal antibodies and the antibodies; corrects the anemia caused by hemolysis

2) *Nursing diagnoses:* newborn: Risk for infection, imbalanced fluid volume; parents: Fear/anxiety

3) *Nursing care measures:* see Plan of care of Infants with Hyperbilirubinemia; measures include keep newborn NPO; check blood compatibility; ensure availability of emergency equipment; assist physician; monitor vital signs, keep track of volume exchange; prevent hypothermia/cold stress; observe for side effects such as bleeding, hypocalcemia, transfusion reaction, and infection

G. Kernicterus, 2, 6, hypotonic, lethargic, suck, Moro reflex, high-pitched cry, opisthotonos, spasticity, hyperreflexia, fever, seizures, 24, half

2. Pregnant woman who is Rh negative (see Hyperbilirubinemia section)

A. *Physiologic basis:* see Rh Incompatibility subsection; if an Rh-negative mother's blood comes in contact with the blood of her Rh-positive fetus, she will form antibodies against Rh-positive blood that can then be transferred via the placenta to the fetus; if a fetus is Rh positive, the presence of these antibodies in its bloodstream will result in destruction of its RBCs (hemolysis)

B. *Meaning of a positive indirect Coombs' test:* indicates that the woman has formed antibodies, probably as a result of her miscarriage and not receiving RhoGAM to prevent antibody formation

C. *Candidate to receive RhoGAM:* woman is not a candidate because RhoGAM cannot be given once antibodies or sensitization has occurred

D. *RhoGAM purpose and use:* prevents sensitization by injecting passive antibodies against the Rh factor that will destroy any fetal RBCs that may have entered maternal circulation

before the maternal immune system is activated; Rh-negative mothers who are indirect Coombs negative should receive RhoGAM after an abortion, after specific invasive tests such as CVS and amniocentesis, during the 3rd trimester, and within 72 hours after the birth of an Rh-positive, direct Coombs–negative newborn

E. *Newborn complications:* see Rh Incompatibility subsection
   • *Erythroblastosis fetalis:* fetus compensates for anemia caused by hemolysis by producing large numbers of immature erythrocytes to replace the RBCs destroyed
   • *Hydrops fetalis:* marked anemia with cardiac decompensation, cardiomegaly, hepatosplenomegaly, hypoxia, generalized edema and effusion of fluid into body spaces; fetal or neonatal death may occur

F. *Prevention of perinatal mortality:* intrauterine transfusions and early birth if the Rh antibody titer rises to dangerous levels and bilirubin is increasing

3. *Care management of newborn born with myelomeningocele:* see Spina Bifida subsection of CNS Anomalies section;
   • Preoperative and postoperative measures including how to position newborn to protect the site, assessment of neurologic function, prevent trauma, rupture, and infection of the site, facilitate bladder emptying
   • Parental support including facilitate attachment process, provide information and emotional care, prepare for surgical care usually in the first 24 hours, make referrals for long-term care for parents and child to help them adjust to and cope with the effects of the congenital anomaly

4. Newborn with a diaphragmatic hernia (see Diaphragmatic Hernia subsection of Respiratory System Anomalies section)
   A. *Clinical manifestations:* severe respiratory distress which worsens as intestine fills with air, diminished breath sounds, heart sounds in the right chest, flat/scaphoid abdomen, bowel in the chest
   B. *Nursing diagnosis:* impaired gas exchange related to inability to fully expand lungs associated with diaphragmatic hernia
   C. *Care measures in immediate postbirth period:*
      • Position: head and chest elevated, affected side down to allow normal lung to fully expand
      • Aspirate gastric contents to decompress gastrointestinal tract
      • Oxygen therapy, mechanical ventilation, and correction of acidosis

5. Newborn with cleft lip and palate (see Cleft Lip and Palate section of Gastrointestinal System Anomalies)
   A. *Nursing diagnoses:* Imbalanced nutrition: less than body requirements, risk for ineffective airway clearance, risk for impaired parent-infant attachment; all of these are related to defective and incomplete development of the lip and palate
   B. *Nursing measures:*
      • Maintain airway patency while ensuring adequate hydration and nutrition using devices that prevent passage of milk into airway.
      • Support and facilitate parental attachment to infant and skill with feeding; prepare parents for discharge.
      • Explain the condition, how it occurs, what it entails, and how and when it will be repaired.
      • Refer to support group.

CHAPTER 40: NURSING CARE OF THE HIGH RISK NEWBORN

Chapter Review Activities

1. B, 2. E, 3. C, 4. A, 5. D, 6. F, 7. T, 8. T, 9. F, 10. T, 11. T, 12. F, 13. F, 14. T, 15. F, 16. F, 17. F, 18. T, 19. T, 20. T, 21. T, 22. F

23. *Purpose of exogenous surfactant administration:* see Surfactant section of Oxygen Therapy; preterm infant born before 34 weeks' gestation has difficulty producing enough surfactant to survive extrauterine life; exogenous surfactant will facilitate alveoli expansion and stability, easing respirations, and enhancing gas exchange until the newborn can produce sufficient quantities on its own; it is administered in several doses via an endotracheal tube directly into the lungs

24. *Kangaroo care:* see Kangaroo Care subsection in Developmental Care section and Fig. 40-15; uses skin-to-skin holding to help preterm newborns interact with parents; benefits newborn and parents by increasing feeling of being in control and allowing better temperature and oxygen stability with fewer episodes of crying, apnea, and periodic respirations; the newborn is in the quiet, alert state longer, thereby enhancing attachment and development; mothers experience increased milk production and fewer feelings of helplessness

25. *Complete the table related to physiologic problems of the preterm newborn:* each physiologic function, along with potential problems, is discussed in its own section of Assessment and Nursing Diagnoses

26. Newborn pain (see Infant Pain Responses section)

A. *Explain CRIES pain assessment tool*: see Table 40-3; scores (scale 0 to 2) crying, requires oxygen for saturation >95%, increased VS, expression, sleepless; the higher the score the worse the pain

B. *Evidence of infant pain memory*: exhibit defensive behaviors when painful procedures are repeated (stiffen, withdrawn when touched); become hypervigilant, gaze at hands of person approaching, not eyes

C. *Consequences of mismanaged pain*:
   - *Physiologic*: increased heart rate and BP, variability in heart rate and intracranial pressure, decrease in oxygen saturation and peripheral blood flow
   - *Behavior*: muscle rigidity, facial expression, crying, withdrawal, sleeplessness

D. *Management strategies*:
   - *Nonpharmacologic*: containment (e.g., swaddling), repositioning, rocking, nonnutritive sucking, use of oral sucrose, distraction, cuddling, music, reducing environmental stimulation
   - *Pharmacologic*: local, regional block, and topical anesthesia, opioids: low-dose, continuous infusion or intermittent bolus of an opioid agonist analgesic such as morphine or fentanyl

27. Respiratory distress syndrome
   A. Pulmonary surfactant, atelectasis, functional residual capacity, ventilation-perfusion, ventilation
   B. Tachypnea, grunting, flaring, retractions, cyanosis, breathing, hypercapnia, respiratory, mixed, hypotension, shock, birth, 6 hours of birth, air exchange, crackles, pallor, accessory muscles, apnea
   C. 72, surfactant
   D. Ventilation, oxygenation, exogenous surfactant, neutral thermal

28. D is correct; seesaw respirations along with retractions, flaring of nares, and expiratory grunting reflect increased effort and work to breathe; A, B, and C are all normal findings consistent with efficient respiratory effort in the preterm newborn.

29. B is correct; A, C, and D are appropriate and important nursing diagnoses, respiration with adequate gas exchange takes precedence especially because adequate surfactant is not produced before 34 weeks' gestation.

30. C is correct; skin temperature decreases before rectal (core) temperature; increase in respirations is an early sign with apnea occurring later; heart rate increases first then decreases as cold stress continues and worsens.

31. A is correct; sterile water is used to lubricate the tube; air, not sterile water, is used to check placement prior to feeding or gastric contents can be aspirated and tested for pH; because newborns are nose breathers the mouth is the preferred route for insertion unless the infant is unable to tolerate.

Critical Thinking Exercises

1. Oxygen therapy for the newborn experiencing respiratory distress (see Oxygen Therapy section of Plan of Care and Interventions)
   A. *Criteria to determine need for oxygen*: increased effort to breathe, respiratory distress with apnea, tachycardia or bradycardia, central cyanosis, PaO_2 less than 60 mm Hg, oxygen saturation less than 92%
   B. *Guidelines for safe and effective administration of oxygen*: observe for signs of complications every 1 to 2 hours with pulse oximeter and arterial blood gases, controlled oxygen concentration, volume, temperature

and humidity; oxygen warm and humidified

C. *Complete table related to oxygen administration methods:* see specific section for each method listed

2. Weaning from oxygen process
   A. *Signs of readiness:* signs of respiratory distress are no longer exhibited, arterial blood gases and oxygen saturation are maintained within normal ranges, newborn displays adequate and spontaneous respiratory effort without difficulty, and exhibits good color and improved muscle tone during increased activity
   B. *Guidelines:* approach carefully from one method to another with close observation for signs of good or poor tolerance of the change; reassure and keep parents informed throughout the process of weaning, pointing out signs that their newborn is breathing effectively and is well oxygenated

3. Meeting nutritional needs of a preterm infant (see Nutritional Care and Gavage Feeding sections)
   A. *Assessment to determine effectiveness of feeding method:* ability to suck and swallow and the coordination of each; signs of respiratory distress during the feeding; length of time for the feeding and the amount ingested; presence of regurgitation, vomiting, or abdominal distention after feeding; daily weight gains and losses and elimination patterns
   B. 15%, 2%, stooling, voiding, evaporative, volume, fluid, malabsorption
   C. *Guidelines to follow when inserting a gavage tube* (see Procedure Box— Inserting a Gavage Feeding Tube and Fig. 40-7); emphasize: tubing choice and measurement of length, insertion without trauma and securing to

maintain placement, checking placement

D. *Nursing diagnosis:* Imbalanced nutrition: less than body requirements related to weak suck associated with premature status

E. *Principles to follow before, during, and after a gavage feeding* (see Procedure Box—Gavage Feeding)
   • Measures to prevent aspiration with proper tube insertion, removal, and position check techniques
   • Instill breast milk or formula at a rate of 1 ml/hour
   • Cuddle, swaddle, talk to infant during feedings; use kangaroo care, involve parents; use nonnutritive sucking
   • Position to prevent aspiration after feeding
   • Assess residual and use residual as part of feeding if less than 25% of feeding
   • Document assessment findings and specifics of the procedure

F. *Advancing to oral feeding:* proceed cautiously, checking for gastrointestinal, nutritional, fluid, and electrolyte signs of tolerance or intolerance for advancement; decrease gavage feedings as ability to suck improves

4. NICU environment (see Environmental Concerns and Placental Support sections of Plan of Care and Interventions)
   A. *Common stressors*
   • *Infant stressors:* continuous exposure to light and noise; administration of sedatives and pain medications; invasive procedures and medications required for treatment; equipment may block vision and ability to make eye contact
   • *Family stressors:* size and compromised and often fluctuating health status of their newborn; difficulty interacting with newborn and making eye contact; increased learning needs regarding status of newborn and care

needs; concern regarding potential disabilities

B. *Cues related to overstimulation or relaxed state:* see Infant Communication section for a description of several cues for each state

C. *Measures to provide a balance of stimuli for the newborn:* see Infant Stimulation section; waterbeds, kangaroo care, bundling, coordinated plan of care to provide for period of interrupted rest and sleep, use pain medications and sedatives as needed, provide diurnal light patterns, decrease noise level, use stroking, talking, mobiles, decals, music, and windup toys for stimulation; reduce inappropriate stimuli

D. *Guidelines for infant positioning:* see Positioning section; change position frequently observing effect of position change on breathing and oxygenation and preventing aspiration; consider boundaries, body alignment, sense of security and comfort when positioning; teach parents

E. *Measures to help family cope with infant's death:* see Anticipatory Grief and Loss of Infant section; support family during visit to infant, encourage expression of feelings, provide privacy and time to be with newborn, arrange for memories according to parents' wishes, facilitate the grieving process, refer to support groups and clergy, arrange for follow-up care

5. Parents of a preterm newborn (see Parental Adaptation to Preterm Infant section)
   A. *Parental tasks:* anticipatory grief, accept failure to give birth to a term newborn, resume process of relating to newborn, learn about ways their newborn is different, adjust home environment to accommodate newborn's needs at discharge
   B. *Nursing diagnoses:* use assessment findings to determine which of these nursing diagnoses are of highest priority for the couple; fear/anxiety, risk for impaired parent-infant attachment, interrupted family processes, anticipatory grieving
   C. *Nursing measures to facilitate progress through developmental tasks:* see Parental Support subsection; be with parents at first visit helping them to see their infant rather than focusing on the equipment; explain characteristics of a preterm infant and the purpose for procedures and equipment; encourage expression of feelings, concerns, and questions; assess their response to the newborn; involve them in the care of their infant as appropriate for them; make referrals to support group and arrange for home care

6. Postterm pregnancy (see Postmature Infant section)
   A. *Rationale for increased mortality:* increased oxygen demands are not met and likelihood for impaired gas exchange occurs, leading to hypoxia and passage of meconium into amniotic fluid; risk for aspiration of meconium into lungs
   B. *Typical assessment findings:* see Care Management section for identification of characteristics including wasted wide-eyed appearance owing to loss of subcutaneous fat and muscle mass; peeling of skin
   C. *Two major complications:* meconium aspiration syndrome and persistent pulmonary hypertension or persistent fetal circulation; see separate subsection that describes each complication

7. Birth of a small for gestation newborn (see Small for Gestational Age and Intrauterine Growth Restriction section)
   A. *Characteristics assessment findings:* head appears large for body; decreased subcutaneous fat and muscle mass

(especially buttocks and cheeks) with the appearance of loose, dry skin and sunken abdomen; thin, dry, yellowish cord; sparse hair and wide sutures

B. *Major complications:* perinatal asphyxia with possible passage of meconium and aspiration, hypoglycemia, polycythemia, heat loss (cold stress)

C. *Physiologic basis for each identified complication:* see separate section for each complication

8. Transport to tertiary center (see Transport to a Regional Center section)

A. *Advantages of transport before birth:*
   - Associated neonatal morbidity and mortality are decreased
   - Infant-parent attachment is supported because separation is avoided

B. *Stabilization of needs prior to transport:* VS, oxygenation and ventilation, thermoregulation, acid/base balance, fluid/electrolyte and glucose levels

C. *Support measures for family:* see Box 40-10; provide information about center (location, visiting hours, phone number, caregivers' names, rules), one parent accompany infant, see infant before transport, get status updates

CHAPTER 41: GRIEVING THE LOSS OF A NEWBORN

Chapter Review Activities

1. *Pregnant woman at 24 weeks of gestation with suspected fetal death* (see Grief Responses section for a description of each phase)
   A. Acute distress and shock
   B. Intense grief
   C. Disorganization
   D. Reorganization

2. Meaning of terms that apply to grief (see Grief Responses section and Box 41-1) *Bereavement (grief):* cluster of painful responses experienced by individuals coping with the death of someone with whom they had a close relationship; cite and describe the stages
   Anticipatory grief: see Chapter 40 for a discussion of anticipatory grief as it relates to the high risk newborn
   Bittersweet grief: grief response that occurs with reminders of the loss: special anniversary dates related to the loss, grief feelings triggered after a subsequent live birth
   Complicated bereavement (see Complicated Bereavement section at end of chapter) extremely intense grief reaction that lasts for a prolonged period

3. *Four tasks of mourners identified by Worden (1991):* see Grief Responses Section; accepting the reality of the loss, working through the pain and adjusting to life without the child, adjusting the environment, moving on; Worden proposes that each task must be accomplished to resolve grief; the nurse should encourage parents to be open regarding feelings and seek support and help from each other and others including family members (e.g., making arrangements); to work through changes at their own pace (e.g., taking down nursery); nurses should also advocate for the parents

4. *Father's grief responses* (see Acute Distress section of Grief Responses):
   - Distressed by maternal grief—may feel helpless as to how to help her; may feel the need to be stoic to meet society's expectations of the strong male for his partner and family
   - May be less able to share deep intense grief; special efforts are required to give them the support they may need
   - Experience a variable response depending on the degree to which he identified with the pregnancy (early vs. late pregnancy loss—miscarriage vs. stillbirth)

5. *Use of the five components of the caring framework developed by Swanson and Kauffman to support grieving parents:* see Communicate Using a Caring Framework section for a description of each component; explain how you would use each of the following to help parents:
   - Knowing—time to understand
   - Being with—acceptance of feelings
   - Doing for—activities of nurse to provide comfort, care, and safety
   - Enabling—offering options for care
   - Maintaining belief—encouraging parents to believe in their ability to heal

6. *Actualizing the loss:* see Helping the Mother, Father, and Other Family Members Actualize the Loss and Creating Memories for Parents to Take Home sections; tangible memories of the baby can help parents actualize (make it a reality) the loss; help them to participate in the options that are most appealing and comfortable for them; use baby's name and words such as dead and died; help parents to tell their story; many other ideas are presented in these sections

7. Complicated bereavement (*see Complicated Bereavement section*)
   A. *Characteristic behaviors:* continued obsession with yearning and loneliness; intense continuing guilt or anger; feelings of inadequacy and low self-esteem; relentless depression or anxiety interfering with role function; suicidal thoughts, abuse of alcohol or drugs, relationship difficulties
   B. *Nursing approach:* refer for counseling to a therapist or counselor that is experienced in grief counseling; be persistent in getting individual or family into counseling, especially to the first visit, enlisting other family members to help

8. A is correct; telling her to be happy that one twin survived may be interpreted

that she should not grieve the loss of the daughter who died—the loss must be acknowledged and the tasks for mourners accomplished; B, C, and D are all appropriate responses by the nurse with B and C helpful in actualizing the loss.

9. D is correct; A and B represent the intense grief phase and C represents the reorganization phase.

10. B is correct; see Box 41-3; note that A, C, and D are in the category of what not to say whereas B represents a response that acknowledges the difficulty of the loss and offers an opportunity for expression of feelings.

Critical Thinking Exercises

1. Family experiencing miscarriage at 13 weeks' gestation
   A. *Approach to individualize support measures:* see Assessment and Nursing Diagnoses section
      - Begin with assessment to determine best approach to take for this couple.
      - Determine nature of the parental attachment with the pregnancy and the meaning of the pregnancy and birth to the parents—their perception of the loss—recognizing that responses of father and mother may differ.
      - Circumstances surrounding the loss—listen to their story.
      - The immediate response of each parent to the loss—do they match?
      - Persons comprising their social network and how can they support them; do the parents want their support?
   B. *Cite questions and observations to gather information required to create an individualized plan of care:* use each of the areas identified in "A" to formulate questions and organize observations

C. *Nursing diagnoses:* see list of Nursing Diagnoses in the Assessment and Diagnoses section; consider assessment findings to determine nursing diagnoses and their priority for a specific family
  - Nursing diagnoses associated with emotional effects of grief: situational low self-esteem, spiritual distress, anxiety, ineffective individual coping
  - Nursing diagnoses associated with impact on family including other child and grandparents: interrupted family processes, ineffective family coping
  - Nursing diagnoses related to the physical effects of the grief process: fatigue, disturbed sleep pattern, imbalanced nutrition
D. *Therapeutic communication techniques to help couple express feelings and emotions:* see Communicate Using a Caring Framework and Helping Bereaved Acknowledge and Express Feelings sections and Box 41-3; examples of therapeutic communication techniques include: encouraging expression of feelings by leaning forward, nodding, reflection, saying "tell me more"; observe nonverbal cues; use touch as appropriate; listen patiently and use silence while couple tell their story; avoid giving advice or using clichés, reassure regarding normalcy of emotions
E. *Analysis of nurse responses:* N, T, N, N, T, T, N, N, T, T

2. *Physical needs of postpartum woman following stillbirth:* see Meet the Physical Needs of the Postpartum Bereaved Mother section;
  - Provide option of staying on maternity unit or transferring to another—discuss the advantages and disadvantages of each option
  - Option for room assignment (away from nursery)
  - Assist with breast care (milk coming in is a reminder of the loss)

- Emphasize the importance of analgesics and comfort measures to help with rest and sleep
- Encourage adequate nutrition, fluids, balance of activity and rest to enhance strength and healing
- Avoid caffeine, alcohol, and tobacco

3. Birth of baby with anencephaly
  A. *Making the decision to see the baby:* See Help Mother and Father and Other Family Members to Actualize the Loss, Create Memories for Parents to Take Home, and Options for Parents sections
    - Tell them about the option to see the baby.
    - Give them time to think about the option so they can choose what is best for them.
    - Come back and ask them their decision; if they are unsure or say no—ask again before discharge.
  B. *Measures to help the couple when they see their baby:*
    - Explain to parents how the baby will look so they know what to expect.
    - Prepare baby making it look as normal as possible: bathe, use powder, comb hair, put on identification bracelet, dress, wrap in a pretty blanket (get help from a funeral director if needed); give parents the opportunity to provide care.
    - Treat baby as one would a live baby when bringing baby to parents: use name, touch cheek, talk about baby's features emphasizing those that are normal, or resemble family members including themselves.
    - Provide time alone with baby and adjust length of time with the baby to meet their needs—observe for cues that tell you they need more time or that they are done.
    - Determine what else they would need to make a memory—foot print, photograph, lock of hair, etc.

4. *Role of the nurse in supporting a pregnant woman at 16 weeks who is told her baby has anencephaly*: see Prenatal Diagnosis with Negative Outcome section;
   - Fully explain anencephaly and discuss her options.
   - Be a good listener encouraging her to express how she feels about the experience including cultural and religious beliefs and values that will guide the option that she will choose.
   - Respect her decision and provide her with follow-up support if she decides to continue the pregnancy or after elective abortion if that is her choice; if elective abortion is her choice determine if she wishes to see the fetus.